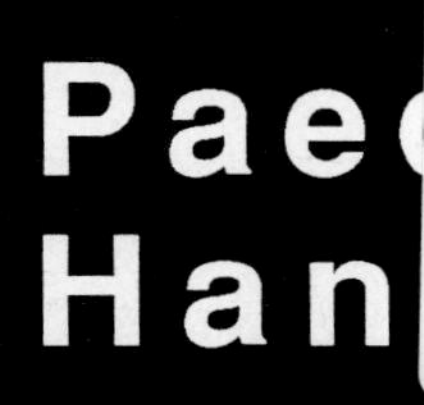

Fifth Edition

Editor
DARYL EFRON

Associate Editor
TERRY NOLAN

b

**Blackwell
Science**

© 1992, 1995 by
Blackwell Science Pty Ltd
Editorial Offices:
54 University Street, Carlton
Victoria 3053, Australia
Osney Mead, Oxford OX2 0EL
25 John Street, London WC1N 2BL
23 Ainslie Place, Edinburgh EH3 6AJ
238 Main Street, Cambridge
Massachusetts 02142, USA

Other Editorial Offices:
Arnette Blackwell SA
1, rue de Lille, 75007 Paris, France

Blackwell Wissenschafts-Verlag
GmbH
Kurfürstendamm 57, 10707 Berlin,
Germany

Blackwell MZV
Feldgasse 13, A-1238 Wien, Austria

All rights reserved. No part of this publication may be reproduced, stored in a retrieval system, or transmitted, in any form or by any means, electronic, mechanical, photocopying, recording or otherwise, except as permitted by the *Copyright Act 1968*, without the prior permission of the copyright owner.

Fourth edition published 1992
Reprinted 1993, 1994
Fifth edition published 1995

Text design by Tom Kurema
Cover design by Brett Petrie
Cover illustration by Michael Leunig
Set by Semantic Graphics, Singapore
Printed in Australia by Brown Prior
Anderson

DISTRIBUTORS

Australia
Blackwell Science Pty Ltd
54 University Street
Carlton, Victoria 3053
(*Orders:* Tel: +61 3 9347 0300
Fax: +61 3 9349 3016)

UK and Europe
Marston Book Services Ltd
PO Box 87
Oxford OX2 0DT
(*Orders:* Tel: 01865 791155
Fax: 01865 791927)

USA
Blackwell Science, Inc.
238 Main Street
Cambridge, MA 02142
(*Orders:* Tel: 800 215 1000
617 876 7000
Fax: 617 492 5263)

Cataloguing in Publication Data

Paediatric handbook.

5th ed.
Includes index.
ISBN 0 86793 337 2.

1. Pediatrics — Handbooks, manuals, etc.
2. Children — Hospital care — Handbooks, manuals, etc.
I. Royal Children's Hospital (Melbourne, Vic.)
618.92

CONTENTS

DEVELOPMENT

PSYCHOSOCIAL PROBLEMS

THERAPY AND NUTRITION

APPENDICES

CONTRIBUTORS

All authors are staff or associates of the Royal Children's Hospital (RCH) unless otherwise indicated

Robert Adler	Chairman, RCH Mental Health Service; Professor, Department of Paediatrics, University of Melbourne
Roger Allen	Paediatrician/Paediatric Rheumatologist, Department of General Paediatrics
Helen Anthony	Clinical Specialist Dietitian, Department of Nutrition
Peter Barnett	Acting Director, Emergency Services, Centre for Community Child Health and Ambulatory Paediatrics
Jennifer Batch	Paediatrician, Departments of General Paediatrics and Endocrinology; Senior Lecturer, Department of Paediatrics, University of Melbourne
Robert Berkowitz	Director, Department of Otolaryngology
Julie Bines	Paediatric Gastroenterologist, Department of Gastroenterology; Physician, Nutrition Support Service
Glenn Bowes	Director, Centre for Adolescent Health; Professor, Department of Paediatrics, University of Melbourne
Doug Bryan	Deputy Director, Department of Child Development and Rehabilitation; Paediatrician, Department of General Paediatrics
Barbara Burge	General Practitioner; Visiting Examiner, Department of Paediatrics, University of Melbourne
Neil Campbell	Director, Department of Neonatology,
Tony Catto-Smith	Director, Department of Gastroenterology
Lex Doyle	Neonatal Paediatrician, Royal Women's Hospital and RCH; Associate Professor, Departments of Obstetrics and Gynaecology and Paediatrics, University of Melbourne

Daryl Efron	Clinical Research Fellow, Centre for Community Child Health and Ambulatory Paediatrics
James Elder	Director, Department of Ophthalmology
Kay Gibbons	Chief Dietitian, Department of Nutrition
Kerr Graham	Chief Orthopaedic Surgeon, Department of Orthopaedic Surgery; Professor of Orthopaedics, Department of Paediatrics, University of Melbourne
Keith Grimwood	Paediatrician and Infectious Diseases Physician, Department of General Paediatrics; Senior Lecturer, Department of Paediatrics, University of Melbourne
Sonia Grover	Adolescent Gynaecologist, RCH Centre for Adolescent Health; Obstetrician and Gynaecologist, Royal Women's Hospital
Karen Hogan	Coordinator, RCH Gatehouse Centre for the Assessment and Treatment of Child Abuse
Geoff Hogg	Director of Clinical Microbiology; Director, Microbiological Diagnostic Unit, University of Melbourne
John Hutson	Director, Department of General Surgery; Professor, Department of Paediatrics, University of Melbourne
Frederick Jarman	Deputy Director, Centre for Community Child Health and Ambulatory Paediatrics
Colin Jones	Director, Department of Nephrology, Victorian Paediatric Renal Services
Andrew Kemp	Director of Clinical Immunology; Paediatrician, Department of General Paediatrics
Julian Keogh	Director, Victorian Paediatric Burns Centre
Geoffrey Klug	Director, Department of Neurosurgery
Margaret Loughnan	Social Worker, Department of Social Work
Lionel Lubitz	Deputy Director, Department of General Paediatrics
James Lucas	Deputy Director, Department of Dentistry
Ernest S. L. Luk	Psychiatrist, RCH Mental Health Service; Associate Professor, Departments of Psychiatry and Paediatrics, University of Melbourne

Peter McDougall Deputy Director, Department of Neonatology

Jim McGill Metabolic Physician, Victorian Clinical Genetics Services

Michelle Meehan Maternal and Child Health Nurse, Division of Community Oriented Paediatric and Adolescent Services

Frank Oberklaid Director, Centre for Community Child Health and Ambulatory Paediatrics; Professor, Department of Paediatrics, University of Melbourne

Bronwyn Parry-Fielder Chief Speech Pathologist, Department of Speech Pathology

George Patton Psychiatrist, RCH Mental Health Service; Senior Lecturer, Department of Paediatrics, University of Melbourne

Peter Phelan Chief Thoracic Physician, Department of Thoracic Medicine; Stevenson Professor and Head, Department of Paediatrics, University of Melbourne

Rod Phillips Paediatrician, Department of General Paediatrics and Centre for Adolescent Health; Senior Lecturer, Department of Paediatrics, University of Melbourne

Harley Powell Senior Nephrologist, Department of Nephrology, Victorian Paediatric Renal Services

Philip Ragg Paediatric Anaesthetist, Department of Anaesthetics

Dinah Reddihough Director, Department of Child Development and Rehabilitation; Paediatrician, Department of General Paediatrics

John Rogers Senior Medical Geneticist, Victorian Clinical Genetics Services

Margaret Rowell Paediatrician, Department of Child Development and Rehabilitation

Frank Shann Director, Intensive Care Unit

Lloyd Shield Director, Department of Neurology

Gerry Silk Clinical Nurse Educator, Division of Community Oriented Paediatric and Adolescent Services

Anne Smith Senior Paediatrician, RCH Gatehouse Centre for the Assessment and Treatment of Child Abuse

Peter Smith Director, Department of Haematology and Oncology; Professor, Department of Paediatrics, University of Melbourne

Michael South Director, Department of General Paediatrics; Senior Lecturer, Department of Paediatrics, University of Melbourne

Russell Taylor Paediatric Surgeon, Department of General Surgery

Jim Tibballs Deputy Director, Intensive Care Unit; Resuscitation Officer; Medical Consultant, Poisons Information Centre

George Varigos Director, Department of Dermatology

John Vorrath Deputy Director, Department of Otolaryngology

Rowan Walker Nephrologist, Royal Melbourne Hospital and RCH; Associate Professor, Department of Medicine, University of Melbourne

Garry Warne Director, Department of Endocrinology and Diabetes

George Werther Deputy Director, Department of Endocrinology and Diabetes

Jim Wilkinson Director, Department of Cardiology

EDITORIAL COMMITTEE

Daryl Efron
Clinical Research Fellow, Centre for Community Child Health and Ambulatory Paediatrics

Terry Nolan
Paediatrician, Department of General Paediatrics; Head, Clinical Epidemiology and Biostatistics Unit; Associate Professor, Department of Paediatrics, University of Melbourne

Keith Grimwood
Paediatrician and Infectious Diseases Physician, Department of General Paediatrics; Senior Lecturer, Department of Paediatrics, University of Melbourne

John Hutson
Director, Department of General Surgery; Professor, University of Melbourne, Department of Paediatrics

Peter Phelan
Chief Thoracic Physician, Department of Thoracic Medicine; Stevenson Professor and Head, University of Melbourne, Department of Paediatrics

Frank Shann
Director, Intensive Care Unit

Michael South
Director, Department of General Paediatrics; Senior Lecturer, Department of Paediatrics, University of Melbourne

Hubert van Doorn
Co-ordinator of General Practice Education

FOREWORD

The *Paediatric Handbook*, produced by the staff of the Royal Children's Hospital, has established itself over the past 30 years as a major source of information for medical practitioners dealing with the health and illness of children. While originally produced with the primary aim of being a ready reference for the junior medical staff of the Hospital, the handbook was rapidly recognised by general practitioners, paediatricians and medical students as a valuable source of information for the diagnosis and management of common paediatric medical problems.

The handbook is based on the management practices at the Royal Children's Hospital, Melbourne, which is one of the largest specialist children's hospitals in the English-speaking world. It has an enviable reputation for its clinical care, teaching and research. The Royal Children's Hospital is the principal paediatric centre for the state of Victoria, the paediatric teaching hospital for the University of Melbourne and the centre for paediatric education for doctors, nurses and the whole range of health care professionals. Many of the staff of the Hospital and of the Department of Paediatrics at the University of Melbourne have contributed to this handbook.

The handbook covers common health problems of newborn infants, children and adolescents. Its aim is to provide practical information and as such should not be seen as a comprehensive textbook. It will be of particular value to those involved in the care of children in hospital.

Fortunately, death in childhood in most developed countries is now an uncommon event, and in Victoria the infant mortality rate has fallen to 4.3 per 1000 live births. Regrettably, there remain preventable causes of death in children; in particular, injuries and infectious diseases which can be prevented by appropriate immunization. In developing countries, infant mortality remains very high from such common disorders as gastroenteritis, acute respiratory infection and malnutrition; often there is a combination of all three. In all countries, childhood morbidity remains high, with important causes being infection, asthma and injury. These conditions receive considerable attention in this handbook, but the emphasis is on management rather than prevention.

The Royal Children's Hospital and its staff are proud of their contribution to child health care in Victoria and beyond. They hope that this handbook will continue to be of value to medical practitioners, medical students and other health professionals, and allow them to better diagnose and treat sick children as well as to further reduce childhood mortality and morbidity.

Peter D. Phelan
Stevenson Professor and Head
Department of Paediatrics
University of Melbourne

PREFACE

The *Paediatric Handbook* of the Royal Children's Hospital is intended as a handy reference to be used by a range of medical practitioners, including general practitioners and other primary care providers as well as hospital residents in secondary and tertiary paediatric centres. Although authoritative, it is not a textbook – discussion of the finer points of pathogenesis and management of conditions is beyond the scope of a handbook. The emphasis is on a problem-oriented, hands-on approach to common and/or important clinical conditions encountered in paediatric practice.

This fifth edition has been comprehensively updated. All chapters have been improved, and many have been extensively revised and expanded, including Neonatal Conditions, Infectious Diseases and Microbiology, Allergy and Immunology, Orthopaedic Conditions, and Infant and Child Nutrition. In addition, several chapters have undergone major rewriting, including Ear, Nose and Throat Conditions, Adolescent Health, and Gynaecologic Conditions.

In recognition of the fact that the delivery of paediatric services is becoming increasingly ambulatory, there has been a shift in emphasis, with the inclusion of important new chapters such as Common Developmental and Behaviour Problems, and Paediatric Health Maintenance. Other new chapters include Rheumatologic Conditions, Pain Management, and The Death of a Child. The handbook now has a much broader base which will ensure its value to a wide range of community practitioners, dealing with issues such as feeding problems (Infant and Child Nutrition) and normal variations and common minor problems of newborn infants (Neonatal Conditions).

Another new feature is the incorporation of many illustrations and diagnostic and management algorithms. These greatly enhance the educational value and 'at a glance' accessibility of the information in several chapters, including Procedures, Common Surgical Problems, Orthopaedic Conditions, Eye Conditions and Renal Conditions. The use of many tables throughout the text further improves the presentation.

The Dermatologic Conditions chapter deserves singling out in that it demonstrates a clear and logical, physical sign-based approach to skin disorders.

Another new aspect is that we have deleted the previous Common Medical Conditions chapter. In this edition these conditions, discussed by general paediatricians, have been included in the appropriate sub-specialty chapters such as Neurologic Conditions, Haematologic Conditions, Gastrointestinal Conditions and Respiratory Conditions.

The Victorian logo that appears in the margin throughout the handbook indicates that information intended primarily for the assistance of Victorian users, but which may also be of interest to readers from other states and countries, has been compiled into the Victorian Information section at the back of the handbook.

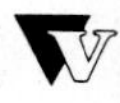

The index has been expanded significantly and carefully to facilitate easy reference.

While every effort has been made to check drug doses throughout the handbook, it is still possible that errors may have been missed. Furthermore, dosage schedules are constantly being revised and new adverse effects recognised. Therefore, the reader is strongly advised to consult the pharmaceutical company's package insert or other product information before administering any of the drugs recommended in this handbook.

We would like to gratefully acknowledge a number of people for their kind assistance. First Dr Frank Shann for permission to reprint his booklet, *Drug Doses, 9th Edition.* Our thanks to the two independent reviewers of the fourth edition, Emeritus Professor Arthur Clark and Dr Greg Rowell, for their helpful comments and suggestions for improvement. Thanks also to Mr Danny Cass for his review of the Common Surgical Conditions chapter, and to Dr David McMaster for his useful contribution. We are indebted to Bill Reid for his excellent illustrations, to Elizabeth Vorrath and Pat Keen for their secretarial assistance, and to Aileen Boyd-Squires and Shirley Green at Blackwell Science for their support throughout the preparation of the manuscript. Particular thanks are extended to Melbourne artist, Michael Leunig, who generously donated the image which appears on the cover.

Daryl Efron
Editor

Terry Nolan
Associate Editor

CHAPTER 1

1

CRITICAL CARE

Jim Tibballs

CARDIORESPIRATORY ARREST

Cardiorespiratory arrest may occur in a wide variety of conditions which cause hypoxaemia or hypotension or both. Examples are trauma, drowning, septicaemia, sudden infant death syndrome, asthma and congenital anomalies of the heart and lung.

The initial cardiac rhythm discovered during early resuscitation is usually severe bradycardia or asystole. The spontaneous onset of ventricular fibrillation in children is uncommon but may occur with congenital heart conditions or secondary to poisoning with cardioactive drugs. Respiratory arrest alone may occur.

DIAGNOSIS AND INITIAL MANAGEMENT

- **Suspect cardiorespiratory arrest when consciousness is lost, or the patient appears pale or cyanosed, or is pulseless or apnoeic**
- Assess circulation by palpation of a carotid, brachial or femoral pulse
- Assess respiration by observing movement of the chest and by feeling for expired breath while positioning the head and neck to maintain an airway. Movement of the chest without expiration indicates a blocked airway
- Whenever possible, treat in a treatment room. Carry the patient there if necessary. If this is not possible, fetch the resuscitation trolley from a treatment room
- Cardiopulmonary resuscitation (CPR) must commence with basic techniques and be supplemented by advanced techniques

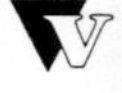

AIRWAY MAINTENANCE AND VENTILATION

- Quickly inspect the pharynx. Clear an airway obstructed by secretions or vomitus by brief suction using a Yankauer sucker. Maintain the airway with backward head tilt, chin lift or forward jaw thrust
- If this fails to permit respiration, ventilate the lungs with a self-inflating

resuscitator (e.g. Laerdal, Ambu, Air-viva) using 8–10 L/min of oxygen. If ventilation cannot be achieved with the resuscitator, use a mouth-to-mask technique

- Intubate the trachea via the mouth if you are able to do this, but do not cause hypoxaemia by prolonged unsuccessful attempts. Select the tube size and insertion distance appropriate to the patient's age: for patients over 1 year, tube size (internal diameter in mm) = age (years)/ 4 + 4. The depth of insertion (after 1 year) is given approximately by the formula: age (years)/2 + 12 cm
- Secure the tube with cotton tape around the neck or affix it firmly to the face with adhesive tape to avoid endobronchial intubation or accidental extubation

Table 1.1 Tube size and insertion distance for paediatric intubation

Age	*Internal diameter (mm)*	*Length at lip (cm)*
Newborn	3.0	8.5
1–6 months	3.5	10
6–12 months	4.0	11
2 years	4.5	12
4 years	5.0	14
6 years	5.5	15
8 years	6.0	16
10 years	6.5	17
12 years	7.0	18
14 years	7.5	19
Adult	8.0	20

EXTERNAL CARDIAC COMPRESSION (ECC)

- *Start ECC if a pulse is not palpable or if it is <60/min*
- Place the patient on a firm surface. Depress the sternum 2–3 cm using two fingers for an infant (<1 year), 3–4 cm with the heel of one hand for a small child (>1 year) or 4–5 cm for a larger child or teenager using a two-handed technique. The site of ECC is the lower sternum for all age groups
- ECC in newborns may be better given by a technique in which the hands encircle the chest, the thumbs compress the sternum anteriorly and the fingers stabilize the vertebral column posteriorly. Avoid pressure over the ribs and abdominal viscera whatever technique is used

- Combine ECC and ventilation for infants and small children in a ratio of 5:1 regardless of the number of persons resuscitating (see Table 1.2). For larger children or teenagers in whom a two-handed technique of compression is required, adequate compression and ventilation may be better achieved with a ratio of 15:2
- If bag-to-mask ventilation or mouth-to-mask ventilation is used, give breaths between compressions; this is best achieved by counting the compressions aloud. This requirement is not as crucial if ventilation is given by bag and endotracheal tube. Whatever technique is used, ensure that ventilation expands the chest adequately and that compression generates a pulse

Table 1.2 Cardiac compression and ventilation

	Large child/teenager	*Small child/infant*
Compression/min	80	100
Ventilation/min	16	20

MANAGEMENT OF CARDIAC DYSRHYTHMIAS

- Determine the cardiac rhythm with defibrillator paddles or chest leads
- Insert an intravenous cannula. Although this is the preferred access to the circulation, do not waste time with repeated unsuccessful attempts, because access can be achieved with the alternative techniques of bone marrow infusion (intraosseous, see p. 26) or endotracheal administration (ETT)
- All drugs and resuscitation fluids can be given via the bone marrow but only adrenaline, atropine and lignocaine can be given via the endotracheal route

The sequential management of life-threatening dysrhythmias is given in Figure 1.1.

OTHER DRUGS

Calcium

Calcium is a useful inotropic and vasopressor agent but it has no place in the management of a dysrhythmia, unless it is caused by hypocalcaemia, hyperkalaemia or calcium channel blocker toxicity. It is not useful and is probably harmful for asystole, ventricular fibrillation or electromechanical dissociation. The intravenous dose is 0.2 mL/kg of 10%

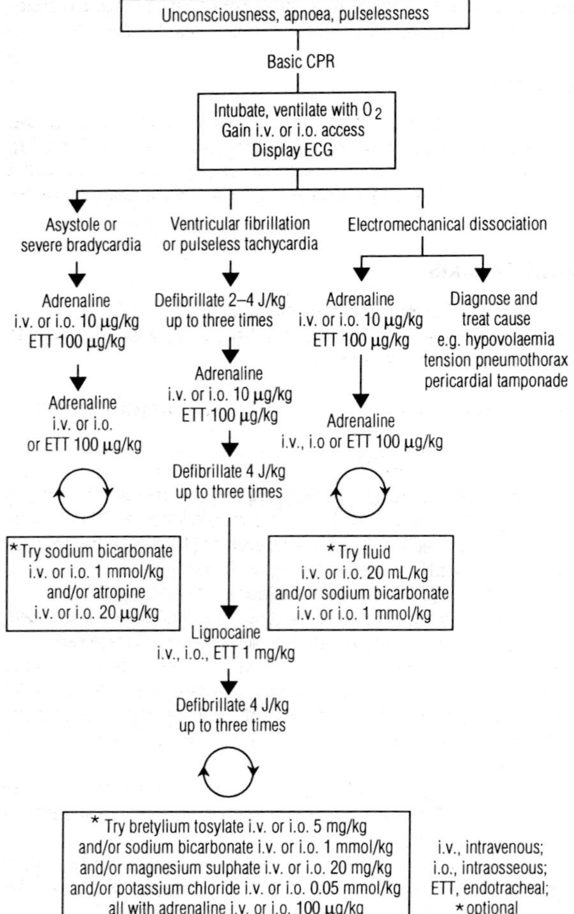

Figure 1.1 Sequential management of life-threatening dysrhythmias

calcium chloride or 0.7 mL of 10% calcium gluconate. Do not administer calcium by endotracheal tube and do not mix it with bicarbonate.

Adenosine

This is the preferred drug treatment for supraventricular tachycardia. Administer as a rapid intravenous bolus in an initial dose of 0.05 mg/kg, increasing up to 0.4 mg/kg if required. Employ synchronized direct current shock (0.5–1 J/kg) if a patient with supraventricular tachycardia is pulseless.

ANAPHYLAXIS

The life-threatening clinical manifestations are:

- Hypotension due to vasodilatation and loss of plasma volume due to increased capillary permeability
- Bronchospasm
- Upper airways obstruction due to laryngeal or pharyngeal oedema

IMMEDIATE TREATMENT

- Vasopressor and bronchodilator therapy. Give *adrenaline* 0.1 mL/kg of 1 : 10 000 solution by slow intravenous injection (over 10 min) or by intramuscular injection. A continuous infusion (10–100 μg/kg per min) may be required if manifestations are prolonged
- Oxygen by mask. Mechanical ventilation may be required
- Intravenous volume expander. Give colloid or crystalloid solution. Give repeat boluses of 10 mL/kg until the blood pressure is restored
- Bronchodilator therapy with *salbutamol* – continuous nebulized (0.5%) or intravenous bolus (5 μg/kg) or intravenous infusion (1–10 μg/kg per min). Secondary therapy with a *steroid*, *aminophylline* and an *antihistamine* may be helpful for prolonged bronchospasm and capillary leak
- Relief of upper airways obstruction: mild to moderate oedema may respond to an inhalation of nebulized *1% adrenaline*, but intubation of the trachea may be required
- Anaphylaxis can be biphasic and the patient may deteriorate again over the next few hours. All patients with anaphylaxis should be admitted to hospital and observed carefully for at least 12 h

HAEMORRHAGIC SHOCK

The normal blood volume is 70–80 mL/kg. A child may lose a substantial volume of blood without developing hypotension. Cardiac output

Table 1.3 Paediatric resuscitation: dose–volume conversions

Age	0	2 m	5 m	1 y	2 y	3 y	4 y	5 y	6 y	7 y	8 y	9 y	10 y	11 y	12 y	13 y	14 y
Bodyweight (kg)	3.5	5	7	10	12	14	16	18	20	22	25	28	32	36	40	46	50
Adrenaline 1 : 1000 (mL)																	
10 µg/kg	0.035	0.05	0.07	0.10	0.12	0.14	0.16	0.18	0.2	0.22	0.25	0.28	0.32	0.36	0.4	0.46	0.5
100 µg/kg	0.35	0.5	0.7	1	1.2	1.4	1.6	1.8	2	2.2	2.5	2.8	3.2	3.6	4	4.6	5
Adrenaline 1 : 10 000 (mL)																	
10 µg/kg	0.35	0.5	0.7	1	1.2	1.4	1.6	1.8	2	2.2	2.5	2.8	3.2	3.6	4	4.6	5
100 µg/kg	3.5	5.0	7.0	10	12	14	16	18	20	22	25	28	32	36	40	46	50
Lignocaine 1% (mL)																	
1 mg/kg	0.3	0.5	0.7	1.0	1.2	1.4	1.6	1.8	2.0	2.2	2.5	2.8	3.2	3.6	4.0	4.6	5.0
Sodium bicarbonate 8.4% (mL)																	
1 mmol/kg	3.5	5	7	10	12	14	16	18	20	22	25	28	32	36	40	46	50

m, month; y, year.

and blood pressure are preserved by tachycardia and vasoconstriction, so hypotension is often a late sign of blood loss.

- Control external haemorrhage by direct wound pressure, arterial vessel pressure or a tourniquet and elevation of the injured area. Investigate and/or surgically explore internal haemorrhage
- Administer oxygen by mask
- Insert a large bore intravenous cannula, preferably in the upper limb. Two cannulae may be required
- Withdraw blood for group and cross-match
- Infuse rapidly 20 mL/kg of a colloid solution (e.g. Haemaccel), or a crystalloid solution if colloid is not available. This may be administered rapidly by syringing with the aid of a three-way tap. Titrate additional volume to the blood pressure and other indices of perfusion
- *If exsanguinating, transfuse urgently with (in order of preference): (i) rapidly cross-matched blood; (ii) uncrossmatched blood of the same group as the patient; (iii) uncrossmatched O negative blood*
- Monitor blood pressure, heart rate, oxygenation and urine output. Warm the blood and measure the central venous pressure, serum calcium and the coagulation and acid–base status if massive transfusion is required. Calcium and fresh frozen plasma may be needed

SEPTICAEMIC SHOCK

Shock due to meningococcaemia is usually accompanied by a purpuric rash.

- Collect blood for culture then give a third generation cephalosporin. Do not delay administration of an antibiotic if a blood sample cannot be collected
- Treat shock with an intravenous colloid solution (20 mL/kg initially—further boluses of 10–20 mL/kg may be needed), and commence infusion of an inotropic agent. *Dobutamine* (5–20 μg/kg per min) may be infused by peripheral vein, but *dopamine* (5–20 μg/kg per min) into a central vein is preferable
- Monitor blood gases. Oxygen and mechanical ventilation may be required
- Defer lumbar puncture until the child has been stabilized

DROWNING

The injury is global hypoxic-ischaemia, and lung damage from aspiration.

- Adequate oxygenation and ventilation are of paramount importance. Mechanical ventilation is required for severe lung involvement, circulatory arrest or loss of consciousness. Lung hypoxic-ischaemic injury is compounded by pulmonary oedema or aspiration of water or gastric contents

- Decompress the stomach, which is usually distended with air and water
- Support the circulation with intravenous infusion of colloid solution and infusion of an inotropic agent (e.g. dopamine 5–20 µg/kg per min into a central vein)
- If signs of cerebral oedema are present (i.e. depressed conscious state) administer *mannitol* 0.25–0.5 g/kg, i.v.
- Correct electrolyte disturbances; hypokalaemia is common. The differences between fresh and salt water drowning are not usually clinically important
- Administer *penicillin* (to prevent the complication of pneumococcal pneumonia)

ACUTE LARYNGEAL OBSTRUCTION

The common cause is laryngotracheobronchitis (croup), and occasional causes are epiglottitis, inhaled foreign body, allergic oedema and trauma.

EPIGLOTTITIS

See also p. 68.

- Complete obstruction may occur in just a few hours. In general, tracheal intubation is required
- Keep the child in a sitting position and administer oxygen by mask. Summon help from an intensivist or anaesthetist. If you are inexperienced, do not attempt intubation unless the child becomes comatose. Intubate orally initially with a relatively small endotracheal tube. It may be hard to see the larynx because of secretions in the pharynx and the swollen epiglottis. Cricoid pressure is very helpful
- If intubation proves to be impossible, attempt to ventilate with a bag and mask—a good technique may achieve adequate ventilation. If ventilation is impossible, perform tracheostomy or cricothyrotomy (see below)

CROUP

See also p. 67. In severe obstruction, give an inhalation of nebulized 1% adrenaline to obtain temporary relief. Obtain anaesthetic help with a view to endotracheal intubation. If this is not available, intubate when the child is going into respiratory failure. Use a small diameter tube with an introducing stylet.

ASPIRATED FOREIGN BODY

See also p. 81.

- Be familiar with first-aid management of choking (back slaps, Heimlich manoeuvre, lateral chest compressions). Do not instrument the airways if the child is coping, but summon an anaesthetist and ENT surgeon
- If complete obstruction occurs, attempt removal of an impacted laryngeal foreign body with forceps—if this is unsuccessful, perform a tracheostomy or cricothyrotomy (see below)
- If respiratory failure is due to a foreign body in the lower trachea or bronchi, attempt ventilation via an endotracheal tube while organizing endoscopic removal

ALLERGIC OEDEMA

Treat with nebulized 1% adrenaline. Refer to an intensivist/anaesthetist for endotracheal intubation, or an ENT surgeon for tracheostomy.

EMERGENCY RELIEF OF A TOTALLY OBSTRUCTED UPPER AIRWAY

- A barely adequate airway can be obtained by inserting a 14 gauge intravenous cannula percutaneously into the trachea via the cricothyroid membrane (which lies immediately below the thyroid cartilage); the patient should be lying straight, with the cannula in the midline and angled towards the feet. Remove the needle of the intravenous cannula; connect the cannula to a resuscitator or a bagging circuit using a connector from a 3.0 mm endotracheal tube. Ventilate with sustained 100% oxygen inspirations; aid expiration by lateral chest compression
- Alternatively, stabilize the thyroid–cricoid region and incise the skin over the cricothyroid membrane. Bluntly dissect into the trachea in the midline. Insert a small tracheostomy tube or an endotracheal tube
- Alternatively, perform percutaneous minitracheostomy

STATUS EPILEPTICUS

A convulsion involving the respiratory musculature and upper airways which does not cease within a few minutes may cause hypoventilation with hypoxaemia and hypercarbia. Administer oxygen and treat with an intravenous anticonvulsant; be prepared to give mechanical ventilation, particularly if the child has meningitis. Some anticonvulsant choices include:

- *Clonazepam* 0.25 mg (<1 year), 0.5 mg (1–5 years), 1 mg (>5 years)
- *Diazepam* 0.1–0.2 mg/kg. May be given per rectum if there is no intravenous access
- *Phenobarbitone* 20 mg/kg slowly, repeated every 15–30 min if required
- *Phenytoin* 15 mg/kg slowly to avoid negative inotropic effect. Slow onset
- *Thiopentone*: titrate dose to effect (usually 2–5 mg/kg). Beware of hypotension

Prolonged convulsions may require large and repeated doses of anticonvulsant drugs and consequently mechanical ventilation. Repeated doses of a single anticonvulsant such as phenobarbitone (where the serum level correlates with the effects) is preferable to using multiple anticonvulsants.

Suspect hyponatraemia as the cause of convulsions in meningitis.

RAISED INTRACRANIAL PRESSURE

Acute intracranial hypertension threatens the blood supply of the brain and may cause herniation of the brain. It is suggested by:

- Deterioration in conscious state (see Fig. 1.2)
- Pupillary dilatation and other cranial nerve signs
- Diminished spontaneous limb movement
- Limb hypertonicity and spasm
- Alteration in pattern of respiration (hyperventilation, irregular respiration)
- Bradycardia and hypertension

Common causes of intracranial hypertension are:

- Acute brain swelling due to cerebral oedema caused by hypoxaemia, infection or trauma
- Space-occupying lesion, such as a haematoma, intracerebral haemorrhage or tumour
- Obstruction of cerebrospinal fluid circulation

A neurosurgeon should be contacted immediately. If it is impossible to treat the cause immediately, reduce the intracranial blood volume by using mechanical hyperventilation to lower the P_aCO_2 and cause cerebral vasoconstriction. (*Note:* Prolonged hyperventilation to P_aCO_2 of <25–35 mmHg may be harmful.) Hypoxaemia and hypotension must be avoided. *Mannitol* may be used to reduce cerebral oedema (0.25–0.5 g/kg, i.v.). Fluids should be restricted to avoid cerebral oedema, but not at the expense of causing hypotension.

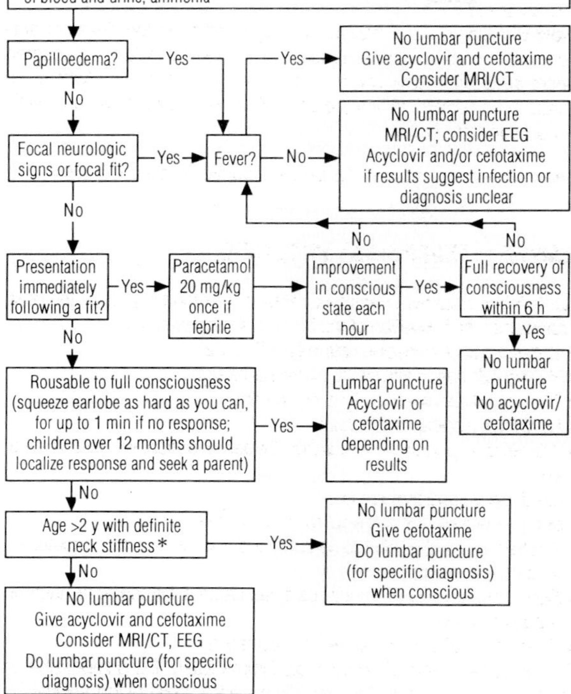

Figure 1.2 A guide to the role of lumbar puncture and the use of chemotherapeutic agents in the unconscious child of unknown cause

CHAPTER 2

POISONING AND ENVENOMATION

Jim Tibballs

POISONING

EPIDEMIOLOGY

Poisoning during childhood occurs mainly among 1–3 year olds following the ingestion of a wide variety of improperly stored agents in the home.

Other circumstances of poisoning are iatrogenic (particularly in infants) or the deliberate self-administration of substances by older children for their recreational use or to manipulate their psychosocial environments. Occasionally, the intention is suicidal.

While poisoning in childhood is frequently minor in severity and mortality is low, serious illness may be caused by prescription and 'over the counter' pharmaceutical drugs and non-pharmaceutical products.

MANAGEMENT

See Fig. 2.1. The principles of management are:

- Resuscitate the patient
- Remove the poison (if indicated)
- Administer an antidote (if one exists)

Recovery is expected in the vast majority of cases if vital functions are preserved, and the complications of poisoning and its management are avoided.

A decision to remove the poison from the body should be dependent upon the degree of severity of the poisoning and the likelihood of success in removing the poison without further endangering the patient. Most poisonings in childhood are minor, and observation alone or non-invasive treatment is indicated.

The severity of poisoning may be assessed by:

- Quantity of the poison(s)
- Preparation of the poison

- Interval since exposure
- Established and expected effects

Removal from the body usually involves a technique of gastrointestinal decontamination but occasionally other methods, such as dialysis, exchange transfusion, charcoal haemoperfusion, plasmapheresis or haemofiltration are warranted.

If the conscious state is depressed, all methods of gastro-intestinal decontamination carry a substantial risk of aspiration pneumonitis. These techniques include induced emesis with Syrup of Ipecacuanha, gastric lavage, activated charcoal and whole bowel washout. The most important factor determining the choice of technique is the conscious state. A guideline for the general management of poisoning using these techniques according to severity of poisoning is shown in Figure 2.1.

Details of management of specific poisons should be obtained from a Poisons Information Centre or from appropriate, up-to-date references.

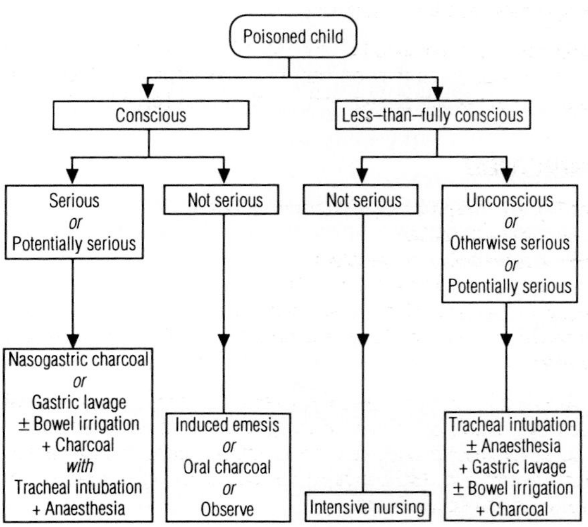

Figure 2.1 General management of the poisoned child

Activated Charcoal

Activated charcoal is more efficacious than induced emesis or gastric lavage and is currently regarded as a 'universal antidote'. It adsorbs most poisons but not metals, corrosives or pesticides. Like other techniques, however, it is contraindicated in the less-than-fully conscious patient or if ileus is present. If aspirated, charcoal may cause fatal bronchiolitis obliterans. Constipation is relatively common. Addition of a laxative decreases transit time through the gut but does not improve efficacy in preventing drug absorption, and it may upset fluid and electrolyte balance. The dose is 1–2 g/kg. Repeated doses of activated charcoal enhance elimination of many drugs, particularly slow-release preparations. A suitable regimen is 0.25 g/kg per h for 12–24 h.

Syrup of Ipecacuanha

Syrup of Ipecacuanha is useful as a first-aid measure in the home or at hospital with early presentation after ingestion of a minor poison. Its usefulness in serious poisoning is limited.

Although Syrup of Ipecacuanha induces vomiting in most children within 30 min of administration, it does not reliably empty the stomach of solids. Moreover, it must be given within 1 h of ingestion to significantly reduce drug absorption. It may cause prolonged vomiting, diarrhoea and drowsiness. The onset of vomiting may be delayed and may mimic the toxic effects of an ingested poison.

Contraindications include:
- Impaired conscious state (risk of aspiration pneumonitis)
- Ingestion of a corrosive, hydrocarbon or petrochemical (risk of additional respiratory tract damage)

Gastric Lavage

Gastric lavage appears to be a logical therapy for ingested poisons, but it too has a limited place in management. Problems include:
- Poor efficacy in preventing absorption when performed more than 60 min after ingestion
- Risk of aspiration pneumonitis in the less-than-fully conscious patient and to a lesser extent in the conscious child
- It is contraindicated after ingestion of corrosives, hydrocarbons or petrochemicals
- In the conscious young child it is psychologically traumatic and difficult to perform, thus predisposing to minor physical trauma

If undertaken, care should be taken to avoid water intoxication and intrabronchial instillation of lavage fluid.

- **Gastric lavage is indicated in serious poisoning when a child is already intubated for airways protection and ventilation.** If potentially serious effects are expected, gastric lavage should only be performed after rapid sequence induction of anaesthesia and tracheal intubation

Whole Bowel Irrigation

Whole bowel irrigation is performed with a solution of polyethylene glycol and electrolytes administered by nasogastric tube. A suitable dosage regimen is 30 mL/kg per h for 4–8 h.

It is useful in delayed presentation and for the management of poisoning by slow-release drug preparations or by substances not adsorbed by activated charcoal or which are irretrievable by gastric lavage.

PREVENTION

- Action should be taken according to the circumstance of poisoning to prevent reoccurrence. Parents should be encouraged to store all medicines in child-proof cabinets and to store toxic substances in places inaccessible to young children
- Psychosocial help should be organized for children who have poisoned themselves intentionally
- Steps should be taken to ensure that iatrogenic poisoning is not repeated

ENVENOMATION

SNAKE BITE

Note: These notes apply to bites by snakes of the genus *Elapids*. Snake bites by species of other genera cause different effects not outlined in this handbook. Please refer to local publications.

- Of the many species of snakes in Australia, the principal dangerous species are from the genera of brown, tiger, taipan, death adder, copperhead and black snakes
- Venoms of these species contain potent *neurotoxins* and *procoagulants* (although death adders do not contain procoagulant). Neurotoxins cause neuromuscular paralysis with respiratory failure,

while procoagulants cause disseminated intravascular coagulation with subsequent haemorrhage due to depletion of clotting factors
- Other less important components are haemolysins, anticoagulants and rhabdomyolysins
- Although not all snakes are venomous and envenomation does not always accompany a bite by a venomous snake, **every snake bite should be regarded as potentially lethal**
- In young children a history of snake bite is often uncertain

Symptoms and Signs of Envenomation

- Early clinical evidence of envenomation is headache, vomiting and abdominal pain; these may be experienced within an hour of a bite
- The bite site may be identifiable by fang or scratch marks surrounded by bruising or oedema. It is important to note, however, that a bite site may be undetectable and occasionally unnoticed by a victim
- Early neurotoxic signs are ptosis, diplopia, blurred vision, facial muscle weakness, dysphonia and dysphagia. Later signs are weakness of limb, trunk and respiratory muscles
- Spontaneous haemorrhage may occur from mucous membranes or from needle puncture sites. Haemolysis and myoglobinuria may contribute to renal failure, particularly if treatment with antivenom is delayed
- The syndrome culminates in respiratory and cardiovascular failure within several hours after envenomation, but may be accelerated in a small child or after multiple bites

Management

Suspected envenomation

- If there is a history of snake bite but no symptoms or signs, the patient should be admitted for close observation, preferably to an intensive care unit
- A test of coagulation should be performed, as it is both a sensitive and reliable indicator of envenomation by major species (*in Victoria*)
- If a pressure-immobilization first-aid bandage has been applied, it should be removed after ensuring that antivenom is available
- The presence of venom can be determined by a venom detection test. A positive test of the washings from the bite site identifies the snake, and a positive test of a biological sample (blood or urine) confirms envenomation

Definite envenomation

A number of measures are required depending on the severity of envenomation:

- Mechanical ventilation and oxygen therapy
- Antivenom (intravenously)
- Blood and coagulation factors (fresh frozen plasma)
- Application of a first-aid bandage. **Do not remove an existing first-aid bandage until antivenom has been administered**
- A venom test

Antivenom Therapy

- Antivenom is required for clinical signs of envenomation, or for symptomless coagulopathy which may cause a serious (e.g. intracranial) haemorrhage
- Specific antivenoms are available against brown snake, tiger snake, black snake, taipan, death adder and sea snakes. A polyvalent preparation contains all of the above named antivenoms (except sea snake)
- Wherever possible, a monovalent preparation should be infused because of a lower incidence of adverse reaction compared with polyvalent antivenom. Premedicate the patient with 0.05 mL/kg of 1 : 10 000 *adrenaline* subcutaneously (or 0.005 mL/kg of 1 : 1000 for larger patients) before the first dose of antivenom to prevent or ameliorate the severity of anaphylaxis. A steroid may prevent serum sickness, which may occur after polyvalent antivenom or after multiple doses of monovalent antivenom
- Selection of antivenom should be based on the result of a venom detection test or upon reliable identification of the snake, as there is little cross-reactivity between antivenoms. However, if antivenom therapy is required before identification, administer antivenom according to location. In Victoria give both brown and tiger snake antivenom, in Tasmania give tiger snake antivenom, and elsewhere give polyvalent antivenom. Infuse over 30 min (faster in life-threatening envenomation)
- The dose of antivenom cannot be predetermined because the amount of venom injected and the patient's susceptibility to it are unknown. Initially administer one ampoule (which contains sufficient to neutralize the average yield) and then titrate additional doses against the clinical and coagulation status. In the treatment of moderate envenomation of children, several ampoules are usually required, while in severe envenomation many ampoules may be required

- Administer antivenom before blood transfusion and coagulation factors to forestall further disseminated intravascular coagulation

SPIDER BITES

Redback Spider

The venom of this spider is potentially lethal but the syndrome of envenomation develops slowly over many hours, and no deaths have been recorded since an antivenom has been available.

Symptoms and signs

- The bite is very painful. Many effects have been recorded hours to days after a bite
- Local immediate effects include erythema, persistent pain, oedema, pruritus, sweating and regional lymphadenopathy
- Systemic effects may be distal limb and abdominal pain, hypertension, sweating, vomiting, fever and headache
- Myalgia, arthralgia, paraesthesia and weakness may last many weeks

Management

- If the effects remain mild and localized up to 24 h after a bite, treatment should be symptomatic only
- Severe local and systemic effects warrant administration of *antivenom* intramuscularly (occasionally intravenously). Premedication with *adrenaline* (0.05 mL/kg of 1 : 10 000 subcutaneously, or 0.005 mL/kg of 1 : 1000 for larger patients) is recommended

White-tailed Spider

Bites by this spider are not fatal, but severe local and extended skin necrosis may develop over several days and require excision, grafting and parenteral analgesia.

CHAPTER 3

PROCEDURES

Peter Barnett and Daryl Efron

Universal precautions should be used during any procedure (see p. 62). Gloves and protective eye wear should be worn, and a hard plastic container should be within easy reach for the disposal of sharps.

VENEPUNCTURE

SITES

- Cubital fossa
- Dorsum of hand
- Others as dictated by availability and/or necessity

TECHNIQUE

- In adolescents and older children, blood can be collected using a needle and syringe, as in adults. In infants and small children, a 23 gauge butterfly offers more stability
- Some visible veins are too small to be used to take blood. A vein that is palpable is more likely to be successful than a non-palpable but visible vein
- In small children it is often best to have the assistant act as both restrainer and tourniquet
- An alternative technique is to snap the hub off a 21 or 23 gauge needle, or cut off the tubing of a butterfly. Insert it into a vein on the dorsum of the hand or foot and allow the blood to drip out directly into the tube. Several millilitres can often be collected this way

INTRAVENOUS CANNULA INSERTION

SITES

- The dorsum of the hand is the preferred site. Use the non-dominant hand whenever possible
- Alternative sites include the anatomical snuff box, volar aspect of the forearm, dorsum of the foot, great saphenous vein or cubital fossa.

Using cubital fossa veins has the disadvantage of requiring the elbow to be splinted

- Scalp veins should only be used when all other possibilities have been exhausted (shaved scalp hair regrows very slowly)

TECHNIQUE

- Be patient and take time to look carefully for the best option. Ensure that the child is warm (especially the extremity in question) and that you have adequate light
- Unless vascular access is required immediately, topical local anaesthetic cream (e.g. EMLA) can be used, but must be applied at least 45 min before the procedure to be effective
- Wrapping small patients in a sheet is often helpful to minimize kicking and wriggling
- If using the back of the hand in infants, grasp the wrist between your index and middle fingers with your thumb over the fingers, flexing the wrist. This achieves both immobilization and compression (see Fig. 3.1)
- Insert the cannula just distal to and along the line of the vein at an angle of 10–15°. When a large vein is entered, a 'flash' of blood will enter the hub of the needle. Advance the cannula a further 1–2 mm along the line of the vein, then remove the needle. Continue advancing the cannula to the required depth. If the cannula is in the vein, blood should flow out along the cannula and continue to fill the chamber. When you are trying to cannulate a small vein, you should not expect a flash of blood to enter the hub of the needle. Insert the cannula and, when you think it may be in the vein, remove the needle

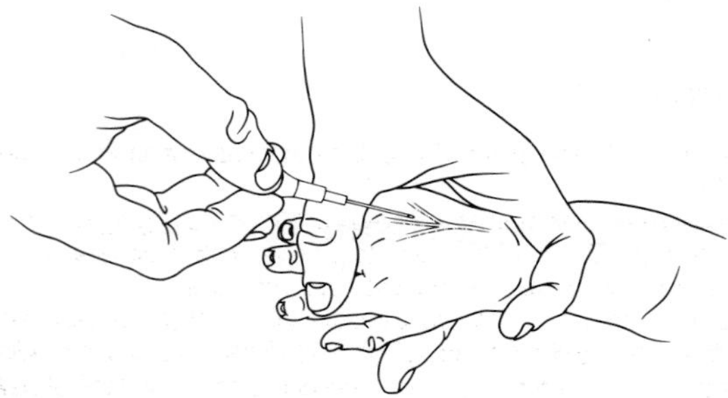

Figure 3.1 Intravenous cannula insertion

and watch for blood moving slowly down the cannula; then advance the cannula along the vein

- Take blood samples at this stage; then strap the cannula securely (using two inverted cross-over straps and another over the top). At this point flush the cannula with saline to confirm intravenous placement. Connect the intravenous tubing and splint the arm to an appropriately sized board (keeping the thumb free). Wrap the whole distal extremity in a crepe bandage

SUPRAPUBIC ASPIRATION (SPA)

INDICATIONS

- Fever with no obvious focus
- Bag urine specimen is suggestive of a urinary tract infection (UTI) on dipstick

Note: Bag specimens should only be used for a dipstick test to *exclude* a UTI; they should not be sent for culture (see Renal Conditions, p. 126). Note that a negative reagent strip screening test does not necessarily exclude infection, particularly in infants under 6 months of age; therefore, an SPA or catheter specimen should be obtained if there is a strong clinical suspicion of UTI.

CONTRAINDICATIONS

- Age >2 years (unless the bladder is palpable or percussible)
- Coagulopathy

TECHNIQUE

- Wait at least 30 min after last void. If doing a sepsis examination, do SPA first
- Position patient with legs either straight or bent in the frog-leg position. In males hold the tip of the penis to prevent voiding. Have a sterile bottle handy for a clean catch in case the child voids
- The site of entry is the skin crease above the symphysis pubis, in the midline. Prep the skin with an alcohol swab. Insert a 23 gauge needle attached to a 2 or 5 mL syringe perpendicular to the abdominal wall (see Fig. 3.2). Pass almost to the depth of the needle, and then aspirate as you withdraw. If urine is not obtained do not remove the

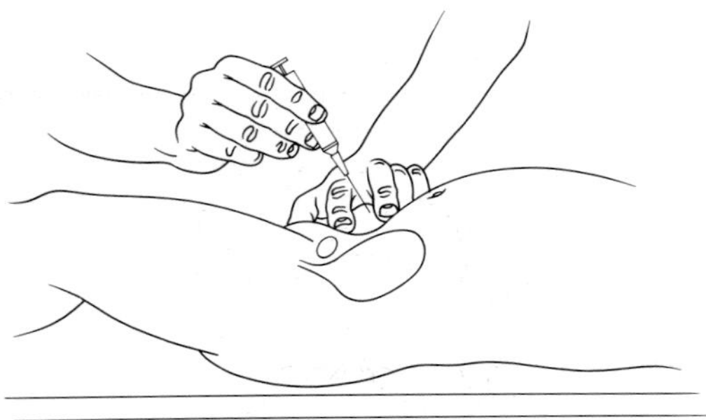

Figure 3.2 Suprapubic aspiration

needle completely; instead change the angle of the needle and insert it again, first angling superiorly and then inferiorly

- In the event of obtaining no urine, either (i) perform urethral catheterization or (ii) wait an hour, giving the child a drink during this time, and then repeat the SPA. It is a good idea to place a urine bag on so that you know whether the child has voided before proceeding with a further SPA

URETHRAL CATHETERIZATION

INDICATIONS

- Suspected UTI
- Acute urinary retention

TECHNIQUE

- An assistant is required to hold the child's legs apart, in the frog-leg position. Prep the area with a water-based disinfectant solution and drape with sterile towels
- For diagnostic catheterization, use a size 5 or 8 feeding tube (depending on the age of the child). For indwelling catheters, use a silastic catheter with inflatable balloon. Lubricant aids insertion
- Using a sterile technique, locate the urethral orifice (see Fig. 3.3). In males the foreskin need not be retracted fully for successful urethral catheterization. Advance the catheter *posteriorly* with care until urine is obtained

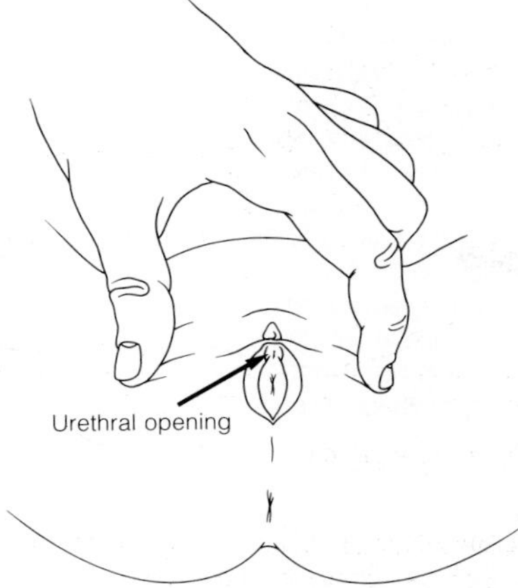

Figure 3.3 Urethral orifice

LUMBAR PUNCTURE

INDICATIONS

- Febrile, sick infant or toddler with no focus of infection
- Fever with meningism
- Prolonged seizure with fever

CONTRAINDICATIONS

- Depressed conscious state, focal neurological signs or coma
- Thrombocytopenia or clotting defect

Note: **If in doubt, do not proceed to lumbar puncture.**

TECHNIQUE

- If time permits, local anaesthetic cream should be used. This must be applied at least 1 h before the procedure
- Positioning of the patient is the key to performing a successful lumbar puncture, and is achieved with the help of an experienced assistant. Restrain the patient in the lateral position. Maximally flex the spine without compromising the airways. Avoid flexing the neck in small

babies as this may cause airways obstruction; flex their shoulders only
- The iliac crests are at the level of L3–4. Use this space or the space below (see Fig. 3.4). Using a strict aseptic technique, cleanse the skin and drape the patient. Local anaesthetic (1% lignocaine) should be used in children older than 6 months. Anaesthetize the area to near the dura (i.e. about two-thirds the length of your chosen lumbar puncture needle)
- The correct needle size is 30 mm for neonates and infants, 40 mm for 1–4 year olds, 50 mm for 4–10 year olds and 60 mm for older children. A 22 gauge is usually appropriate
- Grasp the spinal needle with the bevel facing upwards. Ensure that the patient's back is perpendicular to the bed, and that the needle is perpendicular to the back. Insert the needle through the skin slowly, aiming towards the umbilicus (i.e. slightly cephalad). Continue advancing the needle until there is decreased resistance (having traversed ligamentum flavum) or the needle has been inserted half its length; then remove the stylet and advance the needle about 1 mm. Wait at least 30 s for CSF to appear in the hub. Rotating the needle through 90–180° may allow CSF to flow. Advance 1 mm at a time if no CSF has appeared. If no CSF is obtained when bone is contacted or the needle is fully inserted, withdraw the needle very slowly until

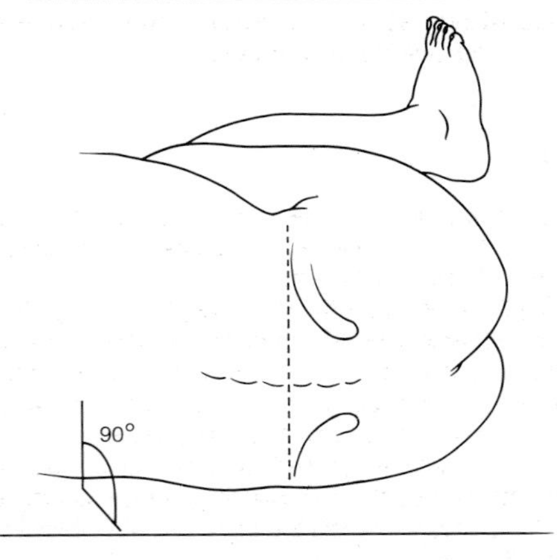

Figure 3.4 Position for lumbar puncture

CSF flows or the needle is almost removed. Then reinsert the stylet, recheck the patient's position and needle orientation and repeat the procedure
- Collect 0.5–1 mL of CSF in each of two tubes, for microbiological and biochemical analysis. Remove the lumbar puncture needle with one quick motion. Press on the puncture site with a cotton ball for about 30 s, then cover with a light dressing

ARTERIAL STAB

INDICATIONS

Suspected hypoxaemia, hypercapnoea or severe acidosis with poor peripheral perfusion.

Note: Acid–base status alone can be assessed by a capillary collection.

SITES

Radial or brachial artery.

Note: Femoral artery is used only in *emergencies* when no other arteries are palpable. ***Never* use the ulnar artery.**

TECHNIQUE

- Clean the skin with an alcohol swab. Using a pre-heparinized 2 mL syringe and a 23 or 25 gauge needle or butterfly, pierce the skin at a 15–30° angle directly over the artery
- On entering the artery, blood will fill the hub; however, gentle aspiration is usually required to fill the syringe. If no blood enters the hub with the needle at its full depth or when bone is contacted, withdraw the needle very slowly while aspirating because blood will often enter the needle on the way out if the artery has been transfixed
- Only 0.5 mL of blood is required for arterial blood gas, sodium, potassium and haemoglobin measurements. After obtaining a specimen, quickly remove the needle and *apply firm pressure to the puncture site for 3–5 min*

INTRAOSSEOUS INFUSION

INDICATIONS

For *emergency* vascular access when efforts to cannulate a vein are unsuccessful.

SITES

Preferred sites of insertion are:

- *Up to 3 years:* proximal tibia (1–2 cm inferomedial to tibial tuberosity) or distal femur in the midline (approximately 3 cm above the condyles) (see Fig. 3.5)
- *Any age:* medial malleolus of the tibia (just above the ankle)

TECHNIQUE

- Prep the insertion site. Inject 1% lignocaine into the area if the patient is conscious. If an intraosseous needle is not available, a short lumbar puncture needle or bone marrow aspiration needle may be used (intravenous cannulae or venepuncture needles are not appropriate).
- Penetrate the skin and then angle the needle at 10–15° from vertical – caudad for proximal tibial insertion and cephalad for femoral or medial malleolus insertion (see Fig. 3.5). Apply downward pressure with a rotary motion to advance the needle. When the needle passes through the cortex of the bone into the marrow cavity, resistance

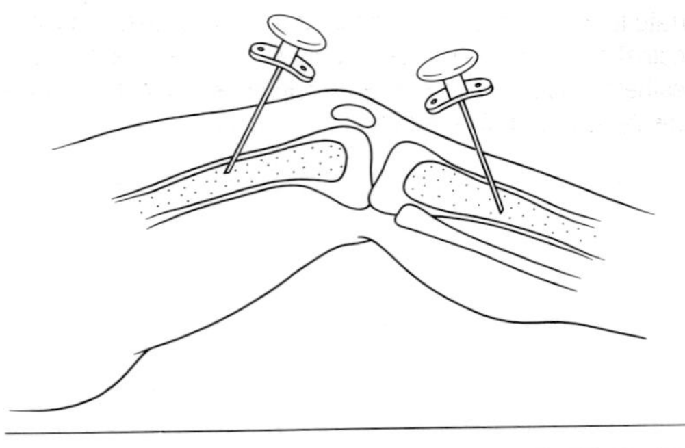

Figure 3.5 Intraosseous needle insertion sites

suddenly decreases. The needle should now stand without support (except in a very young infant)

- Remove the stylet and attach a 5 mL syringe; aspirate to confirm that the needle is in the bone marrow (this is not always possible). Flush the needle with saline to confirm correct placement and then connect intravenous tubing. Often fluids will not flow by gravity into the marrow—a three-way tap and syringe or pressure infusion may be needed
- Watch the infusion site for fluid extravasation. The needle should be removed once intravenous access has been obtained
- Any fluid or drug that can be given intravenously can be administered through the intraosseous route

FEMORAL NERVE BLOCK

INDICATION

Pain relief for proximal femur fractures.

TECHNIQUE

- After skin preparation, palpate the femoral artery below the inguinal ligament. Raise a wheal with local anaesthetic just lateral to the artery
- Introduce a short bevelled needle (such as a lumbar puncture needle or a 23 gauge needle) through this wheal and advance downwards perpendicular to the skin. A characteristic 'pop' or loss of resistance is felt as the needle goes through the fascia lata and again as it penetrates the fascia iliaca (if using a lumbar puncture needle)
- Aspirate to ensure that the needle is not in a blood vessel. Inject local anaesthetic solution (usually bupiva caine in a dose of 2 mg/kg). The anaesthetic should inject smoothly without subcutaneous swelling. Paraesthesia need not be elicited

CHAPTER 4

NEONATAL CONDITIONS

Peter McDougall, Lex Doyle and Barbara Burge

ROUTINE CARE

THE FIRST MINUTES

The newborn baby must start to breathe, the major stimuli being chemical (fall in $P\text{O}_2$ and pH) and tactile (fall in facial skin temperature). The fetal circulation (<10% of cardiac output going to the lungs) must change to the normal circulation (with 100% of cardiac output going to the lungs).

- The *Apgar score* is used to assess well-being at birth. A score of *7–10* at term indicates a well infant – no resuscitation necessary. A score of *4–7* indicates moderate depression – resuscitation includes thermal care, brief tactile stimuli, aspiration of airways, bag and mask ventilation and ongoing assessment. A score of *0–3* indicates severe depression – resuscitation includes thermal care, aspiration of airways, initial bag and mask ventilation and, if poor early response, oral intubation by an experienced physician. Careful attention to circulation may include cardiac massage and intravenous therapy. **Admission to a neonatal intensive care unit is mandatory if spontaneous ventilation is not established by 5 min of age**
- *Heat losses*, particularly evaporative, are huge after birth and can be minimized by drying and wrapping the baby in blankets. This is not necessary for the well, term infant who is being cuddled by the mother immediately after birth. The baby's temperature should stabilize around a core temperature of 37 °C after an hour of age
- The *umbilical cord* should be clamped and cut close to the skin. The cut end and the base of the cord should have an antiseptic solution, such as chlorhexidine in alcohol, applied daily until the cord stump drops off. Observation for omphalitis is important, particularly if these measures are not followed. The plastic clamp is usually removed at 2 days of age
- After the infant's temperature is stable, the skin should be washed with soap and water

THE FIRST HOURS

- Record the colour, heart rate and respiratory rate and effort at frequent intervals – most major causes of respiratory distress will present within the first hours of life
- Often the baby will be very alert and breast feeds are best encouraged at these times

Vitamin K

- Claims regarding the association between intramuscular vitamin K and childhood cancer have not been substantiated by subsequent epidemiologic studies
- An increased incidence of both early and late haemorrhagic disease of the newborn has been observed in Australia in breast fed infants who have received either oral, intravenous, inadequate intramuscular, or no prophylactic vitamin K
- **All infants, regardless of size, maturity or ill-health should receive 1 mg of intramuscular vitamin K.** This has been shown to almost completely eradicate haemorrhagic disease. Do not administer in the delivery ward as other drugs may be given by accident
- Parents who choose to give their infant oral vitamin K should be advised that oral doses need to be given to breast fed infants every 2–4 weeks until 6 months of age to cover the period of risk of haemorrhagic disease

THE FIRST DAY

After an initial period of alertness the infant will often sleep for long periods and may not be too demanding with feeds. In the first 24 h the infant should:

- Be able to *suck and swallow* – if not, consider unrecognized prematurity, neurological or anatomical abnormality, or it may be an early marker of illness (e.g. infection)
- *Pass meconium* – if not, assume low bowel obstruction
- *Pass urine* – if not, observe carefully as voiding is often missed; however, obstructive uropathy is possible

THE FIRST EXAMINATION

Before disturbing the baby the behaviour, general appearance, colour and well-being should be noted.

- *Head and neck:* look for depressed fractures, haematomas, lacerations, red reflex of eye and cleft palate
- *Cardiovascular/respiratory:* respiratory and heart rates, pulses (femorals/brachials), heart and breath sounds
- *Abdomen:* masses (liver, spleen, kidneys, bladder, ovaries), distension, genitalia and hernial areas
- *Hips:* carefully examine for congenital dislocation. Severe deformity of the hip can be avoided by early detection and treatment
- *Weight, length and head circumference* should be measured, and aberrations of growth noted by comparing the measurements with those expected for a baby of the same gestational age

THE FIRST WEEK

After an initial phase of waking frequently until lactation is established, the breast fed baby should establish a regular cycle of waking for feeds, followed mostly by sleeping. However, more mature babies will stay awake after some feeds, even in the first week of life. Bowel actions usually change from black meconium over the first few days, to dark green, yellow-green and finally loose yellow once full breast feeding is established, after 4–5 days of age. However, the colour and frequency of stools varies significantly among breast fed babies.

- *Urine production* is usually low in the first few days, but will increase after feeding has been established, with a urinary frequency of at least once per feed
- More than half of all babies will become *jaundiced* after the first 24 h of age (see later)
- On days 3–5, blood should be sampled to *screen for three diseases:* phenylketonuria (incidence 1 : 10 000), congenital hypothyroidism (incidence 1 : 5000) and cystic fibrosis (incidence 1 : 2500 in Caucasians). Results are available approximately 1 week after sampling. Negative (normal) results are not notified, but the laboratory will contact the baby's doctor regarding the management of children with positive (abnormal) results, and advise on appropriate management, which usually involves immediate referral to a tertiary paediatric hospital for further testing, and treatment if appropriate
- After an initial *weight loss* over the first few days, averaging 6–7% of bodyweight, the baby's weight should stabilize, and then increase towards the end of the first week

THE FIRST MONTH

- Weight gain ranges between 150 and 250 g/week
- Problems usually relate to behaviour (not sleeping enough), weight

(usually not gaining enough) or feeding (usually not drinking enough). These problems are discussed elsewhere in this book (see p. 362)

VARIATIONS OF NORMAL

When the baby is fully examined, normal variants or minor problems may be obvious. The treatment of most of these conditions comprises only explanation to the family and reassurance.

SKIN

- *Naevus flammeus* ('stork-bite'): dilated capillaries on the nape of most babies and on the face (eyelids and forehead) in about one-half. Fades over 6–12 months
- *Milia:* blocked sebaceous glands, particularly on the nose. They disappear over the first month as the outer layer of the epidermis peels off
- *'Mongolian' pigmentation*: bluish areas of increased melanin deposition, mostly over the sacral area, but can be more extensive. Sometimes mistaken for bruising. Present in children born to parents with increased melanin in their skin, irrespective of race. It gradually lightens over a few years as the remaining skin increases its pigmentation
- *Miliaria:* two types – 'crystallina' and 'rubra'. Miliaria crystallina are beads of sweat trapped under the epidermis, and are most prominent on the forehead in babies who are overheated. Miliaria rubra, also called 'heat rash', usually appear after a few weeks of age, fluctuate over 2–3 weeks, and disappear. They are related to increasing activity of the sweat glands, are prominent on the face and in babies who perspire more
- *Dry skin:* the outer layer of the epidermis is thicker in newborn infants because they have virtually been in a water bath for 9 months. The epidermis peels in the uterus, but has to be thicker to do so. After birth, the outer layers of the skin dry out in the air, and the epidermis peels off in sheets, taking up to 1 month to do so. Babies who are more mature have a thicker epidermis and hence drier looking skin after birth. This dry skin never worries the baby, except for occasional cracking and bleeding around the ankles or wrists, and moisturizing creams or lotions are contraindicated as most chemicals can be absorbed through the epidermis into the circulation
- *Puffy eyelids/scalp oedema:* the newborn infant has relatively excessive fluid in the skin after birth. Fluid accumulates easily in the eyelids and, after lying on one side, the lower eye may be more swollen.

Scalp oedema is common in the first few hours after a normal birth, but can persist for several days

- *Bruising/petechiae/subconjunctival haemorrhages:* as the presenting part acts to dilate the cervix in labour, it is commonly noted to be bruised after birth. In addition, when the head appears on the perineum in a vertex delivery, the blood pressure in the head and neck is very high, causing petechial haemorrhages. These disappear quickly after birth if they are in the skin, but can persist for many weeks in the sclera, as scleral blood supply, and hence phagocytic activity, is very low. Subconjunctival haemorrhages occur in up to 25% of babies delivered normally and do not adversely affect vision. Bruising is common after forceps deliveries, particularly over bony prominences, but disappears over the first week of life. Less commonly after forceps deliveries, firm nodules may be noted in the subcutaneous tissue at the same sites. This is subcutaneous fat necrosis. It resolves spontaneously over the first month of life
- *Sucking blisters:* these are common, particularly on the upper lip and at sites that the baby may have been sucking on *in utero* (e.g. the wrist)
- *Breast hyperplasia:* a breast bud is palpable in most term babies, regardless of their gender; in some the breasts can become enlarged during the first week as they respond to the same hormonal changes that occur in the lactating woman, and in some babies milk ('witch's milk') may be observed. The breasts should be left alone and the hyperplasia will subside over several months

BEHAVIOUR

In the first days of life, babies are often in a restless type of sleep (rapid eye movement [REM] sleep), where they breathe erratically, make various noises, including crying, vocalizing and yawning, have many body movements and may seem to be waking up. This behaviour can be very confusing to inexperienced parents.

DEFORMITIES

The skull must change shape (moulding) to enable the baby to be delivered. In addition there may be postural deformities of the face, skull and limbs that are related to the baby's position in the uterus. These gradually improve after birth, but sometimes do not disappear completely — very few people are completely symmetrical, especially in their face.

COMMON MINOR PROBLEMS

- *Hiccups*: occur frequently, especially after a feed. They are not caused by inadequate burping, are harmless and disappear after 10–15 min
- *Snuffles:* most common during or after a feed, after vomiting, or after a prolonged sleep, during which time the baby has not coughed or sneezed to clear the upper airways. Despite the noise, the baby is otherwise quite well, and is able to feed normally. Often thought by parents to be a common cold. The problem diminishes with time as the baby's feeding becomes more efficient and the nasal passages enlarge. Nose drops or other direct treatments of the nose are contraindicated
- *Posseting:* small vomits particularly after feeds. Harmless, as long as not bile-stained (green), blood-stained, projectile, persistent or associated with choking or failure to thrive. Can be minimized by reducing handling of the baby immediately after feeds
- *Bleeding umbilical cord:* occurs as the cord is separating and requires no treatment unless there is also a purulent discharge or cellulitis around the cord indicating infection
- *Umbilical hernia:* present in approximately 25% of babies, resolves in almost all and requires surgery only for cosmetic reasons if persistent beyond 2 years of age
- *Vaginal skin tag:* the vaginal skin commonly protrudes between the labia in newborn girls. It disappears as the vaginal skin shrinks and as the labia become larger
- *Vaginal discharge:* a small amount of vaginal mucus is universal. In some it can be blood-stained for a few days during the first week, as the endometrium involutes and bleeds
- *Urates:* a red–orange discoloration of the napkin, most common when the urine is concentrated (the first few days of life) and sometimes mistaken for blood
- *Clicky hips:* some ligamentous clicking is common in all large joints, including the hips. Can be considered normal in the absence of any abnormal movement of the femoral head, restriction of hip movement, strong family history or breech presentation. However, if there is any doubt, a hip ultrasound is indicated
- *Erythema toxicum* (also called 'toxic erythema' or 'urticaria of the newborn'): a harmless skin condition of unknown aetiology that peaks at 2–3 days of age and is rarely present after the first week of life. New lesions can look spectacular, with a broad erythematous base (up to 2–3 cm diameter) with a 1–2 mm papule which may either disappear or become a pustule. If the fluid in the pustule is examined,

it contains eosinophils and is sterile. Lesions can appear simultaneously anywhere on the body. The major differential diagnosis is staphylococcal skin infection, which usually spreads from one site, with multiple pustules, or even bullae; examination of the fluid in infection reveals neutrophils and Gram-positive cocci, and *Staphylococcus aureus* will grow in culture. The diagnosis of erythema toxicum can usually be made with confidence on clinical grounds alone

JAUNDICE

Jaundice is common in the newborn period and is almost always due to unconjugated hyperbilirubinaemia. Its significance largely depends on the age of the infant at its onset.

THE FIRST 24 HOURS

- *Jaundice in the first 24 h is abnormal*
- It is most likely to be due to Rh or ABO incompatibility between mother and fetus. The severe haemolysis that occurs leads to a rapid rise in serum bilirubin (SBR) over a few hours. The combination of haemolysis and high levels of SBR is the strongest risk factor for kernicterus (bilirubin encephalopathy)
- Rarely it may be conjugated hyperbilirubinaemia, and this needs investigation

Investigations

- SBR: total and direct (conjugated)
- Maternal and baby's blood group
- Direct Coombs' test
- Full blood examination and blood film

Further investigations are indicated if there is no evidence of haemolysis, or if conjugated hyperbilirubinaemia is present.

Management

Jaundice in the first 24 h always requires investigation and paediatric advice should be sought on management. In the event of early discharge the baby should be admitted to hospital immediately.

At this age the following are guidelines for therapy for the term infant with no other illnesses.

- SBR <150 µmol/L: observe and repeat SBR until past peak

- SBR 150–250 μmol/L: phototherapy
- SBR >250 μmol/L: exchange transfusion

Frequent monitoring of SBR levels is essential as rapid changes may occur and clinical assessment of the severity of jaundice, particularly under phototherapy, is unreliable.

DAYS 2–5

The jaundice is almost certainly physiologic if the following criteria are satisfied:

- The jaundice had its onset on days 2–4
- The jaundice is minimal, i.e. confined to the head, neck and upper trunk
- The baby is not low birthweight or preterm
- The baby is well (afebrile, feeding well, alert)
- The baby is passing normal coloured bowel actions and urine
- There are no other abnormalities

It is not necessary to measure SBR or perform other investigations if the above criteria are fulfilled. More than 50% of babies become visibly jaundiced by 2–4 days of age. This usually occurs when the SBR rises above 85–120 μmol/L. In 97% of cases it does not exceed 221 μmol/L and, in a well term baby, kernicterus does not occur at or below these levels.

If the above criteria are *not* fulfilled, an SBR level is indicated. If the unconjugated SBR is >221 μmol/L further investigations should be considered and the baby reviewed. If the baby is unwell, investigations, including a sepsis screen, are mandatory.

Management

A well term infant with no haemolysis is at minimal risk of kernicterus unless the SBR is very high. There are standard indications for treatment available from most major perinatal hospitals based on the infant's age, weight, gestation and level of unconjugated hyperbilirubinaemia. The following are some guidelines:

- If SBR >285 – consider phototherapy
- If SBR >340 – consider exchange transfusion if SBR continues to rise rapidly despite phototherapy

However, sick term infants, in particular those exposed to hypoxic insults, or infants with evidence of haemolysis, are at a higher risk of kernicterus and treatment needs to be started at lower SBR levels. Preterm infants are also at increased risk of kernicterus. This risk increases with decreasing gestation and degree of illness.

PROLONGED JAUNDICE (>14 DAYS)

Prolonged jaundice needs investigating.

- A sudden onset at this age is suggestive of haemolysis due to a red blood cell enzyme abnormality, most frequently G-6-PD deficiency, which can cause rapid haemolysis. Urgent admission to hospital is indicated
- A prolongation of the jaundice from the first few days of life can initially be investigated as an outpatient
- Stool colour must be ascertained, by history and examination. Unpigmented stools (grey) suggest obstruction to bile flow, which requires prompt investigation (imaging, and possibly liver biopsy)

Causes

Raised *conjugated* SBR:

- Biliary atresia
- Neonatal hepatitis
- Choledochal cyst

Raised *unconjugated* SBR:

- Hypothyroidism
- Sepsis
- Red cell enzyme abnormalities

If the above are excluded, the bilirubin is unconjugated, and the baby is well and breast feeding, the likely diagnosis is *breast milk jaundice.* This occurs in 2–4% of breast feeding infants, is not associated with kernicterus and does not need any treatment. Reassurance that breast feeding should continue is very important.

RESPIRATORY DISTRESS

PRESENTATION

Tachypnoea (>60 breaths/min) with associated subcostal and intercostal recession, nasal flaring, expiratory grunt or cyanosis in air.

AETIOLOGY

Common Pulmonary Diseases

Hyaline membrane disease (HMD)/respiratory distress syndrome

- Lung immaturity: more common with decreasing gestation – lack of pulmonary surfactant leads to widespread atelectasis

- Respiratory distress soon after birth: increases in severity and rapid progression to respiratory failure may occur
- Chest X-ray: widespread reticulogranular ('ground glass') appearance with air bronchograms and low volume lung fields

Transient tachypnoea of the newborn/'wet lung'

- Delayed clearing of fetal lung fluid: usually term infants born by elective Caesarean section
- Mild respiratory distress: occasionally prolonged for a few days
- Chest X-ray: coarse streaking of lung fields with fluid in fissures

Bacterial infections

- Group B β-haemolytic streptococcus: commonest cause of bacterial pneumonia in newborn; usually acquired at birth from asymptomatic mother
- Early-onset respiratory distress: frequent associated temperature instability, poor feeding, apnoea and, if not recognized, rapid progression to shock and collapse
- Chest X-ray: consolidation or similar to that of HMD, i.e. not diagnostic

Meconium aspiration syndrome

- Inhalation of thick (particulate) meconium stained liquor at birth
- Persistent pulmonary hypertension and/or birth asphyxia often associated and rapid deterioration common
- Chest X-ray: hyperinflation and patchy consolidation (pneumothorax and pneumomediastinum may follow) or diffuse hazy appearance may be evident

Milk aspiration

Infants unlikely to aspirate feeds unless sick, preterm, neurologically abnormal or an anatomical abnormality present (e.g. oesophageal atresia).

Pneumothorax

Occurs secondary to lung disease or spontaneously after birth: transillumination or needle aspiration of chest may give rapid diagnosis in a severely ill infant with poor breath sounds to auscultation.

Uncommon Pulmonary Diseases

- *Viral infections* acquired after birth (respiratory syncytial virus, rhinovirus, parainfluenza),usually at home, and may cause apnoea in preterm
- *Pulmonary haemorrhage:* preterm infants, small for gestational age, surfactant therapy and birth asphyxia associated
- *Bronchopulmonary dysplasia:* chronic lung disease in infants who have received mechanical ventilation
- *Congenital diaphragmatic hernia:* usually left sided with poor breath sounds and mediastinal shift to the right, scaphoid abdomen
- *Chylothorax:* often bilateral with poor chest movement and breath sounds
- *Pulmonary interstitial emphysema:* extremely low birthweight infants
- *H-type tracheo-oesophageal fistula:* feed related symptoms
- *Congenital lobar emphysema and congenital lung cysts*

Airways Obstruction

- *Nasal:* upper respiratory tract infection, choanal atresia or traumatic deviated nasal septum
- *Oral:* macroglossia
- *Pharynx:* micrognathia with cleft palate (Pierre Robin syndrome)
- *Neck:* goitre
- *Larynx:* vocal cord palsy, subglottic stenosis – inspiratory stridor
- *Trachea:* tracheomalacia – expiratory wheeze

Non-pulmonary

- *Cardiac:* left outflow obstruction (e.g. coarctation) or left-to-right shunt (e.g. large ventricular septal defect)
- *Persistent pulmonary hypertension*

MANAGEMENT

Before Birth

- *Antenatal steroids* in preterm labour: lower the incidence and severity of HMD
- Anticipation of high-risk delivery: transfer to tertiary centre for delivery may be appropriate, particularly for preterm labour

At Birth

Head on perineum: suction of oropharynx if thick meconium or blood is present.

After Birth

- Thick meconium present: under laryngoscopic vision aspirate oropharynx and larynx. Intubate and aspirate trachea if meconium around cords. Avoid positive pressure ventilation until airways are clear
- Diaphragmatic hernia suspected: intubate, as spontaneous breathing or bag and mask ventilation cause gaseous distension of thoracic intestinal contents
- Extremely low birthweight infants should be intubated after birth
- Oesophageal atresia: frequent (10–15 minutely) oropharyngeal suction to keep the airways clear (thereby preventing contamination of the lungs)

General Care

- Temperature control essential: incubator care is necessary
- Avoid enteral feeds if >40% inspired oxygen: give intravenous fluids
- Measure true blood glucose, electrolytes and full blood count
- Sepsis examination should include blood culture as minimum: *penicillin* and *gentamicin* as initial therapy until cultures are reported as clear

Respiratory Care

- Chest X-ray: mandatory for all infants who need >40% oxygen or who are not improving as expected
- *Artificial surfactant*: administered down the endotracheal tube has been shown to improve the outcome of infants with HMD
- Monitoring: cardiorespiratory and transcutaneous $S_{a}O_2$ or $P_{a}O_2$ essential
- Indwelling arterial line: indicated if infant needs >40% inspired oxygen

Oxygen Therapy

- <40%: oxygen delivered into incubator
- >40%: heated and humidified oxygen delivered into a head box
- Nasal prongs: should be avoided in acute early phases of disease
- >50%: should be transferred to a neonatal intensive care unit
- Indications for assisted ventilation: should be considered if more than 50% oxygen required with $P_{a}O_2$ <50 mmHg and/or $P_{a}CO_2$ >50 mmHg

HYPOGLYCAEMIA

DEFINITION

A true blood glucose of <2.5 mmol/L in any baby (see also p. 194). 'Dextrostix' or 'BM stix' are useful for screening purposes. However, if a screening test suggests hypoglycaemia, a true blood glucose should be performed before starting any invasive therapy.

Blood glucose measurement should be done on infants with the following conditions:

- Infants of diabetic mothers
- Large for gestational age
- Small for gestational age
- Preterm
- Birth asphyxia
- Seizures
- Infants receiving intravenous infusions

CLINICAL FEATURES

There are no specific clinical features of hypoglycaemia. The infants may be asymptomatic or exhibit symptoms of apathy, hypotonia, poor feeding, temperature instability, jitteriness or convulsions.

TREATMENT

- For well, asymptomatic infants with a true blood sugar in the range of 1.5–2.5 mmol/L institute early and frequent enteral feeds. However, if there is no response within 2–4 h parenteral dextrose is indicated
- Intravenous dextrose infusion is indicated for symptomatic hypoglycaemia or if the true blood glucose is <1.5 mmol/L. An initial *intravenous bolus of 25% dextrose 2–4 mL/kg* should be followed by an *infusion* of 10–15% dextrose aiming to provide 5–10 mg/kg per min of glucose. The response to therapy should be monitored by frequent blood glucose estimations
- For a 'large-for-dates' infant who has severe hypoglycaemia (<1 mmol/L) it may be very difficult to insert an intravenous line. In these circumstances give 1 unit/kg of *glucagon* intramuscularly
- Further investigation and treatment is necessary for severe intractable hypoglycaemia

NEONATAL SEPSIS

Bacterial sepsis is one of the most common preventable causes of neonatal mortality and morbidity. Bacterial infections may be acquired from the mother's genitourinary tract before or at birth (early onset), and postnatally from the environment by droplet spread or handling (late onset).

AETIOLOGY

The most frequently encountered organisms are:

Early Onset (First 72 h)

- Group B β-haemolytic streptococcus
- *Escherichia coli*
- *Listeria monocytogenes*

Late Onset (After 72 h)

- *Staphylococcus aureus*
- Group B β-haemolytic streptococcus
- Gram-negative enteric bacilli (e.g. *Escherichia coli*, *Klebsiella*, *Pseudomonas*)
- Coagulase negative staphylococcus (level 3 nurseries, related to intravenous lines)

CLINICAL FEATURES

The early symptoms and signs may be minimal but if ignored rapid progression to overwhelming sepsis may occur. The following are important warning signs:

- *A change in an infant's behaviour:* often an early sign of serious infection
- *Respiratory distress:* frequent in early-onset sepsis
- *Fever:* rectal temperature >37.5°C. *Note:* Neonates with bacterial infection often do not have a fever
- *Poor feeding*
- *Apnoea*
- *Seizures*

A careful examination with special attention given to:

- Cardiorespiratory system: signs of respiratory distress
- Abdomen: distension, tenderness with or without cellulitis of the

MEDICINE

abdominal wall may indicate necrotizing enterocolitis. Cellulitis around the umbilicus suggests omphalitis
- The fontanelle may be bulging in meningitis
- Skin: poor circulation or rashes
- Skeletal system: limitation of, or pain, with limb movement suggests septic arthritis or osteomyelitis

INVESTIGATIONS

If one or more of the above warning signs are present it is mandatory to perform a complete sepsis examination. This includes:
- *Full blood examination and differential*
- *Blood culture:* arterial or venous (at least 2–4 mL)
- *Urine:* suprapubic aspiration (SPA). If one SPA fails, do not keep attempting. A catheter specimen should be obtained by inserting a 5 French gauge catheter under aseptic technique. Discard the first two to three drops. A bag specimen is of little value
- *Lumbar puncture:* delay in a sick baby with a bulging fontanelle
- *Chest X-ray* if respiratory symptoms
- *Stool culture* if diarrhoea

MANAGEMENT

Any neonate with a rectal temperature >37.5°C should be investigated and managed in hospital. Empiric broad-spectrum antibiotics given parenterally are generally indicated. Usually this will start with *penicillin* and *gentamicin* for septicaemia or *amoxycillin* and *cefotaxime* for meningitis. The antibiotics will need to be rationalized when cultures are available.

Careful attention to temperature stability, ventilation, fluid and electrolytes, blood pressure, blood glucose and haematology is essential.

NEONATAL SEIZURES

CLINICAL FEATURES

- *Subtle:* deviation of eyes, abnormal sucking, apnoea
- *Tonic:* usually all limbs frequently associated with apnoea and eye deviation
- *Multifocal clonic:* migratory clonic movement of limbs
- *Focal clonic:* localized and may indicate focal brain lesion

- *Myoclonic:* single or several asynchronous jerks of flexion of upper and lower limbs. May precede infantile spasms

DIFFERENTIAL DIAGNOSIS

True neonatal seizures need to be distinguished from:

- 'Jitteriness' (or tremulousness). This has no ocular phenomena, is stimulus sensitive and is stopped with gentle passive flexion of the limbs
- Benign sleep myoclonus. This occurs in the neurologically normal infant and only during sleep. The EEG is normal and no treatment is necessary

AETIOLOGY

An aetiology can usually be found for neonatal seizures.

- *Hypoxic ischaemic encephalopathy:* the seizures occur within 48 h of the hypoxic event and are often initially difficult to control with anticonvulsants
- *Intracranial haemorrhage:* subarachnoid, subdural, periventricular, or intracerebral
- *Metabolic*
    - hypoglycaemia*
    - hypocalcaemia/hypomagnesaemia*
    - hypo- or hypernatraemia*
    - amino/organic acidopathy, hyperammonaemia
    - pyridoxine dependency
    - kernicterus

(* These may occur in isolation or in combination, and are frequently present in hypoxic ischaemic encephalopathy and meningitis.)

- *Infection:* bacterial (group B streptococcus, *E. coli* and *Listeria*) or viral (herpes and enteroviruses) meningitis
- *Drug withdrawal*
- *Developmental brain abnormalities*
- *Autosomal dominant neonatal seizures*
- *Local anaesthetic intoxication*
- *Idiopathic*

MANAGEMENT

Management is aimed at recognizing and treating the cause.

Investigations

- Lumbar puncture
- Blood glucose
- Electrolytes, Ca, Mg
- Cranial ultrasound
- Metabolic screen: indicated when other causes not found
- Cranial CT scan: if focal seizures, birth trauma, uncertain aetiology
- MRI scan: suspected developmental brain abnormality
- EEG: to detect seizure activity and to aid prognosis

Anticonvulsants

- *Phenytoin:* 20 mg/kg, i.v. stat in not less than 20 min
- *Phenobarbitone:* 20 mg/kg, i.v. stat over 10 min. A further 10 mg/kg may be given for refractory seizures
- *Clonazepam:* up to 0.25 mg. This may cause apnoea. Careful monitoring and the availability of mechanical ventilation are essential
- *Pyridoxine:* 100–200 mg, i.v. or oral, should be considered for intractable seizures

Other anticonvulsants, including *thiopentone*, may be necessary.

Most infants are able to be weaned off anticonvulsant therapy within 2 weeks of their last seizure. Some infants who have residual seizures or abnormal neurological signs with an abnormal EEG are treated for months.

General Management

Attention to optimal ventilation, blood pressure control, fluid and electrolyte balance and normoglycaemia is essential.

Admission to a neonatal intensive care unit is indicated in the presence of:
- Apnoea
- Bacterial meningitis
- Poor response to anticonvulsants
- Uncertain aetiology

POSTNATAL DEPRESSION (PND)

Mild to moderate postnatal depression occurs in about 16% of women; a much higher incidence than has been previously believed. **Severe PND can be a risk to the life of both mother and baby.**

All types of depression can have profound effects on the family and on the development of the young child. The diagnosis is not always easy or obvious, so a high level of awareness is needed.

WARNING SIGNS

- Highly anxious about all manner of small things
- Difficult to reassure or keeps presenting to health professionals
- While some babies do cry a lot and need more attention than average, a crying baby can and often does accompany a woman who is depressed. Crying babies can also cause women who are already unsure and vulnerable to become depressed
- Overly 'fussy'
- Leaves her baby crying
- Totally disorganized, not wanting to go out and crying a lot

MANAGEMENT

- Recognition and acknowledgement of the problem
- Appropriate support and counselling
- Medication is sometimes necessary
- Referral to a Mother–Baby Unit or a psychiatric hospital facility may be of benefit

MASTITIS

- Mastitis is common in breast feeding women
- Patients present with aches, pains and fever, and often think that they have 'flu'
- Examination will reveal a tender engorged segment in one or both breasts
- The organism is usually *S. aureus*

MANAGEMENT

- Prompt treatment is important to prevent abscess formation
- Oral antibiotics: *flucloxacillin* 500 mg q.i.d. or *erythromycin* 250 mg q.i.d.
- *Paracetamol* or *aspirin*
- Increased fluids
- Breast feeding should continue as there is no risk to the infant
- Good emptying of the affected breast; the baby is more efficient at this than expression

PROBLEMS OF THE EX-VERY LOW BIRTHWEIGHT (VLBW) INFANT (BIRTHWEIGHT <1500 G)

BRONCHOPULMONARY DYSPLASIA (BPD)

This a common chronic lung disease occurring in infants who have survived mechanical ventilation. It is characterized by oxygen dependency for longer than 28 days. The majority of VLBW infants with BPD are able to be weaned out of oxygen within 4 weeks of the time that they were due to be born. A small number require oxygen therapy for months and some are managed at home in oxygen.

These babies are particularly susceptible to respiratory infections in the first 18 months of life and may deteriorate rapidly.

Warning Signs

- Apnoeic episodes
- Cyanotic episodes
- Poor feeding
- Crackles on auscultation

The presence of one or more of these signs is an urgent indication for admission to hospital.

In the absence of these the infant may be managed at home but the parents need to be informed of the warning signs and the child reviewed frequently.

NECROTIZING ENTEROCOLITIS (NEC)

This an acquired gastrointestinal disease due to infection in the immature small and/or large intestine which has suffered vascular compromise. The result is transmural inflammation of the gut. While many babies recover after conservative management (nil orally, intravenous alimentation, antibiotics) some develop bowel necrosis necessitating bowel resection.

The risks to these babies after discharge from hospital are:

- *Stricture formation:* this can present weeks or months after the initial NEC episode. The presenting features include constipation, failure to thrive and vomiting
- *Gastroenteritis:* this can produce severe dehydration very rapidly, particularly in a baby who has had a bowel resection. It is not appropriate to manage these infants at home with oral rehydration therapy. Admission to hospital is essential

FURTHER COMMON PROBLEMS

- *Umbilical hernia:* does not require treatment
- *Inguinal hernias:* require surgical repair as there is a significant risk of strangulation
- *Otitis media:* associated with prolonged endotracheal intubation and should be considered in babies presenting with fever and irritability
- *Immunization:* an infant should receive the first three doses of DTP, Sabin and Hib vaccines at 2, 4 and 6 months from the actual date of birth, irrespective of the degree of prematurity. *There are no grounds for delaying immunization nor reducing vaccine dose based on size or prematurity*
- *Apnoea:* very common problem until 34 weeks gestation due to immaturity of the respiratory centre and is resolved after the infant reaches this gestation. However, ex-VLBW infants are at risk of further apnoea until the age of 3 months past their due date when undergoing surgical procedures requiring general anaesthesia or if they contract respiratory tract infections (especially respiratory syncytial virus). Close monitoring is advised at these times
- *Capillary haemangiomas* (strawberry naevus): often multiple and appear after birth as raised, red, lobulated and compressible lesions which increase in size over a few months. Most involute over the first 2 years and this starts by grey fibrotic changes appearing in the centre of the lesion. Failure to involute or difficult locations (e.g. around the eye) may be indications for referral to a paediatric dermatologist/ plastic surgeon for consideration of specific therapy

5

CHAPTER 5

INFECTIOUS DISEASES AND MICROBIOLOGY

Keith Grimwood and Geoff Hogg

RATIONAL ANTIMICROBIAL PRESCRIBING

Although the majority of infections are viral, many children receive antibiotics after a visit to the doctor. Reasons include thinking a bacterial infection is still possible, the belief that secondary infections can be prevented by antibiotics and parental expectations of receiving treatment.

Antibiotics do not prevent secondary infection and oral therapy is inadequate treatment of serious bacterial infection. Many children are needlessly given antibiotics, placing them at risk of side-effects. Antibiotics also select resistant organisms, which may spread to other patients or transfer resistance genes to other pathogenic bacteria. *Empiric antibiotic therapy* is prescribed when it may not be possible, or practical, to obtain definitive culture specimens (e.g. otitis media), or when a serious bacterial infection is suspected (e.g. meningitis) and culture results are pending:

- For mild infections, the simplest, safest effective antibiotic against the most likely pathogen should be chosen (e.g. amoxycillin for otitis media)
- For serious infections, potent broad-spectrum agents (e.g. cefotaxime for meningitis) are chosen until the pathogen and its sensitivity is identified. This enables directed therapy for proven pathogens (e.g. in blood, CSF or urine) which should be the most effective, least toxic, narrowest spectrum agent available

The temptation to prescribe the newest antibiotic should be resisted. Theoretical benefits based upon *in vitro* data do not necessarily translate into greater efficacy by more expensive agents, which may have more side-effects and frequently a broad spectrum of action resulting in potential development of resistance or superinfection. Factors used to determine the role of new antibiotics include evidence that the drug has superior clinical efficacy or is safer or cheaper than older, more established antibiotics

THE FEBRILE CHILD WITHOUT A FOCUS

A careful history and examination identifies the source of infection in most patients. A small number, however, present with high fever (>39°C) and no focus is found. While most have a viral infection, a serious infection such as a urinary tract infection (5–8%) or pneumococcal bacteraemia (1–2%) may be present. The challenge is to identify the small percentage of children with a serious infection who, on rare occasions, may develop a severe complication (e.g. 1–5% of children with pneumococcal bacteraemia may develop meningitis).

Most children who present with fever and no identifiable focus appear otherwise well. Ask about past medical and immunization *history*, infectious contacts and travel. Pay particular attention to the following aspects of the *physical examination*:

- General appearance: level of activity and social interaction; peripheral perfusion and colour
- Vital signs: pulse; respiration; blood pressure
- Exclude: full fontanelle; neck stiffness; respiratory distress (grunt, stridor, flare, retractions); abnormal percussion and auscultatory signs in the chest; otitis, mastoiditis, pharyngitis, rhinitis; lymphadenopathy and hepatosplenomegaly; abdominal distension, tenderness or masses; bone and joint tenderness or swelling; skin rashes, petechiae or skin infection

Patients with unexplained fever with *higher likelihood for serious infection* include:

- Neonates
- Immunocompromised (e.g. congenital immunodeficiency, HIV, neoplasms, asplenia, central venous catheters)
- Multiple congenital abnormalities
- Toxic appearing children (e.g. decreasing conscious state, decreasing peripheral perfusion or blood pressure, petechial rash)

These children require hospitalization, with culture of blood, urine, CSF and any septic focus identified on physical examination. Antimicrobial therapy must be discussed immediately with senior medical staff as it is based on the patient's clinical illness and knowledge of the local epidemiological data of potential pathogens and their patterns of antibiotic susceptibility.

In the absence of the above risk factors there is no need for a well appearing febrile child without a focus for infection to undergo laboratory testing or treatment. There is no evidence that oral or parenteral antibiotics prevent the rare occurrence of focal infections from occult bacteraemia; instead, they result in delayed diagnosis, drug side-effects, additional costs and development of resistant organisms. What is required is a careful clinical assessment, review within the next 24 h and parental education.

Parents need to be advised about the *management of fever*:

- Dress the child in light clothing
- Give small, frequent drinks of water or dilute (1 : 4) fruit juices or cordial
- Give paracetamol (15 mg/kg) 4–6 hourly over the next 48 h (max. 90 mg/kg per day) for discomfort or fever >39°C

and *when to seek immediate medical attention*:

- Child looks sicker than previously
- Complains of neck stiffness or light hurting eyes
- Breathing difficulty
- Refusing to drink anything
- Persistent vomiting
- Drowsiness
- Pain
- No improvement in 48 h

CLINICAL SCENARIOS

- The rare child who *appears toxic* or has developed a *focal infection* (e.g. pneumonia, urinary tract infection, meningitis) is treated as discussed in other sections of this handbook
- If upon review the child *remains febrile*, urine and blood cultures should be performed. In the emergency department these tests are often performed at the first visit as patients present later in the illness, or may have already been seen by a medical practitioner
- If the child has *positive blood cultures* and is febrile, or has received prior antibiotics, a full septic examination is required, including repeat blood cultures and lumbar puncture, and parenteral antibiotics are started immediately pending culture results. The most likely organism is *Streptococcus pneumoniae* and the initial antibiotic management is either Penicillin G 30 mg/kg Q4h (normal CSF) or a third-generation cephalosporin if the CSF suggests meningitis (see p. 162)

Patients growing *S. pneumoniae* in their original blood culture, but who are now well, remain afebrile and have not received antibiotics, do not require further investigation or treatment as they have cleared the organism themselves. Parents should, however, be asked to bring the children back for immediate review if they develop further fever within the next 7 days.

Other pathogens such as *Haemophilus influenzae* and *Neisseria meningitidis* carry a significantly increased risk of meningitis, and should be treated with antibiotics most likely to be effective against these bacteria (usually a third-generation cephalosporin and penicillin, respectively) bearing in mind local patterns of resistance.

VIRAL INFECTIONS

ENTEROVIRUS (NON-POLIO) INFECTIONS

Important cause of childhood infections. Wide range of clinical illnesses, including undifferentiated fever, pharyngitis, gastroenteritis, aseptic meningitis, pericarditis, pleurodynia and several forms of viral exanthem (maculopapular, vesicular, petechial, hand, foot and mouth disease).

- *Incubation period:* 3–6 days
- *Infectious period:* at least 1 week after onset of illness
- *Isolation:* contact precautions for 7 days after onset of symptoms
- *Diagnosis:* culture of virus from CSF, blood or respiratory secretions; polymerase chain reaction of CSF is available in some laboratories; as enteroviruses can be excreted in faeces for months, faecal isolates may not be causally related to the patient's illness.
- *Treatment:* symptomatic

EPSTEIN-BARR VIRUS (INFECTIOUS MONONUCLEOSIS)

Fever, exudative pharyngitis, generalized lymphadenopathy, hepatosplenomegaly and atypical lymphocytes in the peripheral blood. Highly variable clinical course, acute phase lasts 2–4 weeks and convalescence may take weeks or months.

- *Incubation period:* 30–50 days
- *Infectious period:* unknown, viral excretion from oropharynx for months
- *Isolation:* none
- *Diagnosis:* Monospot test in blood for heterophile antibody. This test identifies 90% of cases in older children and adults, but lacks sensitivity in children younger than 5 years. Serology is the gold standard
- *Complications:* uncommon (e.g. upper airways obstruction or dehydration from poor oral intake due to grossly enlarged tonsils requiring hospitalization)
- *Treatment:* symptomatic. *Prednisolone* (1–2 mg/kg per day) or *cimetidine* (10 mg/kg 6 h max. 300 mg) for 1–2 weeks may be considered in cases hospitalized for airways obstruction

HERPES SIMPLEX (PRIMARY HERPES GINGIVOSTOMATITIS)

Usually due to HSV-1 in young children. Characterized by fever, irritability, cervical lymphadenopathy, halitosis, diffuse erythema and ulceration within the oral cavity (buccal mucosa, palate, gingiva and tongue) and mucocutaneous junction. Duration is 7–14 days.

- *Incubation period:* 2–14 days
- *Infectious period:* indeterminate; virus can be excreted for at least 1 week, occasionally months. Shed intermittently in the absence of symptoms for years afterwards
- *Isolation:* contact isolation
- *Diagnosis:* immunofluorescence or culture of vesicular fluid
- *Complications:* occasionally, children are hospitalized because of poor oral intake. Auto-inoculation may result in herpetic paronychia, keratitis or genital herpes. Skin infection in children with eczema (*eczema herpeticum*) may be severe. In immunocompromised patients HSV infection can disseminate and is life-threatening
- *Treatment:* symptomatic, oral *lignocaine gel* 3–4 hourly for analgesia, fluids (oral/nasogastric or intravenous) and a soft diet. A child with a severe infection requiring hospitalization *in the first 48 h* may be given *acyclovir* (250 mg/m^2, i.v. 8 h (5 mg/kg, i.v. 8 h if <2 years) or 100–200 mg of oral drug five times per day). Acyclovir is recommended for immunosuppressed children and those with eczema herpeticum

HUMAN HERPES VIRUS 6 (ROSEOLA INFANTUM, EXANTHEM SUBITUM)

Common, acute febrile illness in young children for several days, with occipital lymphadenopathy, then rapid defervescence of the fever and appearance of a red maculopapular rash over trunk and arms for 1–2 days.

- *Incubation period:* 5–15 days
- *Infectious period:* unknown (greatest during period of the rash)
- *Isolation:* none
- *Diagnosis:* serology
- *Complications:* encephalitis (rare)
- *Treatment:* symptomatic

MEASLES ✓

Cough, coryza, conjunctivitis for 2–4 days, then high fever with appearance of a discrete, then confluent, red maculopapular rash, first behind

MEDICINE

the ears and sequentially on to the face, neck, trunk, upper limbs, buttocks and lower limbs over the next 3–4 days. Koplik spots (white spots on a bright red buccal mucosa) appear 1–2 days before the rash and last 3–5 days.

- *Incubation period:* 8–12 days (14 days to appearance of rash)
- *Infectious period:* 1–2 days before onset of symptoms to 4 days after rash
- *Isolation:* respiratory
- *Diagnosis:* serology, nasopharyngeal aspirate immunofluorescence and culture
- *Complications:* otitis media, pneumonia, encephalitis
- *Treatment:* symptomatic
- *Prevention: MMR vaccine*, including within 3 days of exposure in a susceptible immunocompetent child >12 months of age. Consider *normal immunoglobulin* for infants <12 months (0.2 mL/kg, i.m.), and especially for immunocompromised patients (0.5 mL/kg) to a maximum of 15 mL where MMR is contraindicated, given as soon as possible after exposure

PARVOVIRUS B19 (ERYTHEMA INFECTIOSUM, FIFTH DISEASE)

Mild systemic symptoms, fever in 30%, bright red rash on cheeks (slapped cheek) and circumoral pallor for 2–3 days. A few days later a maculopapular, lace-like rash appears on the arms, then trunk, buttocks and thighs. Like rubella, the rash may be pruritic, but unlike rubella it can recur over the next few weeks, especially after a hot bath.

- *Incubation period:* 4–14 days
- *Infectious period:* before onset of rash
- *Isolation:* droplet
- *Diagnosis:* polymerase chain reaction in serum. Serology (IgM) is less reliable
- *Complications:* arthritis; aplastic crisis in children with chronic haemolytic anaemia; fetal hydrops
- *Treatment:* symptomatic

RUBELLA

Mild illness (25–50% subclinical); low-grade fever, posterior triangle and occipital lymphadenopathy, discrete red maculopapular rash, first on the face, chest and upper arms, then abdomen and thighs. Duration 1–5 days.

- *Incubation period:* 14–21 days
- *Infectious period:* 5 days before, 7 days after rash
- *Isolation:* droplet
- *Diagnosis:* serology
- *Complications:* congenital rubella syndrome; arthritis
- *Treatment:* none
- *Prevention:* MMR vaccine

VARICELLA ZOSTER (CHICKEN-POX)

Generalized, pruritic, vesicular rash with a mild fever and systemic symptoms. Duration 3–7 days.

- *Incubation period:* 14–16 days
- *Infectious period:* 1–2 days before, and until rash fully crusted
- *Isolation:* respiratory and contact
- *Diagnosis:* serology or immunofluorescence of vesicular fluid
- *Complications:* second-degree bacterial infection of skin lesions (most commonly *S. pyogenes* or *S. aureus*); neurological—cerebellitis, transverse myelitis, Guillain-Barré syndrome; dissemination (pneumonitis, hepatitis, encephalitis) in patients with abnormal T-cell immunity
- *Treatment: acyclovir* (500 mg/m^2, i.v. 8 h; or 10 mg/kg, i.v. 8 h if <2 years old) in patients with impaired T-cell immunity. *Note:* Acyclovir is not indicated in the immunocompetent child. Antibiotics for second-degree bacterial skin infection (e.g. flucloxacillin). *Analgesia note:* Aspirin is contraindicated because of the association with Reye syndrome
- *Prevention: Varicella vaccine* where available. High-titre intramuscular *zoster immunoglobulin* (ZIG), within 96 h of exposure (6 mL for adults, 4 mL for children 6–12 years, 2 mL for children 0–5 years), for the following patient groups in contact with varicella or shingles:
  - Immunocompromised, susceptible children (e.g. HIV, immunosuppressive therapy [including high dose steroids 2 mg/kg of prednisolone per day], transplantation, lymphoma, leukaemia, severe combined immunodeficiency syndrome)
  - Newborn infant of a mother with varicella within 5 days before, or 2 days after, delivery
  - Hospitalized premature infant whose mother has no history of varicella
  - Hospitalized premature infants <28 weeks gestation or <1000 g regardless of maternal history

Table 5.1 outlines recommended periods of exclusion from school, pre-school and child care for infectious disease cases and contacts.

Table 5.1 Recommended minimum periods of exclusion from school, pre-school and child care centres for cases of and contact with infectious diseases

	Exclusion of cases	*Exclusion of contacts*
Campylobacter	Exclude until diarrhoea has ceased	Not excluded
Chicken-pox	Exclude until fully recovered or for at least 5 days after the eruption first appears. Note that some remaining scabs are not a reason for continued exclusion	Any child with an immune deficiency (e.g. leukaemia) or receiving chemotherapy should be excluded for their own protection. Otherwise not excluded
Conjunctivitis	Exclude until discharge from eyes has ceased	Not excluded
Diarrhoea	Exclude until diarrhoea has ceased	Not excluded
Glandular fever (mononucleosis)	Exclusion is not necessary	Not excluded
Hepatitis A	Exclude until a medical certificate of recovery is received, but not before 7 days after the onset of jaundice or illness	Not excluded
Hepatitis B	Exclusion is not necessary	Not excluded
Human immunodeficiency virus infection (HIV AIDS virus)	Exclusion is not necessary unless the child has a secondary infection	Not excluded
Impetigo	Exclude until appropriate treatment has commenced. Sores on exposed surfaces must be covered with a watertight dressing	Not excluded
Measles	Exclude for at least 4 days after onset of rash	Immunized contacts not excluded. Unimmunized contacts should be excluded until 14 days after the first day of appearance of rash in the last case. If unimmunized contacts are vaccinated within 72 h of their first contact with the first case they may return to school

(Continued)

Table 5.1 *(Continued)*

	Exclusion of cases	*Exclusion of contacts*
Meningitis (bacterial)	Exclude until well	Not excluded
Meningococcal infection	Exclude until well	Not excluded
Mumps	Exclude for 9 days or until swelling goes down (whichever is sooner)	Not excluded
Ringworm, scabies, pediculosis (lice), trachoma	Re-admit the day after appropriate treatment has commenced	Not excluded
Rubella (German measles)	Exclude until fully recovered or for at least 4 days after the onset of rash	Not excluded
Streptococcal infection (including scarlet fever)	Exclude until the child has received antibiotic treatment for at least 24 h and feels well	Not excluded
Tuberculosis	Exclude until a medical certificate from an appropriate health authority is received	Not excluded
Whooping cough	Exclude the child for 5 days after starting antibiotic treatment	Exclude unimmunized household contacts aged less than 7 years for 14 days after the last exposure to infection or until they have taken 5 days of a 14 day course of antibiotics. (Exclude close child care contacts until they have commenced antibiotics)

Source: National Health and Medical Research Council, June 1992.

HIV INFECTION AND AIDS

The *human immunodeficiency virus* (HIV) is the aetiologic agent of the *acquired immunodeficiency syndrome* (AIDS). It is important to distinguish between infection with HIV, which may be asymptomatic during a variable latent period, and the progressive immunologic derangement which leads to AIDS.

PAEDIATRIC RISK GROUPS

Adolescents (as for Adults)

- Homosexual or bisexual males
- Intravenous drug users
- Sexual contacts of persons with HIV or from groups with increased risk for infection
- Transfusion recipients, particularly patients with congenital bleeding disorders who received blood products before 1985

Younger Children

- Infants of mothers who are known to be HIV positive or who are members of a high-risk group (e.g. sex workers, intravenous drug users, bisexual partners)
- Children receiving blood or blood products prior to 1985
- Sexually abused children

CLINICAL FEATURES

Clinical presentations of HIV infection include: prolonged fever; failure to thrive or weight loss >10%; generalized lymphadenopathy; hepatosplenomegaly; parotitis; chronic or recurrent diarrhoea; recurrent otitis; chronic candidiasis and chronic eczematoid rash. Laboratory tests may show lymphopenia, abnormal T-cell subsets and hypergammaglobulinaemia.

Indicator diseases for the diagnosis of AIDS in children include progressive neurological disease, lymphoid interstitial pneumonitis, opportunistic infection (e.g. *Pneumocystis carinii* pneumonia, disseminated *Mycobacterium avium* complex disease, chronic cryptosporidiosis, cytomegalovirus retinitis), recurrent episodes of serious bacterial infection and secondary malignancy (e.g. primary brain lymphoma).

DIAGNOSIS

Patients belonging to one of the high-risk groups **require counselling and informed consent before testing for HIV antibodies.** Testing for HIV infection should be undertaken on a confidential basis.

Specific antibody detection is a sensitive indicator of HIV infection in adults and children, but it is not diagnostic in infants as passively transferred maternal antibody may persist for up to 18 months. The presence of free viral protein (*p24*), a positive *viral culture* or *polymerase chain reaction assay* of non-cord blood confirms the diagnosis of HIV infection.

MANAGEMENT

The management of paediatric HIV should be by physicians, nurses and allied health professionals skilled in the special needs of these patients and their families.

Management of *blood spills* and *needle stick injuries* is discussed in the following section.

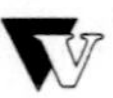

IMMUNIZATION

By 2 years of age <60% of Australian children have received their age-appropriate immunizations. Consequently, outbreaks of vaccine preventable diseases such as pertussis, measles and rubella continue. **Every visit to the doctor should be used as an opportunity to check and update the child's immunizations.** The National Health and Medical Research Council recommends the vaccination schedule (August 1994) shown in Table 5.2.

Every effort should be made to immunize a child, and no child should be denied immunization without serious thought about the consequences for the child and community.

ADVERSE REACTIONS

Immunization is often followed by mild adverse reactions which do *not* contraindicate further immunization:

- Following DTP, 50% of children develop some swelling and redness at the injection site, 20% become febrile and 30% are irritable

- After Hib vaccination, 10% develop transient swelling and redness at the injection site
- MMR vaccine may be followed 7–10 days later by 2–3 days of fever, malaise and occasionally a rash

The routine administration of 15 mg/kg of *paracetamol* just before DTP, and then 4 hourly for up to six doses, reduces the frequency of adverse side-effects.

DTP does not cause permanent brain damage.

Table 5.2 Childhood vaccination schedule

Age	*Vaccine*	*Route*
2 months	Diphtheria, pertussis, tetanus (DPT)	Intramuscular
	Polio (Sabin)	Oral
	Hib vaccine (1 or 2)*	Intramuscular
4 months	DPT	Intramuscular
	Polio (Sabin)	Oral
	Hib vaccine (1 or 2)*	Intramuscular
6 months	DPT	Intramuscular
	Polio (Sabin)	Oral
	Hib vaccine (1 only)*	Intramuscular
12 months	Measles, mumps and rubella	Subcutaneous
	Hib vaccine (2 only)*	Intramuscular
18 months	DPT	Intramuscular
	Hib vaccine (1 only)*	Intramuscular
School entry	DPT	Intramuscular
4–5 years	Polio (Sabin)	Oral
10–16 years	Measles, mumps and rubella	Subcutaneous
School leaving (15–19 years)	Diphtheria and tetanus	Intramuscular
	Polio (Sabin)	Oral

* There are two different schedules for *Haemophilus influenzae* type b (Hib) vaccines: schedule 1 [HbOC (Hibtiter) or PRP-T (Act-HIB)] is given at 2, 4, 6 and 18 months; schedule 2 [PRP-OMP (PedvaxHIB)] is given at 2, 4 and 12 months and is recommended for use in high-risk (e.g. indigenous) populations. single injection for children over 18 months of age.

CONTRAINDICATIONS

There are now *only two absolute contraindications* to further vaccination with DTP:

- Encephalopathy within 7 days (acute, severe illness with prolonged seizures, and/or unconsciousness and/or focal neurologic signs) – but not a simple febrile convulsion. These children should not be given the pertussis vaccine again–they should receive the combined diphtheria–tetanus vaccine instead of DPT
- Immediate, severe allergic or anaphylactic reaction to vaccine. Seek specialist (e.g. immunologist) advice before any further immunizations

The National Health and Medical Research Council in its *Immunization Procedures Handbook* suggests a checklist prior to immunization. Presence of one or more of the conditions in the following list may exclude vaccination, but if there is any doubt consult a paediatrician or public health physician.

MEDICINE

The child:

- Is *acutely unwell* with fever >38 °C and constitutional symptoms
- Is receiving *corticosteroids*
- Has had a *severe reaction* to any vaccine
- Has a history of *severe allergies*
- Has a disease which *lowers immunity* (e.g. leukaemia, cancer, HIV/AIDS) or is undergoing *immunosuppressive treatment*
- Lives with an immunosuppressed patient
- Has recently had a live virus vaccine, immunoglobulin injection or blood transfusion
- Has an *evolving neurological disorder*

Note: **Minor intercurrent infections are not a contraindication to immunization.**

Children suffering from malignant conditions and household contacts of patients with malignancy or immunosuppression should not be given oral polio vaccine to reduce the chance of spread to the child. *Pregnancy* is an absolute contraindication to rubella immunization, and should be avoided for two full menstrual cycles following administration.

Table 5.3 gives guidelines for tetanus prophylaxis in wound management.

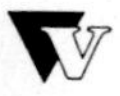

NOTIFIABLE DISEASES

Notifiable diseases vary in different jurisdictions. Readers are advised to consult local authorities for information on local regulations.

Table 5.3 Guide to tetanus prophylaxis in wound management

History of tetanus immunization		*Type of wound*	*Tetanus toxoid, DT**	*Tetanus immunoglobulin*
Uncertain, or less than three doses		Clean minor wounds	Yes	No
		All other wounds	Yes	Yes
	If less than 5 years since last doses	Clean minor wounds	No	No
		All other wounds	No	No
Three doses or more	If 5–10 years since last dose	Clean minor wounds	No	No
		All other wounds	Yes	No
	If more than 10 years since last dose	Clean minor wounds	Yes	No
		All other wounds	Yes	No†

*Two different formulations of DT are available, varying in the amount of diptheria toxoid: 30 Lf for children under 8 years, 2 Lf for adults.
†Tetanus immunoglobulin should be administered for tetanus-prone wounds in this category. Use DT in preference to tetanus toxoid alone.
Source: The Australian Immunisation Procedures Handbook, 5th edn, Australian Government Publishing Service, Canberra, 1994.

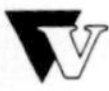

UNIVERSAL PRECAUTIONS FOR PREVENTION OF BLOOD-BORNE VIRUS INFECTION

1. AVOID PENETRATING INJURY WITH POTENTIALLY CONTAMINATED SHARP OBJECTS

- All sharp objects (e.g. needles, scalpel blades, glass, etc.) should be disposed of immediately in Australian Standards Approved (or equivalent) sharps containers.
- Sharps containers should be located in or close to treatment areas; they should not be more than two-thirds full and the lid should be replaced immediately after use
- Needles should not be recapped or removed from syringes manually; needle guards are available for this purpose if removal of the needle is necessary

2. AVOID CONTACT WITH BLOOD OR OTHER POTENTIALLY INFECTED BODY FLUIDS BY (i) THE USE OF PROTECTIVE BARRIERS IF CONTACT IS LIKELY AND (ii) IMMEDIATELY CLEANING UP ACCIDENTAL SPILLS

- All blood, body fluids containing visible blood and objects contaminated with blood should be regarded as potentially infectious
- In general, it is recommended that gloves be worn when undertaking or assisting invasive procedures including venepuncture, insertion of intravenous lines or aspiration of body fluids including lumbar puncture
- Gloves should be worn when attending to patients who are bleeding externally from accidental or surgical wounds, epistaxis, haematemesis, etc.; this includes patients who are menstruating if they require assistance with changing sanitary napkins
- In addition, goggles, mask and a disposable impervious apron should be worn when attending to patients who are bleeding in such a way that splashing of blood is likely to occur
- All blood spills should be cleaned up immediately using rubber gloves, disposable cloths (or paper towelling) and sodium hypochlorite 0.5%. All surfaces in hospitals which are likely to be exposed to blood spills should be able to be thoroughly cleaned or laundered. Disinfectant should be in contact for at least 30 min. For spills, it is often difficult to leave hypochlorite in place for 30 min. An alternative method is to place some 0.5% hypochlorite solution on a wad of paper towels, wipe the spill with this wad, then discard the contaminated paper towels into an infectious waste bag. It may then be necessary to wipe

the area again with hypochlorite, then clean the area with commercial detergent.

- Blood-stained linen that is very wet and saturated with blood which is likely to drip through the linen skip bags, must be placed into a clear plastic bag and securely tied to prevent leakage when handled
- Blood-stained dressings, paper towels, sanitary napkins and other disposable items should be discarded into the yellow Biohazard 'infectious' waste bags and disposed of when no more than two-thirds full

3. MANAGEMENT OF BLOOD/BLOOD-STAINED BODY FLUID EXPOSURE

Initial Response

- Blood should be washed off the skin with soap and water, or from the eyes with water immediately
- Needlestick injury or other significant exposure to blood or blood-stained body fluids is to be reported immediately. Baseline serum from the recipient must be taken at the time, in case it becomes necessary to relate such an incident to the development of a blood-borne viral infection which may occur at a later date. The specimen is for storage only and no serology will be requested, but the source involved in the incident should be noted on the request form

Medical Management: Known High-Risk Source

If the person whose blood was involved is a high-risk source for *hepatitis B virus (HBV)*:

- Check current hepatitis B surface antigen (HBsAg) status of source (this is usually in the patient record)
- Check HBV immunization status of the recipient. If fully immunized for HBV and known to have seroconverted (i.e. antiHBs positive) no further action is required
- If the recipient is not immunized, or is immunized but his/her antiHBs status is not known, and the source is HBsAg positive, blood should be taken from the recipient for antiHBs, and *hepatitis B immune globulin* given within 48 h (preferably 24 h) of the accident
- A course of *hepatitis B vaccine* should be started immediately if the recipient has not seroconverted or been immunized, and antibody status tested again 6 weeks after the last dose. The importance of a full course of immunization should be explained to the recipient

If the person whose blood was involved is a high-risk source for *HIV*:

- Check current HIV status of source
- Collect the recipient's blood and hold for future testing if necessary (with the recipient's informed consent and with strict confidence)

Medical Management: Low- or Unknown Risk Source

If the person whose blood was involved is not known to be a high-risk source, his/her blood should be tested for HBsAg if the recipient has not been fully immunized against hepatitis B. The urgency with which this is done, and whether the source should be tested for HIV, HCV or any other antibody, will be determined by the source's underlying condition and whether there are any other risk factors.

CHAPTER 6

RESPIRATORY CONDITIONS

Peter Phelan

In collaboration with Keith Grimwood

UPPER RESPIRATORY TRACT INFECTIONS

The average child has between 4 and 12 upper respiratory tract infections a year, the peak incidence being between 1 and 6 years.

AETIOLOGY

Viruses are responsible for at least 90% of upper respiratory tract infections. The only common important bacterial pathogen is β-haemolytic streptococcus.

Table 6.1 Clinical features of upper respiratory tract infections

	Viral	*Streptoccocal throat*
Age	Any age	4–15 years
Nasal symptoms	Usually	Infrequent
Cough	Frequent	Rare
Vomiting	Sometimes	Frequent
Level of fever	37–40°C	Usually >38.5°C
Tender, enlarged tonsillar lymph nodes	Not present	Usually present
Exudate on tonsils and pharynx	Sometimes	Frequent

Beware of the child with signs of a mild upper respiratory tract infection who has severe constitutional symptoms. Look for another diagnosis such as meningitis.

MANAGEMENT

Viral

- Symptomatic if necessary. *Paracetamol* if fever >39°C or if the child is distressed
- *Ephedrine nose drops* for nasal obstruction interfering with feeding or sleeping (maximum duration of therapy is 48 h)

Probable Streptococcus

- *Penicillin:* a total course for 10 days is given as Penicillin V orally, 250 mg, b.d. <40 kg; 500 mg, b.d. >40 kg. If the child is very sick, initial therapy may be by injection
- In remote communities, or in situations where compliance may not be reliable, Bicillin all purpose is an acceptable alternative (only for streptococcal tonsillitis). *Note:* This is a very painful injection
- Paracetamol if fever >39°C or the child is distressed

ACUTE OTITIS MEDIA

See also p. 252.

AETIOLOGY

Bacterial pathogens include:
- *Streptococcus pneumoniae*
- *Haemophilus influenzae* species
- *Moraxella catarrhalis*

Respiratory viruses are also common initial pathogens and may be the sole cause of mild otitis media.

DIAGNOSIS

- It is essential to visualize the tympanic membrane to establish a diagnosis of otitis media
- The most useful physical sign is an immobile bulging drum, which confirms the presence of exudate in the middle ear

MANAGEMENT

- Paracetamol for relief of pain or if fever >39°C
- Antibiotics: amoxycillin is used for a total course of 5–10 days. Penicil-

lin by injection may be used initially. Amoxycillin–clavulanate is an alternative

- Failure to respond within 48–72 h signals the need for an ENT opinion, but myringotomy is rarely indicated
- Review after 8–12 weeks to check hearing. It is common for fluid to persist in the middle ear for 4–6 weeks after acute otitis media

LARYNGOTRACHEOBRONCHITIS (CROUP)

CLINICAL FEATURES

- Initial viral upper respiratory tract infection, harsh cough, hoarse voice and stridor
- Children with laryngotracheitis must be admitted to hospital if they have sternal or suprasternal retraction at rest. Persistent stridor at rest without retraction indicates less severe obstruction but children with this sign usually warrant admission
- **The child with laryngotracheitis is likely to deteriorate late at night; therefore the child should rarely be sent home at night, especially if presenting to an emergency department after 2200 h**

MANAGEMENT

- Minimal handling. Nurse in a warm, humid environment. Observe carefully
- Mist is an unproven form of treatment
- **Important signs of hypoxia are restlessness, pallor and increasing pulse and respiration rates.** Cyanosis is a late sign. Exhaustion may be manifested by decreasing respiratory effort
- Ensure adequate fluid intake. Gavage or intravenous fluids are usually contraindicated because of the restraint involved
- Sedation is contraindicated
- Administration of *oxygen* is difficult because of the age of the child. It should be used if the child is hypoxic while arrangements are being made for transfer to ICU or intubation. *Note:* Oxygen should not be used routinely in moderate croup, as it may mask cyanosis, which is an important sign of increasing obstruction
- **Antibiotics have no place in management.** They may be indicated if there is associated infection such as otitis media

The use of *corticosteroids* in croup remains controversial. There is evidence that they reduce the intubation rate and the time of intubation in children with severe croup. If the child's obstruction is severe enough to require a dose of nebulized adrenaline, then this may be a reasonable indication for the use of corticosteroids. There is no proven place for the use of corticosteroids in mild to moderate croup, such as those children being nursed at home or in a general medical ward.

A single intramuscular injection of *dexamethasone* 0.6 mg/kg should be considered in children with severe croup. Steroids should be continued if the child is intubated. *Nebulized adrenaline* may be used to obtain temporary relief of obstruction. Dose: 0.05 mL/kg of 1 : 100 or 0.5 mL/kg of 1 : 1000 (0.1%) solution per dose (diluted to 2.5 mL) by inhalation. Circumstances that may justify its use include:

- Immediately prior to transfer from a metropolitan or district hospital to a major paediatric centre
- While awaiting intubation to be organized
- Unexpected deterioration, particularly late in the course of the illness
- One to two doses may be used in a child with severe croup in the hope of avoiding intubation

Repeated doses may occasionally be used in a child in whom it is desired to avoid intubation (e.g. established subglottic stenosis). It should not be used as definitive treatment and after its use the child must be observed very closely as rebound obstruction frequently occurs

If hypoxia develops, *mechanical relief of obstruction* is required (see Paediatric Emergencies, p. 9).

EPIGLOTTITIS

See also p. 8. The incidence of acute epiglottitis has fallen markedly in countries where immunization against *Haemophilus influenzae* type b is widespread. However, it continues to occur and, **if the diagnosis is not made promptly, the child with it is likely to die.**

CLINICAL FEATURES

This differs from laryngotracheitis in the following ways:

- Most children appear sick because of associated sepsis
- The onset is with fever and lethargy, and symptoms of respiratory obstruction develop after 2–6 h. There may be a history of a preceding upper respiratory tract infection
- The stridor is soft, and the expiratory element is often dominant with a snoring or gurgling quality. Cough is not a prominent feature
- Difficulty in swallowing and excess salivation with drooling are common

All children with suspected epiglottitis require urgent admission to a hospital with facilities to intubate children with acute upper airways obstruction. Following intubation, most should be transferred to a paediatric intensive care unit, preferably by a paediatric emergency transport service. All medical practitioners should know what facilities there are available within their community for dealing with such emergencies.

MANAGEMENT

- *Do not lie the patient flat.* Do not examine the larynx unless an anaesthetist is present and able to intubate
- *Ceftriaxone:* initial dose 100 mg/kg, with a second dose of 50 mg/kg after 24 h
- Alternative: *chloramphenicol,* initial dose 40 mg/kg, i.v. or i.m.; continuing therapy 25 mg/kg 8 hourly, i.v. (75 mg/kg per day) and then orally for a total duration of 4–5 days
- *Rifampicin prophylaxis* for patients at the end of therapy, and for contacts as per *H. influenzae* meningitis (Table 12.2, p. 164)
- *Adequate fluids.* If the patient has an intravenous line, fluids can be given intravenously. Do not give more than 40–60% of maintenance requirements
- *General care:* see p. 67, Laryngotracheobronchitis

WHOOPING COUGH (PERTUSSIS)

Whooping cough continues to be widespread in many communities mainly because of poor uptake of childhood immunization. However, the current vaccines give protection only for 5–10 years and so adolescents and adults can acquire the infection and pass it on to younger children who are inadequately protected.

CLINICAL FEATURES

- Cough of some weeks duration occurring in paroxysms associated with facial suffusion and vomiting. In some children the paroxysm is terminated by an inspiratory whoop
- Between the paroxysms the child will appear normal

DIAGNOSIS

- The diagnosis is dependent on taking a careful history
- Early in the illness, the diagnosis can be confirmed by identifying *Bordetella pertussis* in a nasopharyngeal aspirate

MANAGEMENT

- No pharmacological agents favourably alter the course of whooping cough. *Erythromycin estolate* may reduce the period of infectivity and should be used in children who may pass on the infection to infants under the age of 12 months (who are most at risk from complications)
- **Almost all infants under the age of 6 months** (and some between 6 and 12 months) **with whooping cough require admission to hospital**
- In hospital, careful observation including the use of a monitor is essential. If paroxysms occur frequently and are associated with marked cyanosis, nursing in *oxygen* may be of some help

ACUTE VIRAL BRONCHIOLITIS

CLINICAL FEATURES

- This is an acute viral illness in children usually between 2 weeks and 9 months of age, manifested by cough, wheezy breathing, hyperinflated chest, widespread fine crackles and frequently expiratory wheezes on auscultation
- Some infants can have two or even three episodes of bronchiolitis in the first 2 years caused by different respiratory viruses
- A predisposition to asthma seems to be a risk factor for the development of acute viral bronchiolitis
- If an infant has more than three episodes of wheeze, it is most likely asthma

MANAGEMENT

- Admission indication: increasing respiratory distress manifested by difficulty in feeding
- *Minimal handling.* Careful observation of colour, pulse, respiration and measurement of oxygen saturation by pulse oximetry
- *Oxygen* is the most important agent in the treatment of moderate to severe bronchiolitis. Inspired oxygen percentage should be sufficient to maintain oxygen saturation above 90%
- Continuous positive airways pressure or artificial ventilation in the occasional infant who develops respiratory failure
- *Fluids.* If the baby is unable to feed orally, fluids are given intravenously at about 40% maintenance once any dehydration has been corrected
- *Antibiotics* are indicated only in the rare situation of established sec-

ondary bacterial infection when penicillin is used, or in very severe disease when flucloxacillin and cefotaxime should be given intravenously, while awaiting culture results

PNEUMONIA

CLINICAL FEATURES

- The child with pneumonia usually has tachypnoea, and often an expiratory grunt
- Focal signs in the chest may be difficult to detect
- A diagnosis of pneumonia, especially in younger children, can usually only be made with radiological confirmation

AETIOLOGY

- *Viruses*, especially respiratory syncytial virus and parainfluenzae type 3, are the most common cause in young infants. There is generally only mild to moderate constitutional disturbance. There may be chest hyperinflation and scattered inspiratory crackles
- *Mycoplasma pneumoniae* is the commonest pathogen in children over 5 years old, but it also causes pneumonia in younger children. Typically symptoms develop over several days. Cough is prominent and crackles may be focal or widespread
- *S. pneumoniae* is by far the commonest bacterial pathogen in all age groups. The next is *Staphylococcus aureus* followed by *H. influenzae* (both non-typable and type b). Children are usually unwell and focal signs are present in the chest. Many older children can be satisfactorily managed at home, but **almost all those under 48 months should be admitted to hospital**

MANAGEMENT

- X-ray to confirm diagnosis
- Blood culture; nasopharyngeal aspirate for viruses; Mycoplasma serology. Throat swabs and sputum are of no value for bacterial culture
- Because of inability to make a precise aetiologic diagnosis, antibiotics are recommended, at least initially, unless symptoms are mild and a viral aetiology is highly probable
- Management is determined by age and severity of illness and should follow the algorithm in Figure 6.1.

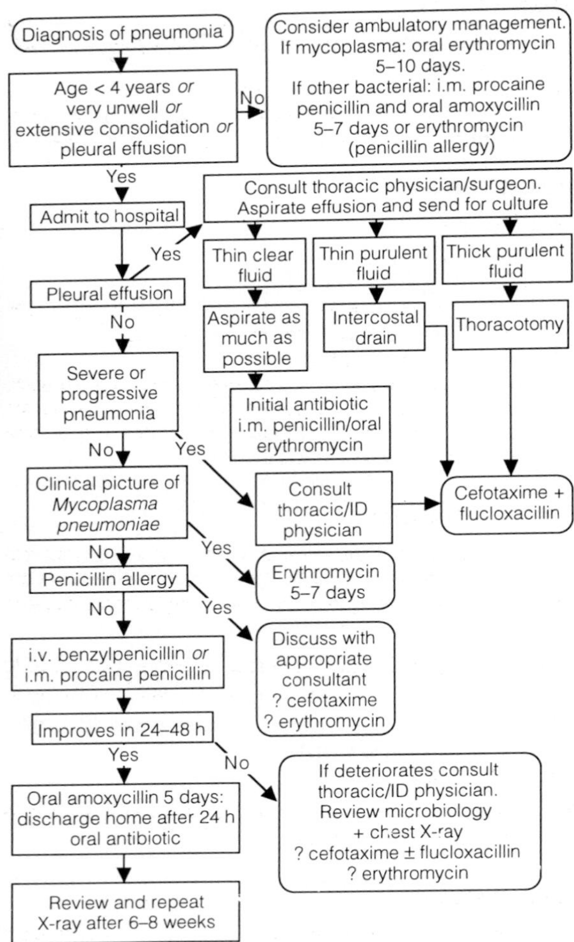

Figure 6.1 Management of pneumonia

General Measures

- Minimal handling; careful observation of colour, pulse and respirations; pulse oximetry
- Increased inspired oxygen concentration
- An adequate, but not excessive fluid intake. If fluids are given intravenously the rate should be 40% maintenance, once any dehydration is corrected

ASTHMA

The aims in the management of asthma:
- To achieve rapid resolution of acute episodes
- To use prophylactic drugs when the morbidity from asthma is sufficient to justify their use in view of potential side-effects
- To prevent exercise-induced asthma

Critical to these issues is the proper assessment of the severity of acute episodes and the degree of morbidity in the long-term, based on the frequency of acute episodes and whether there are interval symptoms between the acute episodes (Table 6.2).

LONG-TERM MANAGEMENT

The aim of long-term management is to control symptoms that interfere with the enjoyment of a normal life-style (Table 6.3). There is no evidence that the use of prophylactic drugs favourably alters the long-term course of asthma.

In this section, significant episodes of acute asthma are considered to be those that require the use of a β_2-sympathomimetic 4–6 hourly for at least 24–36 h.

DELIVERY DEVICES

It is important to use delivery devices that are appropriate to the drug and to the patient's age (Table 6.4).

LUNG FUNCTION

- Children over the age of 7 years admitted to hospital with an acute episode of asthma should, whenever practical, have spirometry performed prior to discharge to check that they are bronchodilator responsive. This is essential in those with troublesome persistent asthma

Table 6.2 Management of acute episodes of asthma

Type of episode	*Treatment*
Mild acute episode Not cyanosed Audible wheeze No use of accessory muscles of respiration Respiratory rate not increased Active More than five to seven words between breaths	One to two doses of inhaled β_2-sympathomimetic with metered dose aerosol, and possibly spacer. May need to continue β_2-sympathomimetic 4–6 hourly for a further 24–36 h
Moderate acute episode Not cyanosed Audible wheeze Use of accessory muscles of respiration Lower rib recession especially in younger children Three to five words between breaths Normal breath sounds Patient wants to sit or lie quietly	Three doses of inhaled β_2-sympathomimetic with metered dose aerosol and spacer or nebulizer over 60 minutes. Observe for a further 30–60 min. Possible outcomes: • Complete clearing of audible wheeze and respiratory distress: continue β_2-sympathomimetic 3–4 hourly for 24–36 h. If further treatment is required, consider a course of oral steroids (e.g. prednisolone 1 mg/kg to 40 mg daily for up to 3 days) • Improvement but not complete clearing: short course of oral prednisolone (1 mg/kg to 40 mg daily for up to 3 days*), continue β_2-sympathomimetic 3–4 h • No improvement after three doses of β_2-sympathomimetic: admit to hospital and treat as severe

Severe acute episode	
Cyanosed in air	Admit to hospital and administer oxygen.
Obvious respiratory distress with	Very frequent or continuous nebulized β_2-sympathomimetic (e.g. 1 mL salbutamol in 3 mL
increased respiratory rate	saline) with nebulizer driven by oxygen.
marked use of accessory muscles of respiration	Corticosteroids—oral, or i.v. if patient is very distressed.
lower rib recession	Methyl prednisolone 1 mg/kg per 6 hourly (max. 50 mg/dose for 24 h), then 1 mg/kg per
Audible wheeze—may be soft	12 h—for a further 24 h if necessary
One to three words between breaths	Then oral steroids 1 mg/kg per 24 h (max. 40 mg) for 3 days*
Wants to lie or sit still	If not settling, transfer to ICU and consider:
Reduced breath sounds	i.v. aminophylline
	nebulized ipratropium bromide—4 hourly
	i.v. salbutamol
	intermittent positive-pressure respiration (IPPR)

*The period of therapy with oral corticosteroids for an acute episode in a patient on moderate to high dose inhaled corticosteroids may need to be longer than the standard 3 days and particularly with high doses, it may be wise to tail off the drug over a further 3–5 days. This certainly should always be the case in patients on maintenance oral corticosteroids.

The only role for β_2-sympathomimetics via a nebulizer is in the management of severe acute episodes. A metered dose aerosol plus spacer is as effective as a nebulizer in all other circumstances.

If nebulized β_2 drugs are used more frequently than hourly, the patient must be seen before and after each dose by a medical officer, and if they are to be used continuously, the patient should be managed in an ICU.

Table 6.3 Long-term management of asthma

Pattern of asthma	*Prophylactic and acute therapy*
Infrequent episodic (75% of asthmatic population) Significant episodes less than every 4–6 weeks Minor wheeze after prolonged exercise No other interval symptoms Normal lung function between episodes	No prophylactic therapy Treat acute episodes as in Table 6.2
Frequent episodic (20% of asthmatic population) Significant episodes more frequently than every 4–6 weeks Wheeze with moderate exercise but usually prevented by prior use of β_2-sympathomimetic Occasional (less than weekly), interval symptoms Normal or near normal lung function between episodes	*Sodium cromoglycate*—as Intal Forte 2 puffs t.d.s. If there is no benefit after 2–3 months: • Simply treat acute episodes *or* • Use inhaled corticosteroids (see below) Treat acute episodes as in Table 6.2
Persistent asthma (5% of asthmatic population)	• If mild symptoms, trial sodium cromoglycate • If it fails, or if symptoms are more troublesome, use *inhaled corticosteroids* (beclomethasone, budesonide). Initial dose: 400–800 μg daily depending on symptoms

Significant acute episodes generally more frequently than 4-6 weeks	Once controlled, reduce dose to minimum necessary to have good quality of life and normal to near normal lung function
	Review dose every 3–6 months
Wheezing or chest tightness with minor exercise not totally prevented by a β_2-sympathomimetic	If control of symptoms is not adequate on seemingly appropriate prescribed therapy, consider inhalation technique and compliance prior to increasing dose
Other interval symptoms requiring a β_2-sympathomimetic more often than two to three times a week (e.g. waking at night, chest tightness on awakening in morning)	• If more than 1000 µg is needed to control symptoms, add *salmeterol*, b.d. • If more than 1200–1500 µg is needed, change to *fluticasone* • If more than 1000 µg fluticasone is needed, add maintenance *oral steroids*
Evidence of airways obstruction between episodes or diurnal variation in peak flow rates >20% (patients over 7 years)	Acute episode: as above except may need a longer course of oral corticosteroids If β_2-sympathomimetic is needed more often than 3-4 hourly, give course of oral steroids If β_2-sympathomimetic is needed more frequently than every 2–3 hourly, admit to hospital

Table 6.4 Delivery devices for asthma management

Age	*Metered dose aerosol (MDI)*	*MDI + small volume spacer*	*MDI + large volume spacer*	*Dry powder devices*	*Nebulizer (severe acute asthma only)*
< 2 years		+ with face mask			+
2–4 years		+ without face mask			+
4–7 years			+		+
> 7 years	+ (inhaled steroids <500 µg/day)		+ (inhaled steroids >500 µg/day)	+ (inhaled steriods <500 µg/day)	+

- Children with presumed infrequent and frequent episodic asthma should have spirometry performed between acute episodes on at least one occasion to check that there is no unrecognized airways obstruction
- Children with persistent asthma should have spirometry performed when seen for consultant review
- Children under the age of 6 or 7 years cannot perform lung function tests reliably
- *Peak flow measures* are unreliable during acute episodes in many children and early adolescents
- It is only patients with persistent asthma who should have a peak flow meter at home. It should be used regularly only to confirm the diagnosis of persistent asthma, when it is being stabilized and when drug doses are being reduced

CRISIS MANAGEMENT

- Action plans based on peak flow measurements are of much less use in children than they may be in adults
- Every patient with asthma should know what to do if they get a sudden severe acute episode. The appropriate action is to take very frequent or continuous β_2-sympathomimetic and to summon an ambulance

OTHER MEASURES

- Exercise-induced bronchoconstriction can be prevented by prior use of an inhaled β_2-sympathomimetic
- Non-pharmacologic measures have never been shown to be effective in the management of asthma in children and adolescents

COUGH IN CHILDREN

Cough is a common symptom in children. The degree to which a family becomes concerned about the frequency and severity of a child's cough seems to be extremely variable. There is often a poor correlation between parental report of cough and objective measures.

Cough is best thought of in the following diagnostic groups:

RECURRENT COUGH

These are episodes of cough lasting a few days to a few weeks with completely asymptomatic periods between. There are two causes: viral respiratory tract infection and asthma.

Viral Respiratory Tract Infection

Cough with a viral respiratory infection, although typically lasting 7–10 days, may persist for 4 or 8 weeks or even longer. Initially it may be loose but later in the course it may become dry. It may be perceived by the family to be worse at night.

Asthma

While cough can be a troublesome symptom of asthma, it rarely occurs without some evidence of airways obstruction (e.g. wheeze). There is considerable doubt as to whether the entity of 'cough variant asthma', in which cough is the only symptom of asthma, exists in children. Be very reluctant to diagnose asthma in the absence of evidence of airways obstruction. The management of asthma is based on severity and duration of airways obstruction, not on cough.

SUBACUTE COUGH

There are a number of entities in addition to post-viral infection in which cough can last some weeks to 2 or 3 months. They include:

- Whooping cough
- Inhaled foreign body
- *Mycoplasma pneumoniae* infection
- Segmental or lobar collapse following an acute respiratory infection
- Tuberculosis
- Psychogenic

Whooping cough and psychogenic cough should be diagnosed on the pattern of the cough. The others will usually be diagnosable on a chest radiograph which is indicated in children with a first episode of cough lasting more than 3–4 weeks, particularly if it has not been triggered by a viral respiratory infection.

PERSISTENT COUGH

This is a cough of many months or even years duration. There may be temporary clearance of the cough with a course of antibiotics but it rapidly recurs once they are ceased. The likely causes are:

- Cystic fibrosis

- Other causes of bronchiectasis: immotile cilia syndrome; agammaglobulinaemia
- Insidious onset bronchiectasis without apparent cause
- Smoker's cough in adolescents

Bronchiectasis probably commences with suppurative bronchitis. If this has been present for <6–12 months, it may be completely reversible without permanent lung damage, following a prolonged course of antibiotics (weeks to months) and physiotherapy.

MANAGEMENT OF COUGH

- The single most important aspect of management is to make a diagnosis and explain its nature to the parents. The effects of passive smoking should be reiterated.
- Almost all cough mixtures are ineffective. The possible exceptions are an opiate cough suppressant which would rarely be used in a child or mixtures with a base of honey or licorice (often with alcohol). These may soothe an irritated throat
- Specific therapy is indicated for asthma, *Mycoplasma* infection, tuberculosis and segmental or lobar collapse. A foreign body must be removed bronchoscopically
- It is often much more difficult to control the cough of asthma than the wheeze

FOREIGN BODY IN THE BRONCHIAL TREE

CLINICAL FEATURES

Symptoms

- Coughing or choking episodes while eating nuts or other solid food or while sucking a small plastic toy or similar object. This story should never be dismissed
- Persistent coughing and wheezing. Remember 'all that wheezes is not asthma'
- Beware of the sudden onset of a first wheezing episode in a toddler in whom there is no history of allergy, especially if it follows a choking episode
- Parents may not volunteer the history of possible inhalation. One of every eight episodes of foreign body inhalation is not witnessed

Signs

- Diminished breath sounds over whole or part of one lung
- Wheeze

INVESTIGATIONS

Chest X-ray is taken in full inspiration and full expiration to exclude obstructive hyperinflation or an area of collapse. Normal X-rays do not absolutely exclude a foreign body.

MANAGEMENT

Admission is indicated for all patients with a suspected inhaled foreign body. If there is any doubt, consult a thoracic physician.

Bronchoscopy

- As radiological examination may be normal, bronchoscopy is necessary in almost every child in whom there is a story strongly suggestive of an inhaled foreign body
- Bronchoscopy in children is difficult and it requires an expert paediatric endoscopist teamed with an experienced paediatric anaesthetist. It should only be done in a major children's hospital
- Once a foreign body has passed through the larynx it is very rare for there to be an immediate threat to life, and referral to the nearest children's hospital is usually quite safe

CHAPTER 7

GASTROINTESTINAL CONDITIONS

Tony Catto-Smith

In collaboration with Lionel Lubitz

ACUTE INFECTIOUS DIARRHOEA

DIFFERENTIAL DIAGNOSIS

It is important that children who present with the acute onset of vomiting, diarrhoea and fever are repeatedly re-evaluated, even after admission to a hospital gastroenteritis ward. Other causes to be considered include:

- Appendicitis
- Intussusception
- Malrotation
- Urinary tract infection
- Otitis media
- Meningitis

ASSESSMENT OF DEHYDRATION

- Dehydration is the most important complication of acute infectious diarrhoea
- Recent change in bodyweight provides the most accurate indication of the degree of fluid depletion. This underscores the importance of accurate weights as a part of clinical assessment
- Starvation produces no more than 1% of bodyweight loss per day. Any change in excess of this is due to water loss
- Recent evidence suggests that signs of ketosis such as Kussmaul breathing and typical ketotic breath are the best clinical indicators of moderate to severe dehydration

For practical clinical purposes, the state of hydration should be evaluated as:

- No, or mild dehydration (<3% bodyweight loss)
- Moderate dehydration (4–6%)
- Severe dehydration (≥7%)

Note: These percentages are approximate and given only as a guide.

MANAGEMENT

General Comments

Treatment is aimed at restoring and maintaining water and electrolyte balance and normal nutrition. The important general principles are:
- Continue breast feeding
- Use oral rehydration
- Feed hungry children
- Avoid drugs: **antibiotics, antiemetics and antidiarrhoeals have no place in the treatment of most cases of childhood gastro-enteritis**

Oral Rehydration

- *Breast feeding:* continue through the illness, supplemented if necessary with an oral rehydration solution by cup, bottle or nasogastric tube
- *Artificial feeding:* commercially available oral rehydration solutions will greatly enhance absorption of water from the small bowel, and can be used to rehydrate children with even moderately severe dehydration, provided they are not shocked
- Vomiting is not a contraindication to oral rehydration. It is best to give small amounts of fluid frequently
- Oral rehydration encourages early return of appetite

Solutions

Sachets containing glucose and electrolyte powder are commercially available and can be added to water as required (e.g. Gastrolyte). They contain glucose, sodium, potassium, chloride and citrate and should be used *to correct dehydration.* Readily available solutions of sugar in water (without salt) can be prepared at home and used for maintenance of hydration in mild or moderate diarrhoea *without dehydration.*

These include:
- Sucrose (table sugar): one teaspoon in 200 mL water
- Cordials: 1 part to 16 parts water
- Lemonade: 1 part to 6 parts water
- Fruit juice: 1 part to 4 parts water

Do not use low calorie lemonade or fruit juice.

Parent Education

The most important message for parents is that **children with diarrhoea need to drink more fluid more often** (because water loss is the main cause of morbidity and mortality).

Fluid is best given in small volumes, frequently. The easiest and safest method is as free water, which may be flavoured with appropriately diluted cordials.

Where diarrhoea becomes significant, electrolyte loss is of increasing concern and it is important to provide an electrolyte source such as a glucose–electrolyte rehydration preparation, or food.

Although home-made solutions and oral rehydration powder are important in the management of childhood gastroenteritis in the home, they are potentially dangerous if made up incorrectly. The fact that a small (appropriate) amount of the oral rehydration powder in solution is good does not mean a larger amount in the same volume of water is better

Specific Treatment Guidelines

Indications for Admission

- Severe illness
- Moderate or severe dehydration
- Very young babies (<6 months old)
- High-risk patients (e.g. ileostomy, short gut, cyanotic heart disease, chronic renal disease, metabolic disorders)
- Diagnosis in doubt
- Family unable to cope

No dehydration

- Children with no clinical features of dehydration can usually be managed as outpatients
- Breast feeding should be continued on demand, and formula-fed infants should be given their normal feeds with extra water. Vomiting babies will tolerate half-strength feeds better than full strength
- Children with mild to moderate diarrhoea can continue on their normal diet with extra water. This can be given as water, cordial, diluted fruit juice or diluted lemonade
- If the child refuses to eat, food may be stopped for up to 24 h; however, *starvation* beyond this may delay recovery

Mild dehydration

- These children may have a history of diarrhoea and vomiting with inadequate oral intake. Urine is usually concentrated but skin turgor and mucous membranes may appear normal
- Children who are dehydrated need to be provided with water and electrolytes to replace their *deficits*, and an ongoing amount of fluid for *maintenance* requirements
- *For practical purposes, the deficit is best determined using a calculation based on percentage of bodyweight*; however, recent accurate bodyweights are rarely available. Children who have minimal or no clinical signs of dehydration (<4%) can be assigned a notional deficit of 3%

The rehydration and maintenance fluid volumes for 24 h should be translated into an easily understood message (e.g. 50 mL every 30 min). Ideally, an oral rehydration solution such as Gastrolyte should be given, but this can be alternated with other appropriately diluted fluids which may be more palatable, such as cordials. It is not usually necessary to admit these children, although **review within 8–12 h is essential.**

Moderate to severe dehydration

- Clinical assessment of percentage dehydration is at best approximate
- Moderate dehydration (4–6%) may be accompanied by dry mucous membranes, sunken eyes and mild oliguria
- Clinical signs of increased degrees of dehydration (7–9%) are more exaggerated, with evidence of ketosis, acidotic breathing, decreased skin turgor and impaired peripheral perfusion
- Most children who are moderately dehydrated can be rehydrated orally, even if they are vomiting. Children who are not shocked should be given a trial of oral rehydration, using adequate volumes of a physiologically balanced fluid by mouth or via a nasogastric tube

The aim is to rehydrate them quickly. A useful rule of thumb for rehydration is to provide a total fluid intake over the first 6 h of between 50 mL/kg (older children) and 100 mL/kg (infants). Thereafter give maintenance fluids or as desired (see Table 7.1).

If the child is tired or cannot keep up with losses, a nasogastric tube should be inserted. Small amounts of fluid should be given frequently, and the child should be reassessed after 4–6 h. Breast feeding should be resumed as soon as oral rehydration is complete, or before if this takes longer than 6 h.

Table 7.1 Maintenance and rehydration fluid requirements for children

Weight (kg)	*Maintenance (mL/h)*	*Moderate dehydration (4–6%) (mL/h)*		*Severe dehydration (≥7%) (mL/h)*	
		1st 6 h	*Next 18 h*	*1st 6 h*	*Next 18 h*
5	20	45	35	70	35
10	35	85	55	135	55
15	50	125	70	200	70
20	60	140	80	220	80
30	70	190	95	300	95
40	80	250	110	400	110
50	90	300	120	500	120

The daily water requirement is relatively high in neonates (150 mL/kg), reducing to 100 mL/kg in older infants and 80 mL/kg per day between 1 and 5 years.

MEDICINE

Severe dehydration with shock

Children who are shocked need immediate resuscitation with intravenous fluids.

Intravenous Therapy

Indications

- Severe dehydration with shock
- Failed oral/nasogastric rehydration
- Gastroenteritis complicated by another problem, e.g. ileostomy or cyanotic congenital heart disease (relative indication)

Resuscitation fluid

If the child is shocked give 10 mL/kg of colloid solution (e.g. 5% albumin, Haemaccel) as quickly as possible to treat circulatory failure. This should be repeated if there are still signs of shock. If colloid is not available, normal saline is adequate.

Replacement and maintenance fluid

- Half normal saline in 4% dextrose with 20 mmol/L of potassium chloride is usually adequate. Sodium bicarbonate is added if there is *persistent* acidosis (acidosis will usually correct itself as the patient is rehydrated)

- Aim to replace the deficit over 24 h if the serum sodium is normal (see Hypernatraemic dehydration below). The maintenance requirement is approximately 4 mL/kg per h up to 10 kg

Example:

- 10 kg child 10% dehydrated
- Deficit 1000 mL = 40 mL/h for 24 h
- Maintenance 4 mL/kg per h = 40 mL/h
- Total 80 mL/h for first 24 h, then 40 mL/h

Oral rehydration solution and breast milk should be offered once the circulation has been restored; it may be possible to remove the drip after a few hours. Appetite is restored more quickly in children given oral fluids.

Biochemical Investigations

Electrolyte and acid–base studies are not required routinely. Indications are:

- Prolonged diarrhoea with severe dehydration
- Disturbance of conscious state or convulsions
- Any child aged less than 3 months
- Any child requiring intravenous fluid

Special Circumstances

Clinical signs of dehydration provide at best an approximation of the degree of dehydration. Assessment is further complicated in patients who have significant *plasma sodium imbalance*, those who are *malnourished* and those who are *obese*.

Hypernatraemic dehydration (Na $>$ 150 mmol/L)

Because of osmotic shifts, **these children may actually be more dehydrated than they clinically appear.** They are at great risk of severe neurological sequelae if rehydration is not carried out appropriately. Rehydration must be slow. Repeated aliquots of 10 mL/kg colloid solution should be given quickly to restore the circulation if the child is shocked, but the remainder of the **deficit should be replaced over at least 48 h** if intravenous fluid is used. As long as rehydration is slow, the intravenous fluid used does not need to have a high sodium concentration; a suitable solution is 1/2 normal saline in 4% dextrose with 20 mmol/L of potassium chloride and 10 mL/L 10% calcium gluconate. Oral replacement should be over at least 24 h.

Consultation with an intensive care unit is recommended for these patients. Serum electrolytes should be measured frequently. As a guideline serum sodium should not fall by >1 mmol/L per h (on average).

Hyponatraemic dehydration (Na<130 mmol/L)

Severe hyponatraemia causing fitting or coma requires consultation with an intensive care unit. Beware of iatrogenic hyponatraemia from fluid (hypotonic) overload.

Malnutrition

Malnourished children may be less dehydrated than clinical examination would suggest. Such infants may be depleted of magnesium and potassium. *Obese infants* may be more dehydrated than the clinical signs indicate.

Drug Therapy

Antidiarrhoeal agents and *anti-emetics* are *not* recommended for children with gastroenteritis. They can have potentially dangerous side-effects. *Antibiotics* have a limited role; they are occasionally required in neonates, severely ill infants, severe shigellosis or prolonged symptomatic *Campylobacter* infection.

SUGAR INTOLERANCE

LACTOSE INTOLERANCE

After infectious diarrhoea, infants may have temporary lactose intolerance. Approximately 50% of formula-fed babies less than 6 months old with infectious diarrhoea requiring admission to hospital are unable to tolerate normal amounts of lactose for at least a week. Lactose intolerance may occasionally persist for some months.

Clinical features of sugar intolerance are:
- Persistently fluid stools
- Excessive flatus
- Excoriation of the buttocks

Typically these infants appear otherwise well.

Diagnosis

Collect the stool fluid in napkins lined with plastic. Dilute five drops of stool fluid with 10 drops of water. Add a Clinitest tablet. A colour reaction corresponding to $\frac{3}{4}$% or more reducing substances indicates that sugar intolerance is present and is probably the main cause of continuing diarrhoea.

Management

- Breast fed babies rarely have clinically significant lactose intolerance, and breast feeding should be continued unless the diarrhoea is persistent and the baby is failing to thrive
- Formula-fed babies should have their feed changed to a full strength lactose-free formula, such as Delact or Digestelac. After 3–4 weeks the usual formula may be reintroduced by substituting for the lactose-free milk in increasing proportions over 2–3 days

Note: A clinical response after change to *soy formula* may indicate either post-infectious lactose intolerance or allergy to cow milk protein.

MONOSACCHARIDE INTOLERANCE

Much less commonly, infants with severe bowel damage secondary to gastroenteritis may be unable to absorb normal amounts of monosaccharide, such as glucose or fructose. Diarrhoea will continue even with a lactose-free formula. Monosaccharide intolerance requires specialist consultation with a gastroenterologist.

GASTRO-OESOPHAGEAL REFLUX

Oesophageal reflux of gastric contents occurs normally and is more frequent after meals. It is regarded as pathological if associated with frequent regurgitation or if it results in clinically significant adverse sequelae. The number of reflux episodes is normally increased in infants compared with older children.

Regurgitated gastric acid with heartburn may result in episodic irritability, but this is usually associated with obvious regurgitation and is rarely 'silent'. Twenty-four hour oesophageal pH monitoring is useful to correlate any episodes of reflux with irritability.

It is important to recognize that vomiting in infants may result from other causes, such as urinary tract infection. These need to be excluded.

COMPLICATIONS

- *Peptic oesophagitis.* This is usually correlated with an increase in the number and duration of reflux episodes. Blood flecked vomitus and anaemia may result

- *Failure to thrive.* Severe cases of gastro-oesophageal reflux may cause loss of calories and anorexia
- *Pulmonary complications.* Recurrent or persistent cough and wheeze may be present and can occur without marked vomiting. These symptoms may result from aspiration of refluxed material (inhalation pneumonia) or through reflex bronchospasm. This mode of presentation requires a high degree of clinical suspicion
- *Peptic strictures* are well recognized in childhood, and present with dysphagia

Specialist advice should be sought if complications are present.

MANAGEMENT

Regurgitation of gastric contents is common in infancy. In most cases, this 'possetting' does *not* result in any adverse sequelae and the most appropriate therapy is parental reassurance. 'Physiological' gastro-oesophageal reflux with regurgitation usually resolves by the age of 9–15 months.

Simple Measures

In the absence of signs of significant oesophagitis, aspiration or growth failure, the following should be suggested:

- The avoidance of excessive handling
- *Posturing* after feeds: the infant should be postured in a cot head-up at or near 30°, preferably on their side. (Although nursing in the prone position has been recommended in the past, there is now evidence that this increases the risk of sudden infant death)
- *Thickening* of feeds: use a proprietary thickening agent

Medication

Note: Medications are not indicated in otherwise healthy, thriving infants with frequent regurgitation.

- *Mylanta* may offer relief of symptoms of heartburn, but there are concerns about long-term use because of its mineral content
- In more severe cases, prokinetic agents such as *cisapride* (0.2–0.4 mg/kg per dose before meals) will reduce the frequency of reflux episodes and improve gastric emptying
- H2 receptor antagonists such as *ranitidine* (2–3 mg/kg per dose before meals) will reduce gastric acidity

However, these agents are not without risk and should not be prescribed without evidence to substantiate the severity of reflux.

Surgery

Fundoplication is indicated for reflux with complications when medical therapy has failed or is inappropriate.

CONSTIPATION

Constipation is common in childhood and is usually associated with abnormalities in control of defecation and occasionally with delayed colonic transit.

Although it is important to consider organic causes of constipation such as Hirschsprung's disease, these are rare.

Apparently painful defecation or blood on the surface of the stools suggests the presence of an *anal fissure*. Children past the toddler age with severe constipation may also develop faecal soiling.

EXAMINATION

- Abdominal palpation will usually reveal abnormal amounts of firm faeces
- The anus should be inspected for a fissure
- The tone of the anal sphincter and the presence of anal stenosis should be assessed
- Rectal examination may be required

INVESTIGATIONS

Investigations are rarely helpful, but an abdominal X-ray may be useful to determine the extent of faecal retention.

Hirschsprung's disease is a rare cause of constipation. Rectal biopsy is unnecessary unless the onset of symptoms dates back to early infancy or there is some other clinical indication (such as considerable abdominal distension or failure to thrive).

MANAGEMENT

- The aim of treatment is to empty the colon and to prevent re-accumulation of abnormal amounts of faeces by regular toileting and with the use of laxatives
- Rectal disimpaction may be required initially
- *Babies:* an adequate fluid intake with prune juice, high-residue cereals and vegetables may be effective. If not, poloxalkol drops (Coloxyl) or lactulose (Duphalac) are usually effective and safe

- *Older children:* a short course of laxatives with the establishment of a *regular toileting regimen* is usually effective

In general the dose of laxative needed is the one that is effective in achieving the passage of at least one soft but formed stool each day. This dose should be gradually reduced with the aim of eventually weaning the patient off laxatives. The longer constipation has been a problem, the longer it takes to achieve this aim. **A common mistake is to give intermittent short courses of treatment which do not allow adequate readjustment of colonic size and sensation.**

When an anal fissure is present stools should be kept soft with a softening agent.

ENCOPRESIS

Encopresis is defined as the involuntary passage of formed or semi-formed stools into the underwear on a regular basis. It is a distressing symptom to the child and family alike.

The majority of children with encopresis have significant faecal retention. The chronic faecal retention is associated with rectal dilatation and insensitivity to the normal urge to pass stool. This is why a structured toileting programme is a most important aspect of management.

INVESTIGATION

A plain abdominal X-ray is often helpful to document the nature and extent of faecal retention, and as a baseline for further treatment.

MANAGEMENT

- The first stage of therapy is to clear the bowel of faeces. An initial cleanout with suppositories (e.g. Durolax), given twice a day for up to 2 days is usually effective in rectal disimpaction
- This should coincide with the commencement of maintenance laxative treatment
- Regular toileting twice to three times daily is essential, with the child being comfortably seated on the toilet for at least 10 min and asked to push during this time. A footstool is often helpful
- Close follow-up is essential with the assistance of behavioural techniques such as a star chart diary to reward regular sitting and successful defecation in the toilet

- A good, normal diet with regular meals, adequate fluids and exercise

should be encouraged. The aim of treatment is to institute good dietary and toileting habits so that the problem does not recur, and then gradually wean the child from medications
- The treatment regimen should be maintained for a minimum of 6 months to ensure resolution of the megacolon

Children with encopresis may demonstrate secondary adjustment difficulties. This usually improves with resolution of soiling.

Sometimes it is clear that disordered family dynamics exists or that there are emotional factors beyond those which one would expect given the symptoms. In these instances there should be careful evaluation of the child and the family, either by the paediatrician or by referral to a psychologist, psychiatrist or family therapist.

RECURRENT ABDOMINAL PAIN

Recurrent abdominal pain affects about 10% of school-age children. There is usually no specific identifiable cause, and it is only infrequently the result of emotional problems. Recent evidence suggests there may be a subgroup with migrainous abdominal pain (associated with pallor, family history). Emotional factors, life-style and temperamental characteristics can modulate the child's response to pain, regardless of its cause

ASSESSMENT

- It is essential to take a careful history, including psychosocial details. It may be helpful to interview the parents alone, the child alone and the family together
- A thorough physical examination is essential. Rectal examination may be helpful
- Full blood count, erythrocyte sedimentation rate (ESR), urine microscopy and culture and a plain abdominal X-ray are appropriate baseline investigations

MANAGEMENT

- The two major causes in childhood are constipation and dysfunctional pain
- Treatment of underlying *constipation* is essential, and management of non-organic issues taken up if necessary
- *'Dysfunctional'* pain may be related to a variation in perception of visceral sensation in the absence of an identifiable organic cause. A detailed consultation and reassurance is often all that is required

- The diagnosis of *psychogenic* recurrent abdominal pain cannot be made simply in the absence of positive findings for an organic disorder. Positive evidence of emotional maladjustment is separately required, and if present should be managed appropriately

CHRONIC DIARRHOEA

An increase in stool frequency or fluid content are often of concern to parents, but do not necessarily imply significant organic disease, although this needs to be excluded. In every child who presents with chronic diarrhoea, the decision must be made as to whether further investigation is required.

The algorithm in Figure 7.1 outlines an approach to the child with chronic diarrhoea.

TODDLER DIARRHOEA

- This is a clinical syndrome characterized by chronic diarrhoea often with undigested food in the stools of a child who is otherwise well, gaining weight and growing satisfactorily. Stools may contain mucus and are passed between three and six times a day, often looser toward the end of the day
- Its onset is usually between 8 and 20 months of age
- There is often a family history of functional bowel disease, such as irritable bowel syndrome
- Treatment is reassurance and explanation. No specific drug or dietary therapy has been shown to be of value in toddler diarrhoea. Some toddlers on high-fructose load (i.e. 'apple juice' diarrhoea) may have diarrhoea that responds to dietary change

COW MILK PROTEIN INTOLERANCE (CMPI)

Symptoms related to ingestion of food or milk may be induced by any one of several components (see also Allergy, p. 99). These may be due to immune or non-immune effects.

Allergic responses to cow milk protein may result in rapid or delayed onset of symptoms. Rapid onset responses are less common, often characterized by the sudden onset of vomiting, and rarely by acute anaphylaxis. Delayed onset responses may be more difficult to diagnose, and present with diarrhoea, malabsorption or failure to thrive, and occasionally intestinal loss of protein or blood.

- CMPI can only be diagnosed with a complete and thorough history, and with **unequivocal reproducible reactions to elimination and challenge**

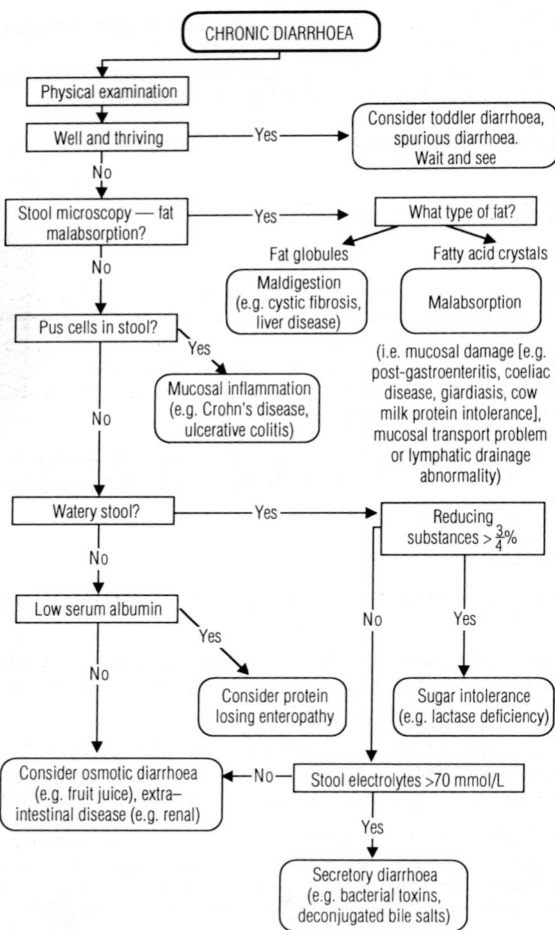

Figure 7.1 Investigation of chronic diarrhoea

- Blood tests and skin testing may help but are not substitutes for clinical assessment
- After a definitive diagnosis is established, cow's milk protein should be removed from the diet and replaced with either soy or a hydrolysed formula
- Most food allergies in infants improve or resolve with increasing age

CHRONIC INTESTINAL INFECTION

GIARDIASIS

Infection with this protozoan is common, particularly in children who attend day-care centres. The clinical spectrum is broad, ranging from asymptomatic cases to frank malabsorption. Younger children are more likely to have symptoms, with diarrhoea, anorexia or failure to thrive. Despite concentration techniques, stool microscopy of a fresh stool may not detect the organism.

Treatment should be with an agent such as *metronidazole* (30 mg/kg per dose (max. 2 g) once daily for 3 days) or *tinidazole* (50 mg/kg (max. 2 g) once only).

NEMATODES

Trichuris trichuria (whipworm) and *Enterobius vermicularis* (threadworm) commonly infect the colon and rectum.

Light infections with *Trichuris* are usually asymptomatic, but large numbers of parasites may result in *diarrhoea*. Infection may be diagnosed by the presence of eggs on stool microscopy.

Enterobius is common and usually presents with *perianal pruritus*. Diarrhoea is not a feature. It can be diagnosed by microscopic examination of clear adhesive tape which has been applied to the perianal skin.

Both organisms can usually be successfully treated with *mebendazole* (doses for >2 years: *Trichuris*, 100 mg, b.d. for 3 days, may repeat in 3–4 weeks; *Enterobius*, 100 mg as a single dose, may repeat in 2–4 weeks). In the case of *Enterobius*, the whole family should be treated.

INFLAMMATORY BOWEL DISEASE

- Crohn's disease is increasingly common in both children and adults
- In childhood, it should be suspected if there is unexplained diarrhoea (with or without blood), malaise, weight loss or abdominal pain

- Laboratory parameters suggesting active disease include anaemia, thrombocytosis, raised ESR and low albumin
- Evaluation and management should be made with the aid of a paediatric gastroenterologist

LIVER DISEASE

BILIARY ATRESIA

Although rare, biliary atresia is important to diagnose early, as the success of treatment depends on the timing of surgery. This condition should be suspected in any infant who has white or grey stools in the first few months of life. Jaundice may be mild in the first 1–2 months. **Prompt and early specialist referral is vital.**

HEPATITIS

If no viral aetiology is found in a child with hepatitis (particularly adolescent females), autoimmune and other causes of hepatitis should be considered. *Autoimmune hepatitis* in childhood usually responds well to corticosteroid therapy, but may have a rapid and fatal course if untreated.

Prevention

Effective vaccination is available for both hepatitis A and hepatitis B.

To minimize the number of carriers in the community (and hence the risk of chronic hepatitis and primary liver cancer later in life) the following groups should be vaccinated against *hepatitis B*:

- Infants born to carrier mothers (HBsAg-positive). This group should also receive hepatitis B immunoglobulin 100 IU (1 mL, i.m.) within 48 h of birth (preferably within 12 h)
- Infants and young children in ethnic groups with a high hepatitis B carrier rate
- Children in high-risk groups, e.g. haemodialysis patients, regular recipients of pooled blood products, household contacts of hepatitis B carriers, residents of institutions for the intellectually disabled, adolescents with multiple sexual partners

Hepatitis A vaccination is recommended for:

- Travellers to highly endemic areas
- Children in high-risk groups, e.g. residents of facilities for the intellectually disabled, adolescent male homosexuals
- Patients with chronic liver disease

CHAPTER 8

8

ALLERGY AND IMMUNOLOGY

Andrew Kemp

An *atopic* (allergic) child is defined as one who produces IgE antibodies to common allergens. Common *environmental allergens* include milk, egg, peanut, house dust mite, cat fur and rye grass.

ALLERGY TESTS

Skin testing and RAST tests identify IgE antibodies. The RAST test is neither more sensitive nor more accurate than skin testing despite being a radioimmunoassay. Neither test proves that the antibodies detected are the cause of the patient's symptoms—the results of the tests need to be interpreted in the light of the patient's history.

When ordering one of these tests the question being asked is: 'Are there IgE antibodies present?' This test will not necessarily answer the question: 'Is this antigen causing the patient's symptoms?'

In immediate food hypersensitivity reactions with a history suggestive of an IgE-mediated reaction, the skin test provides confirmatory evidence. If the skin test is negative one should question the conclusion that this is a true immediate hypersensitivity reaction

ALLERGIC RHINITIS

PERENNIAL RHINITIS

In pre-school and primary school children perennial rhinitis is more common than seasonal rhinitis. Perennial rhinitis occurs at any age.

The contribution of specific allergens to perennial rhinitis is unclear. In some cases house dust mite may be a provoking factor.

Nasal obstruction, and possibly discharge, are the predominant symptoms. Sneezing occurs particularly on awakening in the morning. It is important to consider the possibility of perennial allergic rhinitis in any atopic child. Perennial rhinitis may lead to significant nasal obstruction and snoring at night-time. The existence and symptoms of perennial rhinitis are frequently missed and yet eminently treatable.

Airflow through the nostrils should be assessed and an examination made of the nasal airways in all allergic children. In perennial rhinitis, airflow will be reduced or absent and inspection will reveal swollen turbinates, sometimes completely obstructing the airways.

Management

Topical steroid nasal sprays (beclomethasone or budesonide) are the treatment of choice. Beclomethasone can be given t.d.s. for a week, b.d. for the next week and once a day thereafter. An initial course of treatment should last for 2–3 months.

Antihistamines are not helpful in relieving the nasal obstruction and are not indicated as a first-line treatment.

SEASONAL RHINITIS

Seasonal rhinitis or hay fever is more frequently seen in teenagers and young adults. Rye grass is the common provoking antigen. Children will usually have a strongly positive skin prick test to rye grass.

Symptoms occur in spring and summer when rye grass pollens are present. Nasal symptoms of itchiness of the nose and sneezing may be associated with ocular symptoms of red, watery eyes and itching. The diagnosis is suggested by the seasonal nature.

Management

Topical steroid sprays, and possibly antihistamine. The long-acting non-sedating antihistamines (loratadine, terfenadine, astemizole and cetirizine) are effective but expensive, and most parents find that the cost prohibits their regular use. A useful alternative is hydroxyzine, which can provide long-acting antihistamine activity. Given at night-time as a single dose, the sedative effect does not prove to be a problem.

FOOD ALLERGY

Allergic reactions to food can be considered in two broad groups.

IMMEDIATE HYPERSENSITIVITY REACTIONS

These occur within 1–2 h of ingestion of the food. They are quite common. They typically begin in young infants in the second 6 months of life and frequently resolve by the age of 3 or 4 years.

Common provoking factors are milk, egg and peanut products. Diagnosis is made by a carefully taken history.

Common symptoms of immediate reactions are *erythema* where food touches the lips, *urticaria* which may be facial or generalized, *vomiting* immediately after ingestion of food and occasionally rhinorrhoea, wheezing and anaphylaxis. These reactions can be strongly suspected on the history.

Investigation

In an infant with such a reaction to milk protein, skin testing should also be performed with egg and peanut allergen, as reactions are often multiple. If patients have a history of significant reactions involving the airways, multiple reactions or severe atopic dermatitis one should obtain allergy specialist advice. Practitioners should be wary of advising parents to challenge such children with a suspected food in the home environment as severe reactions and even death have occurred.

DELAYED REACTIONS

These occur within 24–48 h of food ingestion. They are much less common and will often need specialist consultation to truly substantiate.

MEASLES IMMUNIZATION AND EGG ALLERGY

There has been controversy over the appropriate response to measles immunization in view of the vaccine package insert which states that immunization is contraindicated in egg-allergic children.

Measles vaccines are produced in chick embryo fibroblast cell cultures and have not been grown in eggs. The risk of a significant adverse reaction to measles vaccine in egg-allergic children is *extremely low*. No child should have measles vaccine delayed or withheld because of egg allergy. Egg-allergic children should be investigated and managed by practitioners with expertise in this area. Measles immunization should be performed with a single dose of vaccine in a setting where any adverse reaction can be dealt with appropriately. Measles vaccine skin tests and desensitization regimens are not necessary

URTICARIA AND ANGIOEDEMA

Urticarial rashes are raised areas of erythema and oedema, which move over several hours. They are usually itchy.

Angioedema is swelling of deeper tissues and often involves areas of low tension such as eyelids, lips and scrotum. Angioedema is not necessarily itchy.

When faced with the problem of urticaria the lesion should be classified as acute (<6 weeks duration) or chronic (>6 weeks duration). *Acute urticarias* frequently only last a few days.

- The aetiology is unknown but they are often thought to follow viral or sometimes streptococcal infections
- The most important step is to take a history looking for obvious precipitating factors such as drug ingestion (especially aspirin and antibiotics) and immediate hypersensitivity food reactions (in a child <18 months of age). In the great majority of cases no precipitating factor is identified
- Skin test, RAST tests and IgE levels are usually unhelpful and are not indicated

Chronic urticarias can persist or occur intermittently for months.

- The possibility of a *physical urticaria* (e.g. heat, cold, aquagenic) should be considered
- They are rarely caused by IgE-mediated reactions and therefore investigation with skin testing and RAST testing is usually unhelpful
- Some cases may be due to a reaction to chemicals and in persistent cases a preservative- and colouring-free diet may be indicated. The institution of such a diet and interpretation of the results may need specialist advice

ATOPIC DERMATITIS

Atopic dermatitis is not simply an IgE-mediated reaction to ingested allergens (see also Dermatologic Conditions, p. 107). *Immediate* food hypersensitivity reactions can act as exacerbating factors, particularly in young children with severe atopic dermatitis and generalized erythema. The possibility of these reactions should always be considered and investigation is as outlined above.

Delayed reactions to foods may also exacerbate dermatitis in a small proportion of the more severe cases, and this provides the rationale for the use of various forms of dietary manipulation.

There are no skin or blood tests that can reliably identify whether a delayed reaction to a food is occurring. The appropriate test is dietary elimination under supervision with a rechallenge of possible offending foods.

The dietary manipulations necessary in children with severe atopic dermatitis are often complex and difficult to interpret, and specialist advice is frequently required both in the administration of the diet and in the interpretation of results.

The dietary management forms only one component of the management of atopic dermatitis. Appropriate case selection is important, and dietary restrictions should not be instituted in children with mild atopic dermatitis that can be readily controlled with appropriate topical medication.

IMMUNOTHERAPY

There are relatively few indications for immunotherapy in paediatric practice:

- Immunotherapy with purified bee venom is indicated for *life-threatening anaphylactic reactions* to bee stings in children. Referral should be made to a paediatric immunologist or allergist
- In teenagers with *severe seasonal allergic rhinitis* for which a single antigen (usually rye grass pollen) can be identified, immunotherapy may be an option if topical medication and antihistamines are unsuccessful in controlling symptoms

Extreme caution is required in providing immunotherapy to unstable asthmatic patients as deaths have resulted.

GUIDELINES FOR INVESTIGATION AND TREATMENT OF IMMUNODEFICIENCY

WHEN TO SUSPECT IMMUNODEFICIENCY

- It is important to remember that normal, immunocompetent children average five to 10 viral upper respiratory tract infections per year in the first few years of life (even more if the child attends child care or has older siblings). Therefore, recurrent viral infections in a well, thriving child do not suggest immunodeficiency
- A history of recurrent or chronic bacterial infections (e.g. persistently discharging ears, purulent respiratory secretions) or more than one severe pyogenic infection may indicate antibody deficiency
- Severe or disseminated viral infections and/or persistent mucocutaneous candidiasis suggest possible T-cell deficiency
- Infants with chronic diarrhoea and failure to thrive should be investigated for severe combined immunodeficiency

WHICH TESTS TO ORDER

Basic Immunodeficiency Screen

A *full blood count* and *immunoglobulin measurements* (IgG, IgA and IgM) will pick up the vast majority of treatable primary immunodeficiencies (e.g. agammaglobulinaemia, severe combined immunodeficiency, selective IgA deficiency).

Immunoglobulin Subclasses

These should only be considered when there is evidence of persistent or recurrent upper and/or lower respiratory tract suppuration and hypogammaglobulinaemia has been excluded. When considering whether to measure immunoglobulin subclasses, ask yourself: If a subclass deficiency is found, does this clinical condition warrant regular gammaglobulin therapy?

T-cell Numbers, T-cell Function (Mitogenic Stimulation)

These tests are used predominantly in the first 6 months of life to help in the diagnosis of severe combined immunodeficiency and Di George syndrome (absent thymus, hypocalcaemia and cardiovascular anomalies).

Neutrophil Function Tests

Specific defects of neutrophil function (e.g. chronic granulomatous disease) are very rare, and are almost always associated with gingivitis. Look in the mouth before ordering neutrophil function tests.

Others

Chest X-ray for thymic shadow, *functional antibody response* to immunizations (B-cell function), *delayed-hypersensitivity skin tests* (T-cell function) and *complement studies* (meningococcal disease with uncommon serogroups such as X, Y, W135, or in adolescents) may be indicated in certain circumstances. *HIV testing* should be considered.

If in doubt whether immunological function testing is indicated or which test should be ordered, consult with a clinical immunologist before ordering expensive and time-consuming tests.

TREATMENT OF IMMUNODEFICIENCY (PRINCIPLES)

Immunizations

- As a general principle all live vaccines should be avoided unless advised by a specialist
- In certain circumstances measles immunization may be given to patients with a significant T-cell defect (e.g. Di George syndrome or HIV infection) as the risks of wild-type measles infection are considerable while adverse reactions to the vaccine appear to be theoretical
- In cases of combined immunodeficiency and antibody deficiency, immunization with killed vaccines will not promote a significant antibody response
- If the patient is on immunoglobulin replacement therapy, passively acquired antibody will prevent virus infections such as measles and chicken-pox
- Patients of any age with *asplenia* should be immunized with both the Hib vaccine and pneumococcal vaccine

Immunoglobulin Therapy

Immunoglobulin therapy is given when a significant deficiency in antibody production is demonstrated with the development of symptoms, usually in the respiratory tract.

Hypogammaglobulinaemia

Immunoglobulin therapy is generally lifelong.

Immunoglobulin subclass deficiency

If a significant functional antibody deficit is demonstrated *and* the patient has significant symptoms, a trial of immunoglobulin therapy may be used for a restricted period of time. This should only be instituted in conjunction with a clinical immunologist. The finding of a low immunoglobulin subclass level is not sufficient to indicate immunoglobulin therapy.

Use of Blood Products

- If it is suspected or known that the patient has a significant T-cell deficiency, blood products which contain cells (e.g. whole blood, packed red cells or platelets) should be *irradiated* to prevent graft versus host disease
- In infants with severe combined immunodeficiency, attempts should

be made to provide *cytomegalovirus* (*CMV) antibody negative* blood as CMV infection can be a significant problem in such patients

- If possible *Epstein-Barr virus (EBV) antibody negative* blood should also be given as EBV can induce lymphoproliferative states in severely immunodeficient subjects

Bone Marrow Transplantation

Bone marrow transplantation is utilized for severe combined immunodeficiency. The cure rate can be of the order of 80% if the transplant is from a matched sibling, and of the order of 50% if the transplant is only partially matched.

CHAPTER 9

DERMATOLOGIC CONDITIONS

George Varigos and Rod Phillips

INTRODUCTION

The key to accurate diagnosis and hence appropriate management of skin disorders in children is a carefully taken history and astute observation of the rash, particularly focusing on the appearance, site and pattern of development. The examination should attempt to identify the main features of the rash. Working through Figure 9.1 will help select which group of conditions needs to be considered.

ECZEMATOUS RASHES

Consider atopic eczema, allergic dermatitis, contact dermatitis, photosensitivity eruptions, scabies and tinea corporis.

ATOPIC ECZEMA

Clinical Features

Eczema usually begins in infancy, most commonly involving the face, and sometimes the trunk and limbs as well. In older children, the rash may be widespread but is often localized to flexures. Erythema, weeping, excoriation and rarely vesicles may be seen in acute lesions. Chronic lesions may show scale and lichenification. In some children, the lesions are more clearly defined, thickened discoid areas that may intermittently be itchy. There is usually a cyclical pattern of improvement and exacerbation. Weeping and yellow crusted areas which do not respond to therapy may indicate secondary bacterial infection.

Management

- *Education.* Parents need to know that treatments are effective in controlling the disease but they will not cure eczema and that exacerbations are common. There is rarely one allergen as the cause
- *Avoid irritants.* The following may worsen eczema: soaps, bubble

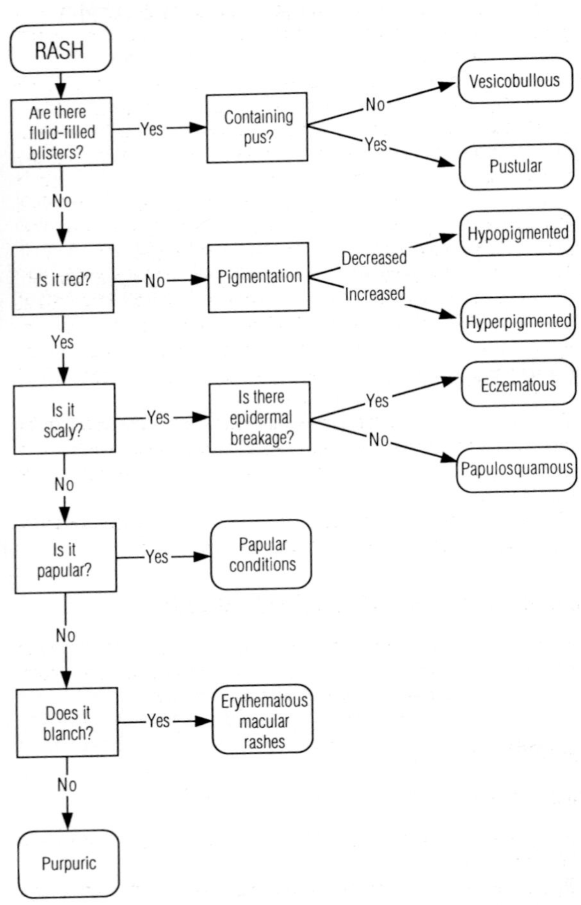

Figure 9.1 Classification of skin disorders in children

baths, prickly clothing, seams and labels on clothing, car seat covers, carpets, overheating or contact with pets. Smooth cotton clothing is preferred
- *Keep the skin moist.* Use a moisturizer such as sorbolene with 10% glycerine, aqueous cream or paraffin ointment as often as several times a day if necessary
- *Treat inflammation.* Steroid creams can be used intermittently with good effect (e.g. 2 days on and 2 days off). Hydrocortisone 1% is usually adequate. If not, moderate potency ointment (e.g. betamethasone 0.02%) can be used for exacerbations in areas other than the face or nappy area. Prolonged use of moderate potency steroids to skin of infants can cause atrophy and adrenal suppression. Oral steroids are rarely indicated in eczema. For chronic eczema on the limbs, zinc and tar combinations are alternatives to steroids
- *Manage itch.* Advise parents to avoid saying 'Stop itching' all the time, to distract the child and to avoid overheating at all times, particularly at night. Bandaging may be helpful, and sedation may be required. Try trimeprazine tartrate, promethazine hydrochloride or chloral hydrate. (Terfenadine (Teldane) should not be used because of occasional fatal interactions if erythromycin is also taken)
- *Treat infection.* Take cultures and treat with simple wet dressings or oral antibiotics (erythromycin, cephalexin or flucloxacillin). For recurrent bacterial infection, use mupirocin nasally to treat staphylococcal carriage if present
- *Diet.* A normal diet is usually indicated. If a child has immediate urticarial reactions to a particular food, that food should be avoided

RED SCALY RASHES (PAPULOSQUAMOUS)

Consider seborrhoeic dermatitis, psoriasis, tinea corporis, pityriasis rosea, tinea versicolor and atopic eczema. Ichthyosis vulgaris is a common cause of generalized scale without itch or redness.

SEBORRHOEIC DERMATITIS

Clinical Features

- Presents in the first months of life, possibly partly due to activity of commensal yeasts
- Red or yellow/brown scaly areas particularly affecting the scalp, forehead and napkin area. The folds behind the ears and around the neck, axillae, groins and gluteal clefts are also commonly affected
- Resolution by the age of 1 year is usual

Management

- Imidazole creams, with hydrocortisone 1% cream or with a mixture of salicylic acid (1%) and sulfur (1%) ointment, b.d.
- Antiyeast shampoos can be helpful. Use carefully to avoid irritation

PSORIASIS

Clinical Features

Psoriasis can occur at any age but is less common than eczema. Lesions begin as small red papules that develop into circular sharply demarcated erythematous patches, with prominent silvery scale. Lesions are often symmetrical and most commonly occur on the extensor surfaces, as generalized guttate (drop-like) lesions, or on the scalp and the anogenital region. Itch can be a problem. Associated features such as nail changes and arthropathy are not usually seen in childhood.

Management

- Treat localized skin plaques with tar-based ointments initially, moving from a low to a higher strength as tolerated
- Thick scalp plaques can be softened with combined salicylic acid and tar ointment and removed with a tar shampoo
- Use hydrocortisone 1% ointment on the face and anogenital region. Topical steroids are generally not used elsewhere in childhood psoriasis because of the possible development of widespread pustular disease on cessation of therapy
- Topical calcipotriol can be used for small areas in children older than 12 years, but insufficient data are available to recommend its use in younger children
- Widespread psoriasis needs referral for possible treatment with one or more of dithranol, etretinate, methotrexate, cyclosporin or ultraviolet therapy, all of which are effective

TINEA CORPORIS

Clinical Features

The typical lesion is a slow growing, sharply demarcated erythematous ring of scaly papules, pustules or vesicles with a clear or scaly centre. There may be one lesion or rarely several lesions distributed asymmetrically on any part of the body. However, tinea corporis can present in a wide variety of ways, particularly if previously treated with steroid ointments. Tinea should be considered in any red scaly rash where the diagnosis is unclear.

Management

- If in doubt about the diagnosis, confirm by collecting scale for microscopy and culture
- Lesions are treated with half-strength Whitfield's ointment or an imidazole cream (clotrimazole, miconazole, econazole) applied twice daily for 4 weeks—then review

RED (OR SKIN-COLOURED) PAPULAR DISORDERS

Consider scabies, papular urticaria, molluscum contagiosum, warts, epidermal naevi (p. 120), angiokeratoma (prominent blood vessels with overlying hyperkeratosis), keratosis pilaris (tiny follicular papules which give a sandpapery feel to the thighs and upper arms) and papular acrodermatitis (red flat-topped papules mainly on the arms, legs and cheeks seen as a response to many common infections).

SCABIES

Clinical Features

An intensely itchy papular eruption develops 2–6 weeks after first exposure to the *Sarcoptes scabiei* mite or 1–4 days after subsequent reinfestation. The characteristic lesion is the burrow, a linear elevation several millimetres in length that is often grey. Burrows are best seen on the hands, especially between the fingers, and on the feet. Papules can occur anywhere including the palms, soles and genitalia. Excoriations and secondary impetigo may be present. There is currently a worldwide pandemic of this contagious disease affecting both adults and children.

Management

- Permethrin 5% cream is effective; however, it is expensive. Cheaper alternatives are lindane 1% (not for infants or women who are pregnant or breast feeding) or benzyl benzoate 25% (irritant for children, can be used for adults), used twice, a week apart
- Treat all family members and any other people who have close skin contact with the family at the same time

- Apply to cool dry skin (not after a bath) from the neck down to all skin surfaces. In infants, apply to the scalp and face as well (not eyes or mouth). Use mittens if necessary to prevent finger sucking
- Leave the cream on for at least 8 h
- Wash the cream off. Wash clothing, pyjamas and bed linen at this time
- The allergic symptoms take a week or two to settle and can be treated with calamine lotion and/or an antihistamine
- Reinfestation is common. The family should notify all social contacts (creche, school, close friends) to ensure all infected people receive treatment

PAPULAR URTICARIA

Clinical Features

This is a clinical hypersensitivity to insect bites. New bites appear as groups of small red papules usually in warmer weather. Older bites appear as 1–5 mm papules, sometimes with surface scale or crust or with surrounding urticaria. Vesicles or pustules may form. Individual lesions may resolve in a week or two or may repeatedly flare up after fresh bites elsewhere. Itch is often intense and secondary infection is common.

Management

- Prevent bites by spraying insecticide in the home, using repellents and treating pets
- Treat itch with an agent such as aluminium sulfate 20% (Stingose), Liquor Picis Carb. 2% in Calamine lotion, moderate potency steroid ointment or antihistamines (promethazine, diphenhydramine)
- Treat secondary infection with topical mupirocin or oral antibiotics

MOLLUSCUM CONTAGIOSUM

Clinical Features

Uncomplicated mollusca are easily recognized as firm pearly dome-shaped papules with a central umbilication. However, presentation to a doctor is often prompted by the development of an immune response or eczematization of surrounding skin. In such cases, recognition can be difficult as these changes can obliterate the primary lesions. A carefully taken history of the initial lesions is usually diagnostic.

Management

- Education. Mollusca are caused by a common virus. A child may develop a few or a great many lesions and individual lesions may last for months. Complete resolution will not happen until an immune response develops, which may take up to 2 or 3 years
- For uncomplicated mollusca, do not use painful therapies such as pricking, lancing or freezing. Aim to stimulate an immune response with aluminium acetate solution (Burows solution, 1:30) for large areas, or benzoyl peroxide 2.5% dabbed on daily to small areas and covered with the adhesive part of a dressing
- Individual inflamed mollusca usually do not warrant antibiotic treatment
- Treat surrounding eczema with a moderate potency steroid ointment

WARTS

Many serotypes of the papilloma virus can cause warts. Different serotypes have a predilection to different areas of skin. Resolution of all warts of the same serotype occur when immunity develops, but this may take years. No treatment is necessary unless the warts are causing a problem to the child (e.g. social embarrassment, pain from plantar wart). Avoid painful and traumatic procedures and never freeze warts in children under 10 years old.

- *Ordinary warts.* Regular paring every 2–3 days with a razor blade or nail file will remove the surface horn. Apply formalin 30% in acetone or a proprietary keratolytic agent containing salicylic and/or lactic acid each day or two as directed
- *Plantar warts.* These are often painful and can appear flat. Pare as for ordinary warts. Apply the affected area of sole for 30 min each night to a small pad of cotton wool soaked in 3% formalin and placed in a saucer on the floor
- *Plane (flat) warts.* These are usually rounded, smooth, flat or slightly elevated, skin-coloured or pigmented lesions. They may occur in lines or coalesce to form plaque-like lesions. If treatment is needed for plane warts on the hands, apply formalin solution as for ordinary warts. Lesions on the face and elsewhere are prone to develop complications with treatment and should be referred
- *Cuminate (genital) warts.* These are soft fleshy warts that occur at the mucocutaneous junctions, especially around the anus, glans penis and external female genitalia. They may be isolated flesh-coloured nodules or may coalesce into large cauliflower-like masses. All patients with cuminate warts should be referred for management.

Note: Genital warts in children should lead you to consider sexual abuse but in the great majority of cases, transmission is by normal intimate parent–child contact. Transmission during childbirth can lead to the development of genital warts in the child even 2 years later.

FLAT RED BLANCHING RASHES

Macular erythematous lesions are most commonly caused by non-specific viral infections or drug reactions. Spider naevi can be seen in children as isolated findings.

HAEMANGIOMAS

Clinical Features

Superficial haemangiomas begin as macular erythematous lesions and become soft, partly compressible, sharply defined, red or purple swellings that can occur anywhere on the body. Deeper haemangiomas may appear as blue or skin-coloured swellings. Most (but not all) haemangiomas are not present at birth; they grow for several months and then resolve fully over several years.

Management

Parents need reassurance about the inherently benign nature of these lesions. Most haemangiomas are best left alone and allowed to involute spontaneously. In some sites, however, haemangiomas can lead to problems such as blindness, destruction of cartilage, respiratory obstruction or death. Urgent assessment by a clinician experienced in this field (within days, not weeks) for possible treatment with steroids, surgery or interferon is needed if any developing haemangioma:

- Is on the eyelid or adjacent to the globe of the eye
- Is deforming structures such as lip, ear cartilage or nasal cartilage
- Begins as an extensive macule that then grows thicker
- Is associated with stridor, thrombocytopenia or multiple lesions

VASCULAR MALFORMATIONS

- These are developmental defects and do not resolve
- They can involve any mix of capillaries (e.g. port-wine stain), veins, arteries (e.g. arteriovenous malformation) and lymphatics (e.g. cystic hygroma)

- Extensive malformations can be associated with sequelae such as soft tissue or bony hypertrophy, bone erosion, haemorrhage, infection and platelet trapping
- Management requires a multidisciplinary approach using expertise from surgical, paediatric, dermatological and radiological fields

URTICARIA

Clinical Features

Urticaria is characterized by the rapid appearance and disappearance of multiple raised red weals on any part of the body (see also p. 101). Individual lesions are often itchy and clear within 1 day. There may be central clearing to give ring lesions. These are not target lesions and do not persist longer than a day (cf. erythema multiforme). The child is usually well but may have associated fever and/or arthralgias (serum sickness). Urticarial episodes usually resolve over weeks or months, rarely longer than 6 months. In most cases of short duration, the cause cannot be determined.

Management

- Investigation is usually not required and does not help determine the cause
- Treat itch with oral antihistamine (e.g. chlorpheniramine)
- For recurrent or chronic urticaria persisting for weeks, look for trigger factors. Consider mast cell degranulating drugs, foods, animals, parasitic infections, heat, cold, physical pressure. Consider investigation with throat swab (for streptococcal carriage), full blood examination (for eosinophilia and anaemia), nocturnal check for threadworms and possible challenge with any suspected agent. Adding cimetidine to the antihistamine may help

Urticaria may be the first sign of anaphylaxis. If there is associated angioedema (prominent subcutaneous swelling) or wheeze, continued observation and appropriate treatment is required (see p. 5).

PURPURIC RASHES

Children who present with petechiae or purpura can have a wide range of underlying conditions.

SEPTICAEMIA

Suspect septicaemia (usually meningococcal) in a child with recent onset of fever and lethargy. Skin lesions may be erythematous macules progressing to black, scattered petechiae or extensive purpura. If in any doubt, take blood cultures, give antibiotics and arrange admission (see also p. 7).

LEUKAEMIA

Suspect leukaemia in a child with generalized petechiae or purpura in the absence of trauma. Look for tiredness or pallor. If in doubt, obtain an urgent full blood examination (see also p. 152).

HENOCH-SCHOENLEIN PURPURA

See also p. 214

Clinical Features

Non-itchy, painless macules, papules or urticarial lesions with purpuric centres occur in a symmetrical distribution mainly on the buttocks and ankles, occasionally on the legs, arms and elsewhere. There may be associated abdominal pain, arthralgia or haematuria. Renal involvement leading to chronic renal failure is rare, but can occur irrespective of the severity of the rash and other symptoms, and may be delayed until weeks or months after the onset of the illness.

Management

- If warranted by symptoms, consider analgesia, bed rest and crutches
- Follow-up for at least 12 months: check blood pressure and urinalysis for blood and protein

CHILD ABUSE

Twisting, compression, pinching and hitting can all cause petechial or purpuric lesions (see p. 333). Look for bruises of bizarre shapes and different ages, evidence of bony fractures and an abnormal affect.

IDIOPATHIC THROMBOCYTOPENIC PURPURA (ITP)

Bruises, petechiae or purpuric lesions appear over a period of days or weeks, mainly in sites of frequent mild trauma (see also p. 148). The child is otherwise well. Full blood examination will show a low platelet count.

TRAUMA AND VASOMOTOR STRAINING

- In some ethnic groups, it is common to treat a febrile or unwell child by rubbing or suctioning the skin with a variety of implements. This produces bizarre circular and linear patterns of petechiae which can alarm the unwary
- Petechiae can appear around the head and neck in normal children after coughing or vomiting. Restraining a small child for a procedure such as a lumbar puncture can also lead to the development of petechiae on the upper body

VESICULOBULLOUS RASHES

IMPETIGO (SCHOOL SORES)

Atopic eczema (p. 107), irritant dermatitis, contact dermatitis, tinea (p. 110), scabies (p. 111), papular urticaria (p. 112), sunburn, child abuse (p. 333), varicella, herpes simplex and enteroviral infections (p. 51) can all present with blisters.

Clinical Features

Impetigo presents as areas of ooze and honey-coloured crusts on the face, trunk or limbs. Occasionally, the primary lesions are bullous. Lesions are rounded and well demarcated and may be single, grouped or widespread. Onset and spread may be rapid or occur over days. In the more chronic cases, there is often central healing with peripheral spread to give annular lesions. Impetigo may be secondary to pruritic conditions such as eczema, papular urticaria or lice. Generalized impetigo may mask underlying scabies.

Management

- Swab for cultures (*Staphylococcus aureus* and/or *Streptococcus pyogenes*)
- Bathe off crusts
- Apply topical antiseptics or give oral antibiotic (erythromycin, flucloxacillin or cephalexin)
- Isolate the child from other children or from sick adults unless all lesions are covered or treated
- Treat any underlying condition such as scabies

ECZEMA HERPETICUM

Clinical Features

Herpes simplex virus infection in children with eczema is common, but most cases are misdiagnosed as either an exacerbation of the eczema or bacterial infection. Grouped vesicles may be prominent but more often, vesicles are rudimentary or absent and the infection presents as a group of shallow 2–4 mm ulcers on an inflamed base. The infected area may not be painful or itchy and does not respond to standard eczema therapy. Untreated, resolution usually occurs in 1–4 weeks but dissemination may occur. Recurrences may be at different sites.

Management

- Collect fluid and loose epithelium for herpes immunofluorescence and culture
- Local disease in an otherwise well child requires regular observation but does not usually need antiviral therapy. Referral for assessment may be appropriate
- A child with fever or multiple sites of cutaneous herpes infection may need admission to hospital and treatment with intravenous acyclovir. Oral acyclovir is not appropriate for disseminated disease
- Eye involvement should be managed with topical and/or systemic acyclovir and urgent referral
- Underlying eczema can be treated with moisturizer or wet dressings

SINGLE BLISTERS

In a child who presents with a single blister as an isolated finding, consider enterovirus (e.g. hand, foot and mouth disease), herpes simplex virus, insect bite, cigarette burn, friction, impetigo and spider bite. The latter can grow over days to become a non-tender blister of many centimetres diameter.

PUSTULAR RASHES

ACNE

Clinical Features

Acne mainly affects the forehead and face but other sebaceous gland areas (neck, shoulders and upper trunk) can be involved. Early lesions are blackheads, whiteheads and papules. In more severe cases there may be pustules or inflammatory cysts that can lead to permanent scarring.

Management

- Acne is treatable. No person with acne should be told it is an inevitable part of adolescence. Effective acne therapies are now available and should be used sufficiently aggressively to control the disease
- For mild disease, use topical benzoyl peroxide 2.5–5%. Other topical agents include antibiotics (clindamycin, erythromycin or tetracycline), isotretinoin (not in pregnancy) or azelaic acid. These can be used singly or in combination and improvement may be seen in 2–8 weeks. All of these topical agents have side-effects with which practitioners must be familiar
- Treatment of moderate acne often involves the addition of long-term antibiotic therapy requiring continued reassessment. In unresponsive moderate acne and in all cases of severe acne, referral to a specialist for oral isotretinoin therapy is needed
- Consider underlying endocrine disorders if acne begins before puberty

HYPOPIGMENTED LESIONS

In hypopigmented lesions, look for fine scale. If scaly, consider tinea versicolor or pityriasis alba. If not scaly, consider tinea versicolor, post-inflammatory loss of pigment, halo naevi or vitiligo.

TINEA VERSICOLOR

- Probably caused by increased activity of commensal yeasts
- Multiple oval macules, usually covered with fine scale and sometimes confluent, appear on the trunk or upper arms. The lesions may appear paler or darker than surrounding skin
- Treatment with anti-yeast shampoos is effective. For example, apply selenium sulfide 2% (Selsun shampoo), leave on for 2 h then rinse, treat weekly for 4 weeks, then monthly

PITYRIASIS ALBA

This is extremely common. Single or multiple, poorly demarcated hypopigmented 1–2 cm macules are seen on the face or upper body. Lesions are not itchy but often have a fine scale, which relates to mild eczema. Treat the eczema before summer and tanning will occur.

VITILIGO

Vitiligo is characterized by sharply demarcated, often symmetrical areas of complete pigment loss. Eventual repigmentation in childhood vitiligo is common and is helped by strong steroids. In troublesome cases, specialist advice regarding treatment (e.g. corrective cosmetics, psoralen therapy) is helpful.

HYPOPIGMENTED STREAKS, WHORLS AND LINES

These are often congenital as a result of genetic mosaicism but may not be noticed until the child gets sun exposure. Rarely, there are associated abnormalities of other organ systems, especially eye, musculoskeletal and central nervous systems.

HYPERPIGMENTED LESIONS

In addition to the lesions described below, consider tinea versicolor (p. 119), café-au-lait spots, warts (p. 113), Spitz naevi and hyperpigmented streaks, whorls and lines (as for hypopigmented streaks, whorls and lines).

MELANOCYTIC NAEVI

During childhood, most children develop multiple pigmented lesions, which may be freckles, lentigines, naevus spilus, congenital melanocytic naevi, acquired melanocytic naevi or rarely, melanoma. Lesions present at birth, covering large areas or causing concern may need specialist assessment for diagnosis, surgery, laser treatment and/or long-term follow up.

POST-INFLAMMATORY HYPERPIGMENTATION

Particularly in dark-skinned people, many inflammatory skin disorders may heal to leave diffuse, hyperpigmented macules that can persist for months or years. No treatment is satisfactory.

EPIDERMAL NAEVI

- Linear or whorled patterns of warty hyperkeratosis and epidermal hypertrophy
- Can be congenital or appear during childhood

- Some variants (e.g. sebaceous naevi) have significant malignant potential and should be removed
- Treatment, if needed, is surgical but relapses are common

ANOGENITAL RASHES

Virtually all anogenital rashes seen in infants wearing nappies are primarily caused by reaction with urine or faeces (irritant napkin dermatitis). Soaps, detergents and secondary yeast infection may contribute. In older children, threadworms (*Enterobius vermicularis*) are a common cause of an itchy anogenital rash. Look for the worms at night and treat with pyrantel or mebendazole. A repeat dose 2 weeks later helps reduce the high rate of reinfestation.

Consider also rare causes such as malabsorption syndromes (diarrhoea, erosive dermatitis and failure to thrive; p. 96), zinc deficiency (sharply defined anogenital rash with associated perioral 'eczema'), Langerhans cell histiocytosis, psoriasis (p. 110) and Crohn's disease (p. 97).

IRRITANT NAPKIN DERMATITIS

Clinical Features

This is the most common cause of napkin dermatitis in infants and typically presents as confluent erythema sparing the groin folds. Variant presentations include multiple erosions and ulcers, scaly or glazed erythema, and satellite lesions at the periphery. Satellite lesions are suggestive of *Candida* infection.

Management

- Keep the area clean and dry. Leave the nappy off whenever possible
- Gel-based disposable nappies or a non-wettable undernapkin can be helpful. Cloth nappies should be thoroughly washed and rinsed
- Use topical zinc cream for mild eruptions
- Add hydrocortisone 1% cream if inflamed. Do not use stronger steroids
- Antifungal therapy is often not needed even if *Candida* is present

CANDIDA *NAPKIN DERMATITIS*

This occurs secondary to antibiotic use and irritant napkin dermatitis. Treat with a combination of topical antifungal cream (e.g. clotrimazole 1%) and hydrocortisone 1%.

MEDICINE

PERIANAL STREPTOCOCCAL DERMATITIS

Streptococcus pyogenes infection.

Clinical Features

- Localized, well-demarcated erythema that covers a circular area of 1–2 cm radius around the anus
- If not treated, may remain for months
- May have painful defecation, fissures and constipation

Management

- Culture to confirm the presence of *Streptococcus pyogenes*
- Treat with oral antibiotics (penicillin, erythromycin) for a minimum of 2 weeks. Several weeks therapy may be required. Intramuscular benzathine penicillin can be used if there are concerns about compliance

LICHEN SCLEROSIS ET ATROPHICUS

Presents as an asymptomatic or itchy area of atrophy, white shiny skin, purpura and/or telangiectasias often in the perivulval region of girls aged 3 years or older. Cases have been misdiagnosed as sexual abuse. Management is with moisturizers or brief courses of moderately potent steroid ointment. About 50% of cases resolve spontaneously.

HAIR PROBLEMS

There are three common causes of hair loss in children: tinea capitis, alopecia areata and traumatic alopecia.

ALOPECIA AREATA

Clinical Features

Typically one or more oval patches of hair loss develop over a few days. Some hairs may remain within the patches. Occasionally, the hair loss is diffuse. The scalp appears normal and does not show scaling, erythema or scarring. Most cases in childhood resolve spontaneously but progression to total scalp or body hair loss or recurrent alopecia can occur. Regrowth can occur decades later.

Management

- For isolated small patches present for weeks without further progression, no treatment is needed
- For recent or progressive hair loss, treatment with moderate potency topical steroids for a few weeks may help. In difficult cases, other therapies including contact sensitization, irritant agents and more potent immunosuppression need to be considered

TRAUMATIC ALOPECIA

Clinical Features

This condition is usually caused by rubbing (as on the occiput of many babies), cosmetic practices (e.g. tight braiding) or hair pulling as a habit (trichotillomania). Trichotillomania may be largely nocturnal and parents are often unaware of it. Affected areas are usually angular and on the anterior or lateral scalp. The areas contain hairs of different lengths and are never completely bald.

Management

- Recognition of the problem and careful explanation to the family is often sufficient
- Trichotillomania does not indicate significant psychological problems are present. It is a habit similar to thumb sucking or nail biting and a low-key approach similar to that used in those conditions is appropriate

TINEA CAPITIS

Clinical Features

Tinea capitis is usually caused by *Microsporum canis* contracted from cats or dogs. It is characterized by patches of hair loss with some short, lustreless, bent hairs a few millimetres in length. Redness and scaling are present in the patch. Hair loss without any of these features is not likely to be fungal.

Management

Confirm the diagnosis if possible by greenish fluorescence of the hair shafts with Woods light (not present with some fungi) or by microscopy and culture of hair and scale. Treatment usually comprises griseofulvin orally 10–15 mg/kg for 4–6 weeks or until non-fluorescent. Optimal dosage regimens for newer antifungals (terbinafine, itraconazole) have not yet been determined. Children may attend school providing they are being treated.

KERION (INFLAMMATORY RINGWORM)

This represents an inflammatory scarring immune response to tinea. It is an erythematous, tender, boggy swelling discharging pus from multiple points. These swellings appear fluctuant but skin incision should be avoided. Treatment is with oral griseofulvin, often with antibiotics for secondary infection, and a brief course of oral steroids to suppress the immune response.

HEAD LICE

Infestation of the scalp with *Pediculosis capitis* is associated with itching. Eggs (nits) can be seen attached to the hairs just above the scalp surface. Epidemics of head lice regularly sweep through primary schools in all areas.

Management

- Suitable treatments include pyrethrin 0.165% (e.g. Pyrifoam), malathion 0.5% and permethrin 1% (e.g. Nix, Lyclear cream rinse)
- Wash the hair with soap and water. Thoroughly moisten the hair with the treatment and leave for 10 min. Rinse well and comb out with a fine-toothed comb. Reapply 1 week later to kill eggs that have subsequently hatched
- Reinfestation is common. Regular physical inspection and combing of the hair is as important as chemical treatment

NAIL PROBLEMS

Congenitally abnormal nails are usually atrophic and can be the presenting feature of rare inherited conditions such as ectodermal dysplasias, dyskeratosis congenita, pachyonychia congenita, congenital malalignment of the great toenails and the nail–patella syndrome.

Acquired nail disease is usually a result of fungal infection, ingrown toenails, or twenty nail dystrophy. It may also be seen in association with diseases such as psoriasis, alopecia areata and lichen planus. Nail biting and picking can lead to marked pitting of involved nails.

TINEA UNGUIUM (ONYCHOMYCOSIS)

Clinical Features

- Dermatophyte infection may affect one or more nails
- White or yellow patches develop at the distal and lateral nail edges. The rest of the nail may become discoloured, friable and deformed with accumulation of subungual debris
- Tinea is often also present on the adjacent skin

Management

- Confirm the diagnosis by microscopy and culture of nail clippings
- In mild cases, treatment with physical debridement and antifungal ointment (e.g. clotrimazole, terbinafine) may be effective
- Oral griseofulvin is fungostatic. Much more effective agents including oral terbinafine, oral itraconazole and amiolfarone lacquer are becoming available

TWENTY-NAIL DYSTROPHY

This condition occurs in preschool children and is characterized by all 20 nails becoming ridged, roughened, opalescent and fragile. Alternative diagnoses such as inherited disorders and fungal nail infection (which never involves all 20 nails symmetrically except in immunodeficient children) can usually be readily excluded. The child remains well, no treatment is needed and resolution may gradually occur over many years.

10

CHAPTER 10

RENAL CONDITIONS

Colin Jones, Harley Powell and Rowan Walker

Significant renal disease in childhood usually presents in one of the following ways:

- Antenatal ultrasound abnormality of the urinary tract
- Urinary tract infection (UTI)
- Proteinuria (including nephrotic syndrome)
- Haematuria
- Hypertension
- Acute renal failure
- Chronic renal failure

ANTENATAL ABNORMALITIES

See Figure 10.1

URINARY TRACT INFECTIONS

Diagnosis

Urine infections may be diagnosed on midstream urine specimen (MSU), catheter specimen (CSU) and suprapubic aspirate (SPA).

Bag urine specimen collection

This is suitable for children up to 3 years who cannot void on request, from whom a specimen is required to exclude a UTI. If the bag specimen tests positive for either leucocytes or nitrites on a 'ward test' strip, a definite specimen (SPA or CSU) should be taken.

- Pyuria is neither sensitive nor specific for infection in infants
- A bag urine specimen that has no growth excludes a UTI; however, a UTI cannot be diagnosed from a bag specimen
- In sick infants or those where the suspicion of UTI is high (e.g. renal tract anomaly, previous UTI), a bag specimen should not be taken, as it only delays the diagnosis. A SPA or CSU sample should be obtained

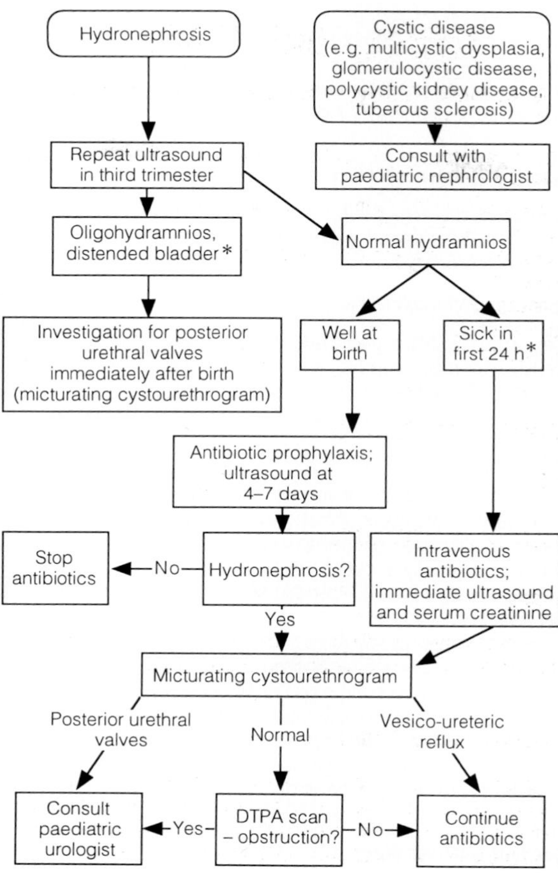

*Consult a paediatric nephrologist or urologist early in all cases

Figure 10.1 Antenatal abnormalities

Midstream urine specimen collection

This can be obtained from children who are able to void on request (usually by 3–4 years). The child's genitalia are first washed with warm water. In girls the labia should be separated. The child is asked to void. After discarding the first few millilitres, a specimen is collected. A pure growth of $>10^4$ organisms/mL indicates infection.

Suprapubic aspirate collection

Aspirated urine should be sterile, hence any growth of bacteria indicates infection. (See Procedures, p. 19, for collection technique.)

Catheter specimen collection

These are useful in infants after a failed SPA, or in older children who are unable to void on request. A pure growth of $>10^3$ organisms/mL indicates infection. (See Procedures, p. 19, for collection technique.)

Management

- Most infants <12 months of age with a UTI and older children with acute pyelonephritis (fever, vomiting and loin/abdominal pain) require intravenous amoxycillin and gentamicin
- In older children without pyelonephritis, a 5 day course of oral antibiotics is usually sufficient. Antibiotic sensitivity should be checked when available (usually 48 h)
- Prophylactic antibiotics should be commenced immediately after the treatment antibiotic course has finished
- Two days after commencing prophylactic antibiotics, a further urine specimen should be obtained to ensure treatment has been effective
- Prophylactic antibiotics should be continued until the minimal initial investigations have been performed, and a decision is then made on the basis of the anatomy of the urinary tract (see Fig. 10.2)

Intravenous antibiotic doses

Amoxycillin: 25–50 mg/kg per dose, 6 hourly
and
Gentamicin: 2.5 mg/kg per dose (max. 100 mg), 8 hourly

While gentamicin has in the past usually been administered using an 8 hourly regimen, there is increasing evidence that single daily dosing may

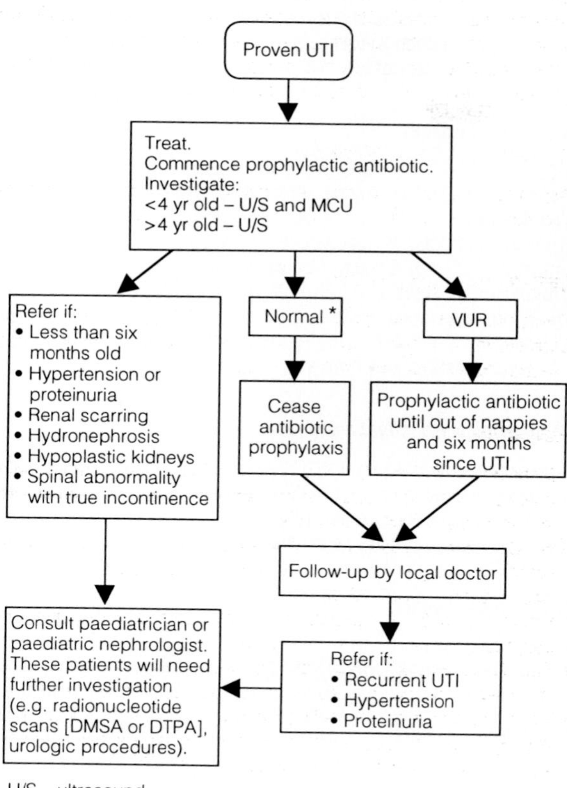

U/S ultrasound
MCU micturating cystourethrogram
VUR vesicoureteric reflux
* A normal U/S does not exclude scarring

Figure 10.2 An outline of the management of a proven urinary tract infection (UTI)

be as/more efficacious in Gram-negative infection, and associated with less toxicity.

Serum gentamicin levels should be taken after the fourth or second dose (at 24 h); trough level should be <2.0 mg/L (8 hourly dosing) or <1.0 mg/L (daily dosing) to avoid toxicity.

Oral antibiotic doses

- *Cotrimoxazole. Treatment:* (sulfamethoxazole 200 mg/trimethoprim 40 mg in 5 mL) 0.5 mL/kg, b.d. *Prophylaxis:* (200/40 mg in 5 mL) 0.25 mL/kg daily
- *Amoxycillin/potassium clavulanate. Treatment:* 10/2.5 mg/kg (maximum 500/125 mg), 8 hourly. *Not appropriate for prophylaxis*
- *Nitrofurantoin. Treatment:* 1.25 mg/kg per dose, 6 hourly. *Prophylaxis:* 1.25 mg/kg per dose, nocte
- *Cephalexin. Treatment:* 10 mg/kg (maximum 250 mg), orally, 6 hourly. *Not appropriate for prophylaxis*

Minimal Initial Investigations

Forty per cent of children with UTI have renal tract abnormalities including vesico-ureteric reflux (VUR, 35%), reflux nephropathy (renal scarring, 12%), pelviureteric junction (PUJ) or vesico-ureteric junction (VUJ) obstruction (together 4–6%) and other congenital abnormalities.

All children <4 years

- Renal ultrasound
- Micturating cystourethrogram (MCU)

All children >4 years

- Renal ultrasound
- Further investigation(s) as indicated by the ultrasound

The flow-chart in Fig. 10.2 outlines further investigations.

PROTEINURIA

ISOLATED PROTEINURIA

See Figure 10.3.

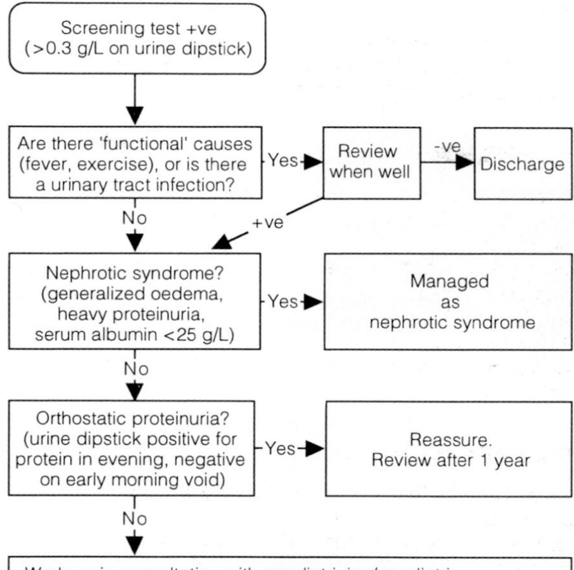

Work up in consultation with paediatrician/paediatric nephrologist:

History

- Family history of renal disease, deafness
- Medications (e.g. gold, penicillamine, probenecid, amphotericin)
- Other symptoms related to urinary tract or systemic disease

Examination

- Height, weight, blood pressure

Urinalysis (including specific gravity), *microscopy and culture*

Renal function

- Serum creatinine, electrolytes
- 24 h urine collection for protein

Further investigations may be indicated
(e.g. renal ultrasound, protein electrophoresis, C3, serum lipids renal biopsy)

Figure 10.3 Isolated proteinuria

NEPHROTIC SYNDROME

Diagnosis

The diagnosis of nephrotic syndrome is made on the basis of proteinuria (>40 mg/m^2 per h on a recumbent urine, usually >3 g/1.73 m^2/day), generalized oedema, hypoalbuminaemia (<25 g/L) and hypercholesterolaemia (>4.5 mmol/L).

Management

Exclude life-threatening complications:
- Sepsis (peritonitis)
- Symptomatic hypovolaemia (cool extremities, postural hypotension)
- Symptomatic thrombo-embolism (e.g. venous sinus thrombosis: convulsions, reduced conscious state; deep venous thrombosis; pulmonary embolism)
- Symptomatic oedema (marked ascites, respiratory distress with pleural effusions, skin breakdown)

Admit to hospital: for initial assessment, as well as patient and family education.

Treatment (*Note:* Minor variations in protocol may exist between different centres):
- *Prednisolone.* Administer according to the following dosage schedule:
  - 60 mg/m^2 per day as single dose up to maximum of 80 mg/day until remission of proteinuria (to trace or negative on urinalysis) for 4 days
  - 45 mg/m^2 per day for 8 days
  - 60 mg/m^2 per alternate day for 8 days (four doses)
  - 45 mg/m^2 per alternate day for 8 days
  - 30 mg/m^2 per alternate day for 8 days
  - Reduce by 5 mg every 8 days until finished
- *Phenoxymethyl penicillin:* twice daily to prevent pneumococcal sepsis while oedematous
- *Aspirin:* 10 mg/kg per alternate day to reduce incidence of arterial/venous thromboses

Note: The long-term prognosis of nephrotic syndrome is dependent upon response to prednisolone.

Treatment of complications

- *Symptomatic oedema.* Concentrated albumin 1 g/kg, i.v. over 4 h with frusemide 1 mg/kg at 2 and 4 h after start of the infusion

- *Circulatory insufficiency*. Concentrated albumin 1 g/kg, i.v. over 4 h. (Frusemide only if circulation markedly improved at end of infusion—dangerous in hypovolaemic patients)
- *Thrombo-embolism*. Systemic anticoagulation with heparin, followed by warfarin for 3–6 months
- *Sepsis*. High dose antibiotic therapy to cover pneumococcus, *Haemophilus influenzae* and *Escherichia coli* (e.g. cefotaxime 50 mg/kg, i.v. 6 hourly). In suspected *primary peritonitis*:
  - Peritoneal tap to establish diagnosis
  - If early diagnosis and minimal symptoms, antibiotic therapy alone may suffice
  - Usually requires laparotomy for peritoneal lavage

Additional treatments

If the patient does not respond to steroids, refer to a paediatric nephrologist for consideration of *cyclophosphamide* or *cyclosporin A* treatment.

Indications for Renal Biopsy

- Age <1 year
- Failure to respond to prednisolone within 3–4 weeks treatment using 60 mg/m^2 per day, either at diagnosis or with relapse
- Nephritic/nephrotic syndrome (increased blood pressure, moderate haematuria, renal impairment without evidence of peripheral circulatory insufficiency)
- Low C3

Relapse

Most (75%) patients relapse.

- Usually precipitated by febrile illness or allergic reaction
- Four days of heavy proteinuria (>100 mg/dL) distinguishes relapse from transient proteinuria associated with a febrile illness
- Treat as for initial diagnosis, with use of penicillin and aspirin if patient becomes oedematous

Referral to paediatric nephrologist

- Nephritic/nephrotic syndrome
- Complications
- Failure to respond to steroids in 2–3 weeks
- Frequent relapsing nephrotic syndrome or steroid dependence

HAEMATURIA

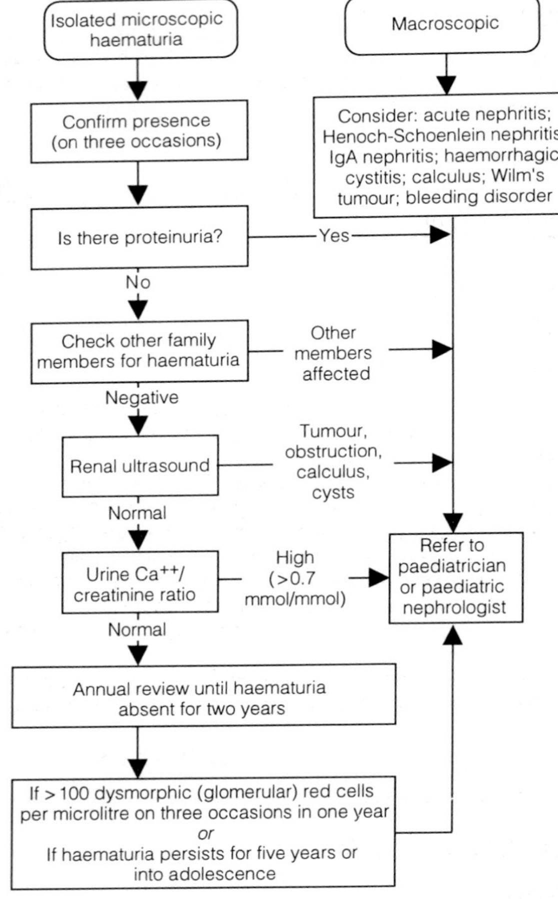

Figure 10.4 Haematuria assessment

HYPERTENSION

MEASUREMENT

- Use a cuff with a bladder that covers at least 75% of the arm's length
- Take in the right arm, with the patient sitting; if initially increased, retake after resting quietly

Definition

The 95th percentiles for BP at different ages in childhood are as follows:

- Newborn: 95/70
- 0–6 years: 115/75
- 6–13 years: 120/80
- 13–16 years: 135/85
- 16–18 years: 140/90

Cautions

- As in adults, treatment of the asymptomatic child should not be based on a single BP measurement. BP should be repeated on three occasions to confirm sustained elevation
- BP 'tracks' poorly (i.e. only 20–40% of children with BP higher than the 80th percentile still remain in that group 10 years later). Children placed on medication for essential hypertension should undergo a trial of no treatment after their BP has been controlled for 9 months
- There are no proven advantages of lowering blood pressure in terms of modifying adult cardiovascular risk in normal children
- BP reduction probably lessens the progression of renal impairment in those with renal disease
- Hypertensive children should be referred to a paediatrician or paediatric nephrologist for investigation as outlined in Tables 10.1 and 10.2

Causes of Hypertension and Recommended Treatment

See Tables 10.1 and 10.2.

ACUTE RENAL FAILURE

Definition

Acute change in glomerular filtration such that the renal solute load (electrolytes, other ions, and nitrogenous wastes) cannot be excreted.

There are two main forms:

Table 10.1 Hypertension in childhood

Cause of hypertension	*Usual severity*	*Drug treatment of choice*
Primary hypertension	+	Non-pharmacological Control weight A or B, then C
Secondary causes		
Renal (75%)		
Post-infectious glomerulonephritis	+ +	*Frusemide*, C
Chronic glomerulonephritis	+	A or B or C
Obstructive uropathy	+	A or B or C
Polycystic kidney disease		
Autosomal recessive	+ + +	A then B
Autosomal dominant	+	A then B
Reflux nephropathy	+	A then B
Renovascular	+ + +	B then C
Haemolytic uraemic syndrome	+ +	*Nifedipine* (blocks veratoxin entry)
Cardiovascular (15%)		
Coarctation of the aorta	+ +	B
Endocrine (5%)		
Phaeochromocytoma	+ +	*Phentolamine* + B
Hyperthyroidism	+	Thyroid treatment
Congenital adrenal hyperplasia	+	Corticosteroid
Primary hyperaldosteronism	+ +	*Spironolactone* Surgery
Cushing syndrome	+ +	*Spironolactone* Surgery
Other (5%)		
Neuroblastoma	+	
Neurofibromatosis	+ +	
Glucocorticoids	+	
Increased intracranial pressure	+	

A, angiotensin-converting enzyme inhibitors; B, beta-blocker; C, calcium channel antagonist.

Table 10.2 Neonatal hypertension

Hypertension	*Cause*
Renovascular (80%)	Nearly all renal artery/vein thrombosis
CNS (10%)	Infection, haemorrhage
Coarctation (5%)	
Others (5%)	Including steroid, ocular phenylephrine, theophylline, calcium

- *Oliguric:* acute reduction in urine output to <0.5 mL/kg per h. This form is more complex to manage (see Fig. 10.5)
- *Polyuric:* often subacute and clinically inapparent, until fluid intake is reduced and the patient becomes dehydrated due to an inappropriately high urine output

Causes

Pre-renal

- Dehydration (e.g. gastroenteritis)
- Shock
- Sepsis
- Nephrotic syndrome

Renal

- Crescentic glomerulonephritis: acute post-infections; membrano-proliferative; Henoch-Schoenlein purpura; antineutrophil cytoplasmic antibody-associated haemolytic uraemic syndrome
- Acute tubular necrosis
- Crush injury (myoglobinuria)
- UTI with septicaemia
- Nephrotoxin (e.g. gentamicin)

Post-renal

Obstruction, especially to a single kidney. The cause is usually apparent from the clinical context of the illness.

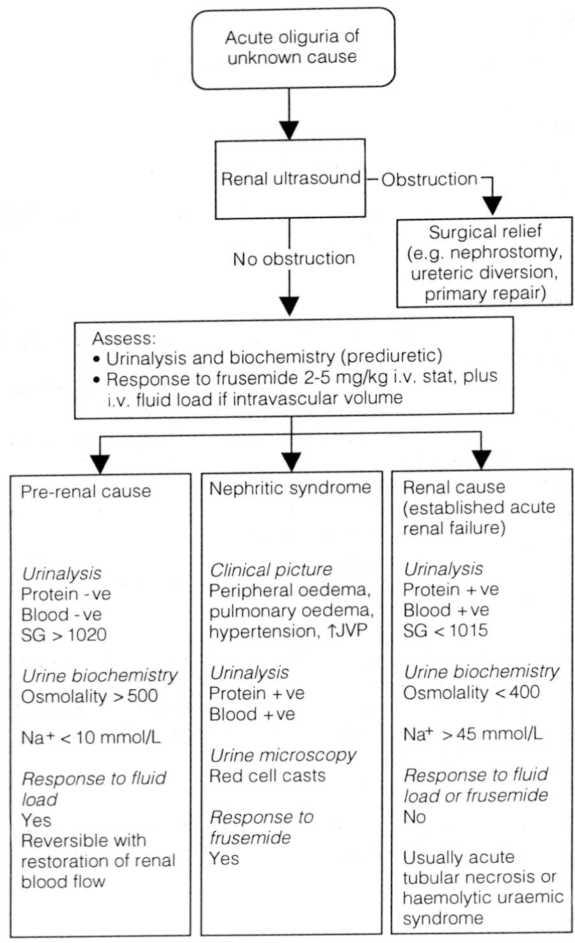

Figure 10.5 Differentation of types of oliguria

Management

Water

Limit to insensible losses (300 mL/m^2) plus urine output.

Sodium

- Principle: intake = urine sodium + other sodium losses
- Oliguric: minimal Na^+ intake
- Polyuric: need to measure urine $[Na]^+$ volume of urine. Generally about 75 mmol/L required

Potassium

No intravenous or oral intake until losses of K^+ established. *Hyperkalaemia:*

- Repeat venous or arterial serum K^+ urgently. **Arrange haemofiltration or dialysis with patient in established renal failure.**
- ECG: peaked T waves, wide QRS, increased PR interval, decreased P and R waves, ST segment depression, prolonged QT interval.
- If K^+ >7 mmol/L with ECG changes:
  - 10% *calcium gluconate* 0.5 mL/kg, i.v. over 3–5 min (do not mix with bicarbonate). Works in seconds
  - *Insulin* plus concurrent *glucose* infusion: 0.1 U/kg rapid acting insulin and 2 mL/kg 50% dextrose. Works in minutes
  - Arrange dialysis urgently
- If K^+ >7 mmol/L, no ECG changes:
  - *$NaHCO_3$* 1–3 mmol/kg (shifts K^+ intracellularly); risk of hypocalcaemic tetany with decreased pH. Works within hour
  - *Dextrose* 0.5 g/kg per h (10% dextrose at 5 mL/kg per h) until blood glucose reaches 14 mmol/L (shifts K^+ intracellularly). Works within hour
  - Arrange dialysis urgently
- If K^+ >6 mmol/L:
  - Na^+–K^+ exchange resin, e.g. *Resonium A*, 1 g/kg, p.o. (action within 6–12 h) or p.r. (action within 30 min; may repeat Q1–2h)
  - Arrange dialysis

Acidosis

Correct with bicarbonate (mmol = base deficit × weight × 1/3) over 4 h provided:

- Patient is not severely hypocalcaemic (HCO_3 may lower Ca and cause convulsions)
- Accompanying Na load does not cause fluid overload (hypertension, pulmonary oedema)

Hypocalcaemia

This is usually due to increased serum phosphate.

- Low phosphate diet
- Calcium carbonate (phosphate binder)
- Symptomatic hypocalcaemia may require intravenous calcium gluconate
- Danger of metastatic calcification if Ca × PO_4 product is >5–6
- If increased phosphate, consider dialysis

Uraemia

- Acute rise in serum urea to >30 mmol/L may cause CNS symptoms
- Protein restriction and high-quality protein food
- High carbohydrate diet

Indications for dialysis/haemofiltration

- Fluid overload (hypertension or pulmonary oedema) not responding to frusemide
- Hyperkalaemia
- Severe metabolic acidosis
- Progressive uraemia
- Dialysable nephrotoxin
- Hyperammonaemia
- Reduction of intravascular volume of facilitate total parenteral nutrition or blood transfusion

CHRONIC RENAL FAILURE

Presentation

- Known renal disease
- Growth failure
- Rickets
- Anaemia: normochromic, normocytic
- Laboratory test: increased serum creatinine, increased urea, increased phosphate, metabolic acidosis

- Radiological studies: small kidney, with other renal disease, e.g. obstruction uropathy
- Proteinuria
- UTI

Management

Investigation of the cause and treatment of chronic renal failure should be performed in conjunction with a paediatric nephrologist.

11

CHAPTER 11

HAEMATOLOGIC CONDITIONS AND ONCOLOGY

Peter Smith

In collaboration with Michael South

ANAEMIA

The initial investigation is a full blood count and film. Further investigations are determined by the blood film appearance. Remember that there is a variation in the lower limit of normal haemoglobin (Hb) at different ages (see Reference Ranges, Appendix 1).

Where possible, treatment is deferred until a definitive diagnosis is made. Transfusion is avoided in nutritional anaemias if possible.

IRON DEFICIENCY ANAEMIA

Iron deficiency is common among Australian children. However, it is often subclinical, and only leads to anaemia in the small proportion with severe deficiency. Iron deficiency may be present in 10–30% of children in the high-risk groups. *Iron deficiency can lead to reduced cognitive and psychomotor performance, even in the absence of anaemia.*

Malabsorption and gastrointestinal bleeding (except in association with cow milk) are rare causes of iron deficiency in childhood.

Suspect iron deficiency in the at-risk groups (see Table 11.1); take a careful history including diet.

Suspect iron deficiency *anaemia* if there is pallor (although remember this physical sign is only reliably detected when the Hb is <70–80 g/L), listlessness and irritability. Eating or chewing unusual items (geophagia and pica) are rare features. Severe anaemia may cause cardiac failure.

Prevention of Iron Deficiency

- Introduce iron-containing solids from 4 to 6 months
- Avoid cow milk in the first 12 months (small amounts allowed in custards, cereals, etc.)
- Avoid excessive intake of cow milk up to 24 months

Table 11.1 High-risk groups for iron deficiency

Group	*Additional risk factors*	*Mechanisms*
<6 months of age	Prematurity Low birthweight Multiple births Maternal iron deficiency	Inadequate stores
6–24 months of age	Exclusive breast feeding after 6 months	Inadequate intake
	Delayed introduction of iron-containing solids	Cow milk may cause microscopic gut blood loss
	Excessive cow milk	
Adolescents	Females Poor diet	Menstruation Rapid growth spurt
Aborigines Migrant families Socially disadvantaged Vegetarians/fad diets	Poor diet Excessive cow milk	Inadequate intake

MEDICINE

- Ensure formulas (if used) and cereals are iron-fortified
- Consider supplementation in high-risk groups (e.g. prematurity)

Good Sources of Iron for Children

- Infant milk formulas
- Fortified breakfast cereals
- Meat (including red meat, chicken and fish)
- Green vegetables (especially legumes, e.g. peas and beans)
- Dried beans and fruit
- Egg yolk

Note: Foods high in vitamin C, including citrus fruit, strawberries, cauliflower and broccoli will increase iron absorption from non-meat sources.

Investigation and Management

In most patients two investigations usually suffice: the *full blood examination* (FBE) and *serum ferritin. Note:* Ferritin is an acute phase reactant and may be misleadingly normal/high during an intercurrent illness.

MEDICINE

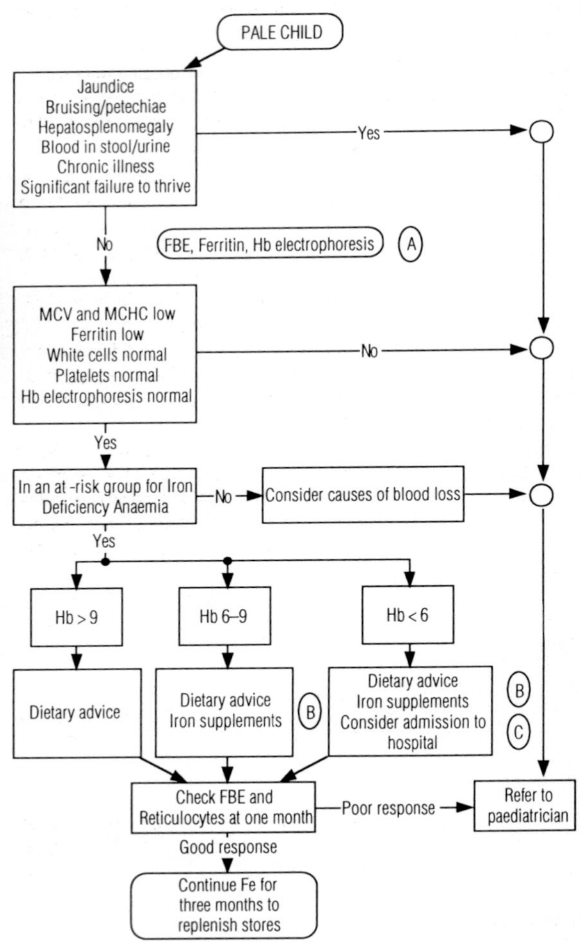

Figure 11.1 Approach to the pale child (see p. 145).

In *mild iron deficiency*, the FBE is normal but the ferritin is reduced, which demonstrates low iron stores. Dietary advice is usually all that is needed in this group.

In *iron deficiency anaemia* the ferritin, Hb, mean corpuscular volume (MCV) and mean corpuscular Hb concentration (MCHC) are low (see Appendix 1). Remember that iron deficiency anaemia due to poor diet may be associated with other macro- or micronutrient deficiencies.

See Fig. 11.1. *Note:*

A Consider *haemoglobinopathy* in children of African-American, Mediterranean, South-east Asian, and Arabic descent, especially if there is a family history, or with normal ferritin and/or anaemia resistant to iron therapy. Order Hb electrophoresis

B *Supplemental iron* is best given as *ferrous gluconate* mixture (daily dose = 1 mL/kg of the 300 mg/5 mL preparation), and should be continued for 3 months after the Hb has returned to normal to replenish stores. The stools may become black/grey. Dietary advice must always be given. **Iron overdose can be fatal, and supplements should be stored in a locked cabinet**

C *Parenteral iron supplementation* is rarely indicated in children. *Blood transfusion* is also rarely indicated. It may be used if a very anaemic child requires urgent surgery, or if significant cardiac failure is present. Transfusion should be slow and aimed only to raise the Hb to 60–80 g/L (see Formulas for Calculation of Blood Transfusion Volume Required, p. 149)

THALASSAEMIA MAJOR

Transfusion

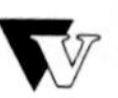

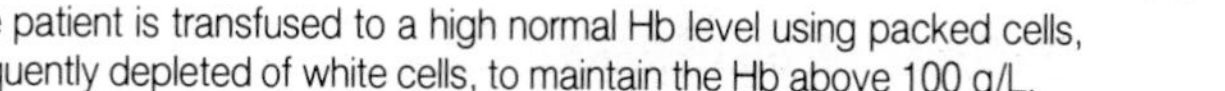

The patient is transfused to a high normal Hb level using packed cells, frequently depleted of white cells, to maintain the Hb above 100 g/L.

Desferrioxamine

This is usually given with each unit of blood transfused. A dose of 0.5 g is used. Subcutaneous infusions administered by a constant infusion pump are given overnight for 5–6 days/week.

Immunization

Pneumococcal and *Haemophilus influenzae* type b immunization (ideally pre-splenectomy) and penicillin prophylaxis (125–250 mg, b.d. indefinitely) is given to all patients who have had a splenectomy.

SICKLE CELL DISEASE

Patients may present with a crisis which may be haemolytic, infarctive, aplastic or splenic sequestration. Splenic sequestration is a medical emergency, the child presenting with hypovolaemic shock, anaemia and acute splenic enlargement. Most patients in crisis require admission. Consultation with the clinical haematologist on duty is essential in the management of these patients.

DRUG-INDUCED HAEMOLYSIS

This may present at any age, including the newborn period, with anaemia and/or jaundice. The FBE will show a normocytic, normochromic anaemia. Characteristic features on the blood film include a reticulocytosis, spherocytes and fragmented red cells.

Drugs which produce haemolysis when taken by subjects with erythrocyte glucose-6-phosphate dehydrogenase deficiency or haemoglobin H disease include:

- *Antimalarials:* chloroquine; primaquine; quinacrine; quinine
- *Antipyretics and analgesics:* acetylsalicylic acid; quinidine
- *Nitrofurans:* nitrofurantoin; nitrofurazone
- *Sulfones:* sulfamethoxazole
- *Other drugs:* aminosalicylic acid; chloramphenicol; dimercaprol (BAL); methylene blue; naphthalene; phenylhydrazine; probenecid; trinitrotoluene; vitamin K (water-soluble analogues; Synkavit)

Fava beans (broad beans) may also produce haemolysis in patients with this deficiency.

COAGULATION DISORDERS

INVESTIGATION OF A CHILD WITH SUSPECTED BLEEDING DISORDER

Screen for Haemostatic Problem

- Platelet count
- Activated partial thromboplastin time (APTT)
- Prothrombin time (PT)/international normalized ratio (INR)
- Fibrinogen
- Bleeding time (not if platelet count is very low)

Special Tests to Identify a Specific Disorder

These may be arranged depending upon the results of tests listed above and after discussion with a haematologist. Such tests might include specific coagulation and function assays, von Willebrand Factor assay or platelet function studies.

HAEMOPHILIA (FACTOR VIII DEFICIENCY)

Dose (Desired Levels of Factor VIII for Control of Haemorrhage)

In general, 1 unit of *Factor VIII concentrate*/kg raises Factor VIII levels by 2%. Thus 15 units/kg will increase Factor VIII by 30% and 25 units/kg by 50%.

Most bleeding can be controlled with a single dose calculated to increase the Factor VIII level to 30–50%. Remember a minor head injury can become serious: the Factor VIII level should be raised to 100% and the child admitted for observation.

Recombinant human Factor VIII has recently become available; however, it is expensive and its use is restricted to particular indications. Please consult the appropriate local guidelines.

Mouth Bleeding

Use *tranexamic acid* tablets. For children less than 25 kg: 250 mg, t.d.s.; 25–35 kg: 500 mg, t.d.s.; 35–50 kg: 750 mg, t.d.s.; over 50 kg: 1 g, t.d.s.

General Measures

These are applicable to all congenital bleeding disorders.

- *Analgesia*. Do not give aspirin. Avoid narcotic analgesics
- *Do not give intramuscular injections*. Splinting of limbs reduces pain

Consult with the haematologist on duty on the need for joint aspiration. Beware of risk of Volkmann's ischaemic contracture in forearm bleeds, and of femoral nerve palsies with retroperitoneal bleeds tracking underneath the inguinal ligament.

VON WILLEBRAND DISEASE

This responds to *cryoprecipitate*, or less predictably, to *Factor VIII concentrates*. Some patients respond to *desmopressin*. The half-life of von Willebrand's factor is approximately 4 h, but Factor VIII levels con-

MEDICINE

tinue to be increased for 48–72 h after infusion of cryoprecipitate. Further doses are given if bleeding recurs.

CHRISTMAS DISEASE (FACTOR IX DEFICIENCY)

This is treated with *Prothrombinex* (prothrombin concentrate). Each 10 mL of Prothrombinex contains approximately 200 units of Factor IX.

- *Requirements:* as in haemophilia
- *Dose:* in general 1 unit Factor IX/kg increases the Factor IX level by 1.6%
- *Frequency:* injections at 24 h intervals (half-life for Factor IX = 24 h)

RARE BLEEDING DISORDERS

When the diagnosis of the disorder is in doubt, treatment with *fresh frozen plasma* (20 mL/kg) until the precise defect is known.

IDIOPATHIC THROMBOCYTOPENIC PURPURA (ITP)

In young children this usually presents with bruising and petechiae following an apparent viral infection. Gradual onset in an older child, particularly a female over 10 years of age, suggests a higher chance of chronic disease. With the acute form, more than 80% undergo spontaneous remission within 8 weeks.

Management

- If the clinical presentation and FBE/blood film suggest classical ITP (i.e. no pallor, hepatosplenomegaly or lymphadenopathy; no anaemia, leucopenia or blasts), a bone marrow biopsy is *not* necessary
- Careful observation without specific treatment may be appropriate in many cases. If the patient and family have been seen by a consultant paediatrician and are assessed as having a good understanding of the necessary precautions, and adequate follow-up is assured, admission may not be required. However, if there are any concerns regarding parental education/reassurance, it is often helpful to have the child in hospital for 24 h
- The indications for treatment, as well as the best form of treatment for children with acute ITP, remain controversial. Patients with active bleeding (e.g. mucosal, gastrointestinal) should receive treatment to increase their platelet count rapidly. Some authorities also recommend treating patients with a platelet count $<10 \times 10^9$/L and a florid petechial rash

- When treatment is indicated, the choice lies between *high-dose intravenous immunoglobulin* (1 g/kg over 8–12 h, once, or daily for 2 days) and *corticosteroids* (prednisolone 2 mg/kg/day for 2 weeks, then tapered)
- Splenectomy is reserved for patients with severe chronic thrombocytopenia and should be accompanied by the usual precautions (see Thalassaemia Major above). Consultation with a paediatric haematologist is recommended

USE OF BLOOD COMPONENTS

Many forms of anaemia do not require transfusion. Removal of the cause of the anaemia and replacement of the deficiency will frequently produce a rapid rise in the Hb and avoid the need for transfusion.

WHOLE BLOOD

Used to maintain the blood volume during acute blood loss and for transfusion of patients with sickle cell anaemia in crisis.

PACKED RED CELLS

Used in preference to whole blood in the treatment of anaemia. Packed cells are especially indicated for cardiac failure, renal disease, liver disease and autoimmune haemolytic anaemia.

LEUCOCYTE DEPLETED AND/OR WASHED CELLS

For patients with demonstrated leucocyte or platelet antibodies.

FRESH BLOOD

Fresh blood (less than 3 days of age) is used in neonates.

Formulas for Calculation of Blood Transfusion Volume Required

This assumes a haematocrit of 33% for whole blood and 66% for packed cells.

- Whole blood (mL) = wt (kg) × g% Hb rise required × 6
- Packed cells (mL) = wt (kg) × g% Hb rise required × 3

PLATELETS

Indicated for bleeding associated with thrombocytopenia, especially in leukaemia and aplastic anaemia. *Dose:* 6 units/m^2.

The normal life span for platelets is 10 days, but the effective life span of transfused platelets may be greatly shortened in the presence of bleeding or infection. Transfusion may be required every 1 or 2 days for control of bleeding or more frequently if there are clinical indications. Platelets should not be refrigerated and should not be infused through a filtration set.

COAGULATION FACTORS

See coagulation disorders, p. 146

- Factor VIII concentrate
- Cryoprecipitate
- Prothrombinex (see Factor IX deficiency, p. 148)

FRESH FROZEN PLASMA

Each pack contains approximately 300 mL. Dose 10–20 mL/kg.

Indications

- Emergency therapy of congenital bleeding disorders
- Congenital bleeding disorders not responsive to cryoprecipitate or Prothrombinex
- Post-extracorporeal circulation

STABLE PLASMA PROTEIN SOLUTION (SPPS)

Contents

- 86% albumin and 14% globulin as a 5% solution, i.e. 5 g plasma protein in 100 mL
- Sodium: 130–150 mmol/L
- Potassium: 4–6 mmol/L
- Calcium: 1.5–2.5 mmol/L

May be used to expand blood volume in shock.

Table 11.2 Blood transfusion reactions

Type	*Symptoms and signs*	*Treatment*	*Prevention*
Pyrogenic	Pyrexia, rigors, anxiety and restlessness	Slow rate of flow Antihistamines	If not better in 30 min, discontinue transfusion
Allergic	Usually pyrexia and rigors, urticaria, facial and laryngeal oedema, dyspnoea Cyanosis and peripheral collapse	Discontinue transfusion Adrenaline Antihistamines Hydrocortisone, i.v.	Prophylactic antihistamines Use appropriate leucocyte- poor or washed cells
Haemolytic	Pyrexia, rigors, lumbar pain, pain in vein, jaundice, haemoglobunuria, haemoglobinaemia, oliguria later	Obtain expert advice Check all labels Take blood samples Save urine Discontinue transfusion	Careful grouping and cross-matching Care in storing blood Check labels prior to transfusion
Infected blood	Pyrexia, pain in limbs and chest, pallor, dyspnoea headache, shock	Discontinue transfusion Save donor blood Treat shock Antibiotics	Care in collecting Storage of blood at correct temperature Observation of expiry time
Circulatory	Pulmonary oedema, dyspnoea, headache, venous distension, heaviness in limbs Possibly pyrexia and rigors	Slow rate of flow Diuretic (frusemide) Digoxin Venesection if extreme	Use of packed cells Give all fluids very slowly If in doubt, give frusemide

MEDICINE

ALBUMIN

Contents

- 20% albumin in 10 or 100 mL of buffered solution
- Sodium: 46–58 mmol/L

Use is restricted to hypoproteinaemia and raised intracranial pressure. The solution has an osmotic equivalent of up to four times that of SPPS. Hence, if isotonicity is required, the administration of an appropriate volume of fluid should follow.

- 5% albumin in 50 or 500 mL of buffered solution
- Sodium: 140 mmol/L

This solution may be used to expand blood volume in shock.

IMMUNOGLOBULINS

Normal γ-globulin

This is obtained from *pooled serum*. Indications:

- *Hypogammaglobulinaemia*. Loading dose of 400–600 mg/kg is given. This may be repeated if IgG levels remain low. Maintenance doses are given every 4 weeks to maintain IgG levels above the fifth percentile. Dose adjustment should be made in consultation with the immunologists. Major reactions to pH modified intravenous globulin are not common. Consult with an immunologist if these occur
- *Infectious hepatitis contacts*. 0.2 mL/kg, i.m. (maximum 5 mL)
- *Measles contacts*. 0.2 mL/kg, i.m. daily in children less than 12 months and 0.5 mL/kg, i.m. for immunocompromised children (maximum 15 mL; split dose and give in two separate sites)

Hyperimmune γ-globulins

Varieties currently available are:

- *Anti-Rh (D)* for prophylaxis of Rh haemolytic disease in the newborn
- *Tetanus* for both prophylaxis and therapy (see p. 61)
- *Varicella* (zoster immune globulin) for prevention of chicken-pox when it may be life threatening, e.g. in immune deficiency states. Must be given within 96 h of exposure. Dose: 2 mL (0–5 years), 4 mL (6–12 years), 6 mL (adult)

ONCOLOGY

The management of paediatric cancers is a specialized field within the discipline of paediatrics and is best undertaken under the supervision of a specialist in a paediatric tertiary referral centre.

PRESENTATIONS OF CHILDHOOD MALIGNANCIES

The possibility of a malignancy should be considered in children presenting with any of the following symptoms and signs:
- Combinations of pallor, bruising, petechiae, fever, bone pain
- Lymphadenopathy—marked or persistent/progressive
- Hepatosplenomegaly
- Any unusual mass
- Persisting, severe headache associated with vomiting or visual disturbance
- Ataxia or other neurologic signs
- Unexplained weight loss

These children should be referred to a centre of paediatric expertise for investigation and management.

EMERGENCIES IN ACUTE LEUKAEMIA

Complications of acute leukaemia or its treatment are the immediate cause of most early deaths rather than the leukaemia itself. It is important that they be recognized early and treated vigorously to ensure the patient's survival.

The most likely complications are infection, haemorrhage, toxic drug reactions, hyperuricaemia and other metabolic disturbances.
- Cultures are taken and appropriate broad-spectrum intravenous antibiotics are used to treat infection
- Platelets and blood transfusions are used to treat haemorrhage
- Adequate hydration, allopurinol, biochemical monitoring and attention to fluid balance are used to treat hyperuricaemia

FEBRILE NEUTROPENIA

Any child receiving chemotherapy who has a fever must be considered likely to be neutropenic and should have a white cell count performed. If the child's total neutrophil count is less than 0.5×10^9/L then blood and urine cultures should be taken, and broad-spectrum intravenous antibiotics (e.g. pipericillin and gentamicin, or ceftazidime) should be given to prevent overwhelming septicaemia.

NAUSEA AND VOMITING

Nausea and vomiting are well described complications of chemotherapy. The use of new generation anti-emetics will ameliorate this problem for most children.

- For children receiving intensive chemotherapy agents such as *cis-platinum*, *cyclophosphamide*, *ifosfamide* or high-dose *anthracyclines* it is better to use a new generation anti-emetic such as *ondansetron* prophylactically
- For children receiving a less emetogenic programme such as a standard acute lymphoblastic leukaemia (ALL) induction, a trial of an agent such as *metoclopramide* is recommended as it is likely to be effective and is much less expensive

CONSTIPATION

Constipation is a common side-effect of *vincristine* when used regularly such as in an ALL induction. Children who have gone more than 2 days without a bowel motion should be given an aperient. The use of micro-enemas in stubborn cases should be undertaken with care so as not to induce anal mucosal trauma in a neutropenic child.

PAIN

As much as possible should be done to minimize pain and distress in children with cancer.

- Procedures should be performed after careful explanation to parents and child and the use of appropriate sedation, analgesia and/or anaesthesia
- At presentation, pain of active disease usually responds to appropriate major analgesia, e.g. intravenous *morphine* and application of the appropriate treatment protocol. Localized pain related to disease in relapse will often respond to local palliative radiotherapy. More generalized chronic pain usually requires major analgesia (e.g. with sustained release morphine or parenteral morphine), which can be delivered intravenously or subcutaneously by constant infusion
- For older children, a patient-controlled device should be considered
- For severe refractory pain consultation with a pain clinic, anaesthetist or neurosurgeon may be indicated (see p. 393)

LONG-TERM EFFECTS

Before commencing any chemotherapeutic programme it is essential to discuss long-term effects of treatment. These can be classified under the headings of effects on growth, development, fertility and risk of second neoplasm. The likely long-term effects in a given child will depend upon the modalities and intensity of treatment.

- *Radiation treatment* given to a young child will invariably inhibit growth of the part irradiated. Similarly, irradiation of gonads will invariably lead to infertility. Cranial radiotherapy may lead to hypothalamic–pituitary dysfunction later in life

- The effect of *chemotherapy* on these parameters will also depend upon the agents used and the intensity of treatment. Less-intensive treatment with antimetabolites has little effect on growth and development and minimum effect on fertility. Intensive treatment with agents such as alkylating agents is likely to have a more serious effect on fertility. Risk of second malignancies is increased by the use of agents such as radiotherapy, alkylating agents and epipodophyllotoxins

12

CHAPTER 12

NEUROLOGIC CONDITIONS

Lloyd Shield, Geoffrey Klug and Keith Grimwood

FEBRILE CONVULSIONS

- *Febrile convulsions (FC) are usually brief, generalized convulsions associated with a febrile illness, in the absence of any CNS infection or past history of afebrile seizures*
- They occur in 3–4% of children aged 6 months to 5 years, and are recurrent in 25–30%
- In otherwise healthy children they are not accompanied by an increased risk of intellectual disability, cerebral palsy, other neurological disorders or death

MANAGEMENT

- A continuing convulsion (>10 min duration) may be terminated by *i.v. diazepam* (see p. 11)
- General temperature lowering measures such as removing clothing and administering *paracetamol* may be helpful
- A careful search for the cause of fever is conducted. Most will be due to viral respiratory infections
- Lumbar puncture need not be performed routinely following a simple FC, but meningitis should be considered in any unwell child, especially when there is a persistently depressed conscious state, and in children with multiple or prolonged convulsions. The younger the child the higher should be the index of suspicion of meningitis

Recurrence of FC is more likely if the seizure occurs in early infancy and if there is a family history of FC. As FC are benign and anticonvulsants may have significant side-effects and do not prevent subsequent epilepsy, these drugs are not routinely recommended for children with recurrent FC. In some circumstances parents may be taught to administer rectal diazepam.

Less than 3% of children with FC develop *epilepsy* later in life. Risk factors include:

- Previous abnormal neurological development

- History of epilepsy in first-degree relatives
- Prolonged (>15 min) FC
- Focal features present during, or after, the FC
- Multiple convulsions during a single febrile episode

When counselling parents, one should remember that many will have felt that their child nearly died. The excellent long-term prognosis and low risk of epilepsy need to be emphasized. Advice on the management of future febrile illnesses and FC is given. A follow-up visit is recommended to review FC, and minimize the development of fever phobia in the parents.

EPILEPSY

PRIMARY GENERALIZED EPILEPSY

- This term describes the group of childhood epilepsies characterized by recurrent *generalized tonic–clonic seizures* and/or *absence seizures* of unknown (presumed genetic) aetiology
- The first seizure is usually between 4 and 16 years age, in an otherwise normal child
- The prognosis is generally good for seizure control and remission in later childhood or adulthood

PARTIAL (FOCAL) SEIZURES

Partial seizures arise from a localized area of cortex in one cerebral hemisphere, and are often due to underlying structural pathology. Metabolic disturbances (e.g. hypoglycaemia and hypocalcaemia) may also produce partial seizures.

Two common forms of partial epilepsy are temporal lobe epilepsy and benign focal epilepsy of childhood.

Temporal Lobe Epilepsy

- Temporal lobe epilepsy is more common than is generally realized
- Complex partial seizures are the main seizure type, and usually manifest by arrest of activity, staring, autonomic features, mouthing movements, semipurposeful motor activity and altered conscious state, sometimes preceded by epigastric or olfactory auras
- Seizures typically occur in clusters, and are often difficult to treat. These children frequently have learning and behavioural problems
- Investigation for structural pathology is important

MEDICINE

Benign Focal (Partial) Epilepsy of Childhood

- Onset is typically in mid-childhood
- Seizures are commonly nocturnal or early morning. They are usually focal motor or sensory phenomena related to the face, mouth or jaw. Generalized tonic–clonic seizures may also occur
- EEG spike discharges typically occur in the centrotemporal region
- Prognosis is excellent as the seizures are usually infrequent, readily controlled on carbamazepine if treatment is required, and remit in the teenage years

BREATH HOLDING ATTACKS

See p. 168

STATUS EPILEPTICUS

See p. 9

ANTICONVULSANT THERAPY

Indications for Commencing Anticonvulsants

The decision to investigate and treat a child following a seizure depends on many factors. Many children have only a single convulsion, and treatment would not normally be commenced unless there are clinical features to suggest an increased risk of recurrence. These include:

- The seizure was prolonged (>10 min)
- The seizure was partial
- There is evidence suggesting organic cerebral damage, such as intellectual disability, a history of birth injury, head injury or previous meningitis

If seizures are recurrent, maintenance anticonvulsants are generally indicated (see Table 12.1).

Principles of Anticonvulsant Therapy

- Most patients can be controlled as well on one anticonvulsant as with two or more; polypharmacy should be avoided if possible
- Introduce or change one anticonvulsant at a time, except in emergency situations
- **Start low and go slow** to avoid side-effects during introduction
- Give anticonvulsants an adequate trial before withdrawal

Table 12.1 Guidelines for use of the common anticonvulsants

Drug	*Status epilepticus*	*Generalized tonic-clonic seizures*	*Partial: simple or complex*	*Typical absence (petit mal)*	*Myoclonic/ tonic/atypical absence*	*More common or severe side effects*	*Oral dosage*
Carbamazepine (Tegretol)	–	+ + +	+ + +	–	–	Drowsiness, irritability, GIT	10–15 mg/kg per day
Clobazam (Frisium)	–	+ +	+	+ +	+ + +	Drowsiness, irritability	5–30 mg/day
Clonazepam (Rivotril)	+ + +	+ +	+ +	+ +	+ + +	Irritability and behaviour disorder, increased secretions	0.1–0.2 mg/kg per day
Diazepam (Valium)	+ + +	–	–	–	+ + + (i.v. only)	Drowsiness, respiratory depression	Intravenous 0.1–0.2 mg/kg slowly
Ethosuximide (Zarontin)	–	–	–	+ + +	+	Gastrointestinal disturbance, thrombo-cytopenia	20–40 mg/kg per day
Gabapentin (Neurontin)	–	+ +	+ + +	–	–	Drowsiness, dizziness, ataxia, fatigue	>12y: 600–1800 mg/ day, 5–15 mg/kg per dose 8 hourly
Lamotrigine (Lamictal)	–	+ +	+ + +	+	+ +	Skin rash in 3%: may be severe. Increased risk if rapid introduction or on sodium valproate	See Pharmacopoeia for details of regimes

(Continued)

MEDICINE

Table 12.1 *(Continued)*

Drug	*Status epilepticus*	*Generalized tonic-clonic seizures*	*Partial: simple or complex*	*Typical absence (petit mal)*	*Myoclonic/ tonic/atypical absence*	*More common or severe side effects*	*Oral dosage*
Nitrazepam (Mogadon)	–	–	–	–	+ +	Drowsiness, increased bronchial secretions	Increase slowly from 1.25 mg/day
Phenobarbitone	+ +	+ + +	+ + +	–	–	Cognitive, irritability, overactivity or drowsiness	3–5 mg/kg per day
Phenytoin sodium (Dilantin, DPH)	+ +	+ + +	+ + +	–	–	Gum hyperplasia, ataxia, nystagmus, serum-sickness like illness, cognitive	5–8 mg/kg per day
Sodium valproate (Epilim)	+	+ + +	+	+ + +	+ + +	Nausea, anorexia vomiting. Rarely severe hepatotoxicity	20–50 mg/kg per day
Vigabatrin (Sabril)	–	+ +	+ + +	–	–	Excitation, agitation, drowsiness, dizziness, headache, weight gain, mild GI upset	30–80 mg/kg per day *or* **3–9 y: 1 g/day** **Over 9 y: 2 g/day**

*This table shows the relative effectiveness of each drug against each of the major seizure types. It does not represent a comparison of one drug against another. Sodium valproate should be used with caution in children under 3 y, particularly if multiple anticonvulsants are being used and underlying cerebral pathology is present. Cognitive side effects may be seen with all anticonvulsants, particularly benzodiazepines, barbiturates and phenytoin.

- Individuals vary greatly in dosage requirements and tolerance. Young children and infants typically require relatively large doses
- If seizure control is inadequate or non-compliance or clinical toxicity is suspected, check anticonvulsant blood levels

Depending on the type of epilepsy, several years free of seizures are generally required before anticonvulsants are withdrawn. This is done gradually over several months.

WEAKNESS OF ACUTE ONSET

The acute onset of symmetrical limb weakness usually has a peripheral neuromuscular or spinal cord origin. Toxins (e.g. snake or tick bite), metabolic disturbance, systemic illness and psychogenic causes need to be considered under appropriate circumstances.

Two key questions require urgent consideration:

- Is there a treatable cause?
- Is there respiratory or pharyngeal dysfunction of sufficient degree to warrant management in an intensive care unit?

MYASTHENIA GRAVIS

- This diagnosis should be considered in any child with relatively acute onset limb weakness, particularly if accompanied by ptosis, eye movement disorder, pharyngeal or respiratory insufficiency
- A diagnostic/therapeutic trial of parenteral *anticholinesterase* is warranted if myasthenia is a possibility

GUILLAIN-BARRÉ SYNDROME

- This condition is often not recognized in its early stages when there may only be an 'ataxic' gait
- The child should be transferred to a tertiary referral centre at the time of diagnosis, as *respiratory weakness may occur rapidly*, and plasma exchange or γ-globulin need to be commenced early if they are to be effective
- Similarly a child with suspected *infant botulism* should be transferred urgently to a centre capable of undertaking long-term ventilation

SPINAL CORD COMPRESSION

- Brisk deep tendon reflexes or extensor plantar responses may not be

MEDICINE

prominent early, and a sensory level is often the most important clue to a myelopathy

- **Confirmation or exclusion of trauma, tumour, abscess, haematoma or skeletal anomaly is an urgent priority**
- Spinal imaging is required even when *acute 'transverse' myelopathy* is suspected

BACTERIAL MENINGITIS

Bacterial meningitis is a medical emergency.

CLINICAL FEATURES

- In infants, the presenting symptoms and signs are non-specific, and may include only lethargy, irritability and vomiting
- In older children, headache, vomiting, drowsiness, photophobia and neck stiffness are present

DIAGNOSIS

- Diagnosis is confirmed by lumbar puncture. **However, when a child is either comatose, demonstrates focal neurological signs, has prolonged seizures or signs of raised intracranial pressure, lumbar puncture must be delayed because of the risk of coning.** Identification of the pathogen will then rely upon blood culture and urine antigen results
- Antibiotic therapy must be given immediately after the collection of appropriate cultures

Cerebrospinal Fluid (CSF) Findings

- In bacterial meningitis, the CSF is typically cloudy. It usually has $> 100 \times 10^6$/L white blood cells, predominantly neutrophils, with raised protein and low glucose concentrations
- Organisms are frequently seen by Gram stain or their antigens may be detected within the CSF. However, these findings may be absent, and any abnormalities in the presence of raised CSF neutrophils must be viewed cautiously
- If the CSF is contaminated with blood, a ratio of 1 white blood cell to 500 red blood cells is allowable
- The normal CSF protein level is up to 0.4 g/L. Allow 0.01 g/L for every 1000 red blood cells in blood contaminated CSF

- Glucose levels in CSF should be >2.5 mmol/L, or >50% of the blood glucose value
- The CSF culture will confirm the diagnosis

ANTIBIOTIC TREATMENT

Age >3 Months

The incidence of bacterial meningitis has fallen dramatically since the introduction of the conjugated *Haemophilus influenzae* type b (Hib) vaccines. The major pathogens are now *Streptococcus pneumoniae*, *Neisseriae meningitidis* and to a lesser extent, Hib. Third-generation cephalosporins are still given as initial empiric therapy in the fully immunized child because of developing resistance to penicillin shown by some strains of *S. pneumoniae* and *N. meningitidis*.

Initial therapy

Cefotaxime 50 mg/kg 6 hourly or ceftriaxone 50 mg/kg 12 hourly.

Continued therapy

Adjust antibiotic treatment according to culture and sensitivity results to complete a minimum 7–10 day course of therapy; e.g. Penicillin G 30 mg/kg 4 hourly, amoxycillin 50 mg/kg 4 hourly or continue with either cefotaxime or ceftriaxone (dosages as above).

Age 1–3 Months

Organisms responsible for meningitis in this age group can be either neonatal pathogens (e.g. group B streptococcus, *Escherichia coli*, *Listeria monocytogenes*), or those more commonly detected in older children (*S. pneumoniae*, *N. meningitidis*, Hib).

Initial therapy

Amoxycillin and cefotaxime or ceftriaxone (dosages as above).

Continued therapy

Adjust treatments according to culture results and sensitivities. In Gram-negative bacillary meningitis, therapy is continued for at least 3 weeks after CSF sterilization. See Table 12.2 for prophylaxis regimens.

Table 12.2 Prophylaxis regimens

Organism	*Antibiotic*	*Comments*
H. influenzae type b	Rifampicin 20 mg/kg as a single daily dose (600 mg max.) for 4 days*	Give to index case and all family contacts if the index case is <2 years or the household includes other children <4 years of age who have not been fully immunized against Hib[†] If more than one case occurs at a single day care centre, rifampicin prophylaxis is recommended if contact children have not been fully immunized[†]
N. meningitidis	Rifampicin 20 mg/kg as a single daily dose (600 mg max.) for 2 days*	Give to index case (if treated only with penicillin) and all intimate, household or daycare contacts. Give to any staff who gave 'mouth-to mouth' resuscitation
S. pneumoniae	None	No increased risks to contacts

*Half dosage in neonatal contacts. *Note:* As rifampicin lowers chloramphenicol levels, children treated with this drug are given prophylaxis at the end of therapy. Otherwise it is important that rifampicin is given early to both the index case and contacts, especially for *N. meningitidis* disease because of the rapidity with which secondary cases develop. Rifampicin decreases the efficacy of oral contraceptives. Pregnant meningococcal contacts may be given ceftriaxone 250 mg, i.m. as a single dose of prophylaxis. However, nasopharyngeal carriage of Hib is not eradicated by a single injection of ceftriaxone. As prophylaxis is not infallible, any febrile household contact should seek urgent medical attention.

[†]A child is considered fully immunized against Hib disease following: (i) at least one dose of conjugate vaccine at ⩾15 months of age; (ii) two doses of conjugate vaccine at 12–14 months of age; or (iii) two or more doses of conjugate vaccine at <12 months of age, followed by a booster dose at ⩾12 months of age. In households with one or more infants <12 months of age (regardless of immunization status) or with a child aged 1–3 years who is inadequately immunized, all household contacts should receive rifampicin prophylaxis following a case of invasive Hib disease that occurs in any family member.

Neonatal Meningitis

See Neonatal sepsis (p. 41).

GENERAL MEASURES

- After any fluid resuscitation for shock, *fluid restriction* is an essential principle of management because of the risk of the syndrome of inappropriate antidiuretic hormone secretion (SIADH). A patient who is not in shock, and whose serum sodium is within the normal range, is given 50% of maintenance fluid requirements as initial management (see also p. 347). If SIADH is present, restrict fluids to insensible losses (250 mL/m^2 per day) plus urine output to a maximum of 50% of maintenance requirements. This is approximately 10 mL/kg of fluid per day. Fluid administration is subsequently adjusted according to clinical status and serum sodium concentration
- Control of seizures is vital. Careful attention is paid to the child's respiratory rate, both before the selection and following the use of an anticonvulsant
- Early consultation with an intensive care unit is necessary for any child who is experiencing deterioration in conscious state, haemodynamic instability or seizures
- Fever persisting for >7 days, or a secondary fever commonly results from: nosocomial infections (usually viral), subdural effusions, other suppurative lesions or immune-mediated disease (e.g. late-onset sterile arthritis). Uncommonly, fever may also arise from inadequately treated meningitis, a parameningeal focus or drugs. Management, including a repeat lumbar puncture, must be individualized

Although widely practised, routine administration of *dexamethasone* is **not recommended.** Studies of dexamethasone have drawn criticism, and any possible benefits are confined to patients with Hib meningitis. Since the introduction of immunization, Hib meningitis has become uncommon. Reports of dexamethasone delaying CSF sterilization in *S. pneumoniae* meningitis is of additional concern.

All patients require *hearing assessment* 6–8 weeks after discharge, or sooner if hearing loss is suspected.

More than one in four survivors have mild disabilities adversely affecting school performance and behaviour. Consequently, all children surviving bacterial meningitis should be reviewed during their early school years.

MEDICINE

CHRONIC AND RECURRENT HEADACHE

- *Migraine* is the most common cause of recurrent or chronic headache in childhood
- In adolescence, *muscle contraction* (tension-type) headache is also important
- Although rare, *raised intracranial pressure* and *systemic illness* must also be considered
- Careful history, examination and follow-up will usually yield the correct diagnosis

HISTORY

- Determine the location of the headache, and its quality, duration, frequency and time of onset
- Identify trigger factors, associated symptoms (e.g. nausea or vomiting) and disruption to normal activities
- Inquire whether the symptoms are progressive and if there is a family history of migraine or cerebral tumours, recent head injury, development of visual, gait or co-ordination difficulties, or changes in personality or intellectual functioning
- Take a detailed social history

Distinguishing Features

- Migraine without aura is usually a frontotemporal or bilateral headache and in older children is frequently accompanied by nausea and vomiting, followed by lethargy or sleep. Marked pallor is common
- Migraine headaches with aura or prolonged neurological symptoms are uncommon
- Migraine has a fluctuating temporal pattern, while tension-type headache tends to be persistent but usually does not interfere with sleep
- *Recurrent morning headaches, headaches which are intense, prolonged and incapacitating or which show a progressive change in character over time suggest intracranial pathology.* These patients, or those with abnormal examination findings, the rarer variants of migraine or those who do not respond to simple treatment measures, require paediatric referral

EXAMINATION

- Measure head circumference and blood pressure

- Auscultate the skull for intracranial bruits; palpate over the sinuses, cervical spine and teeth
- Perform a thorough neurological examination, including examination of the visual acuity and fields, eye movements, optic fundi, co-ordination and gait
- Assess the child's growth and pubertal status; inspect the skin for neurocutaneous stigmata

MANAGEMENT

- Reassurance of the child and parents is an important part of management
- In migraine, trigger avoidance, stress management and early use of *paracetamol* during an acute attack is frequently all that is required
- Prophylactic therapy for those with severe or frequent attacks is best done in consultation with a paediatrician

NON-EPILEPTIC PAROXYSMAL EVENTS

- Many children referred for assessment of epilepsy do not have epilepsy, but some other non-epileptic paroxysmal disorder
- In differentiating epileptic from non-epileptic events the description of the event is important, but equally important is a description of the circumstances in which the event occurred and the details of what the child was doing immediately before the event
- Many non-epileptic paroxysmal disorders can be diagnosed positively on history alone, although in some circumstances more detailed investigations such as video-EEG monitoring may be required

Table 12.3 lists some of these events and their salient features.

HEAD INJURIES

ASSESSMENT

History

It is essential to determine the nature of the injury, its severity, the time of occurrence and the clinical course prior to consultation.

General and Neurological Examination

- These findings will provide a baseline for further assessment and must be carefully recorded

Table 12.3 Non-epileptic paroxysmal events

	Breath holding attacks	*Shuddering*	*Benign paroxysmal vertigo*	*Infantile self stimulation*	*'Day dreams'*	*Night terrors*	*Nightmares*	*Syncope*
Age	Infancy	Infancy	Preschool	Preschool	School	Preschool/ school age	All ages	School/ adolescence
Circumstances	Always upset	Anytime/ anywhere	Anytime/ anywhere	Anytime/ anywhere	Commonly school, watching TV, times of inactivity	First third of sleep (non REM)	Second half of sleep (REM)	Always triggering factor
Frequency	Varies greatly	Sometimes many per day	1 month or less	Daily or less	Varies but not large numbers per day	Nightly or less. Rarely more than one per night	Nightly or less	Occasional
Onset	Sudden, with or without crying	Sudden	Sudden	Sudden	Vague	Sudden	Sudden	Gradual
Recovery	Slow if hypoxic seizure occurs	Rapid	Rapid	Rapid	Vague. May be 'snapped out'	Returns to sleep	Remains asleep	Gradual
Duration	Seconds to minutes	Seconds	1–5 minutes	Minutes to hours	Seconds to minutes	Minutes	Minutes	Seconds to minutes

Impairment of consciousness	Usually	No	No	No	Apparent but not real	Apparently awake but does not respond	Asleep	Yes
Observations	Cyanotic or pale, limp, may develop opisthotonus/ seizure	Rapid shivering movements maximal in head, trunk and arms	Frightened, pale, holds onto objects to maintain balance or falls	Posturing with stiffening and while lying on side or supine, leaning against firm edge. Irregular breathing, flushing, sweating	Blank staring but no motor automatisms or blinking despite long episodes. Not precipitated by hyperventilation	Screaming, crying inconsolably, may get out of bed. Appears terrified	Nil	Can usually describe light headedness, dizziness or loss of vision. Tonic or tonic/ clonic seizure may occur at end
Post event impairment	Mild unless hypoxic seizure occurs	No	No	No	No	No recollection of event	Good recall of events	Minimal
Main differential	Epilepsy	Epilepsy	Epilepsy	Seizures/ abdominal pain, movement disorder	Absence seizures	Frontal lobe epilepsy	Night terrors	Epilepsy Cardiac

- *Cervical spine injury* must also be diagnosed or excluded as it may occur in association with head injury

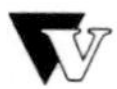

Radiological Examination

- Skull X-ray is not performed routinely in patients presenting with head injury, nor is it used to determine whether or not a child requires admission. If a child is assessed as being clinically unwell following a head injury, they should be transferred immediately to a centre with paediatric neurosurgic expertise; transfer should not be delayed by taking a skull X-ray
- In general **if the child is unwell enough to warrant a skull X-ray then the child should be in hospital under observation.** There is no place for a skull X-ray 'just in case'. The only exception is the child with a large scalp haematoma who is otherwise perfectly well, where a *depressed skull fracture* cannot be excluded clinically
- Cervical spine X-ray is necessary when there is a suggestion that the spine has been damaged, and as a routine in all patients with severe head injuries
- A CT scan is indicated in all patients with significant head injury, particularly if there is the possibility of an intracranial haematoma, as suggested by severe headache and vomiting, depressed conscious state or focal neurologic signs

BLUNT HEAD INJURY

This form of injury is due to an impact on a flat surface which produces an acceleration–deceleration type of injury.

Effects

- *Scalp haematomas are common:* in the infant or young child it may be responsible for a significant reduction in the circulating blood volume
- *Skull fracture:* significant injuries may not necessarily have a skull fracture, but the majority do. Conversely, a skull fracture may not be associated with significant brain injury. The fracture is usually linear and it may extend to the skull base. Involvement of the nasal, paranasal or middle ear spaces implies that the injury is compound, with the risk of infection. Check for CSF rhinorrhoea or otorrhoea
- Concussion: the duration of unconsciousness is an indicator of the severity of the concussion
- *Localized brain damage:* this is due to either local deformity at impact (which is not generally an important factor except for some injuries in

infancy), or surface laceration of the brain due to brain movement within the skull
- *Intracranial haemorrhage:* subarachnoid and subdural haemorrhages are usually due to surface laceration of the brain. In extradural haemorrhage, a dural vessel is torn by distortion at or near the point of impact, especially if on the lateral aspect of the head

Clinical Course

Most patients rapidly recover from the effects of concussion in 12–24 h. Delay or reversal of recovery suggests haemorrhage, brain swelling, infection or an extracranial complication – most commonly an impairment of ventilation (hypercarbia>brain swelling).

Management

Mild

- A brief loss of consciousness (<5 min) suggests a mild injury, and these patients can be sent home after an initial 4 h observation in emergency
- Adequate explanation must be given to the parents and they must be given written information regarding signs suggesting deterioration, and indications for re-presentation (see below)
- The patient should be reviewed the following day, either by the LMO or in emergency

Mild blows on the side of the head are potentially serious, and these patients should be admitted.

Serious

A more serious head injury is indicated by:
- Longer period of unconsciousness
- Deterioration in conscious state, behaviour or vital signs
- Neurological defects
- Bleeding or CSF leak from nose or ear
- Severe bleeding from a scalp wound
- Superficial haematoma on the side of the head may be associated with an extradural haematoma even if no fracture is seen on X-ray

Children with these signs will require admission and must be observed carefully for at least 48 h.

Delayed presentation

These are in four categories:

- Symptoms and signs as described for potentially serious head injuries – admit
- Patients with a wide linear fracture and a large scalp haematoma – admit
- Patients presenting with a skull X-ray showing a narrow linear fracture, but who do not require admission on clinical grounds – discuss with the neurosurgical registrar
- Apparently well patients – send home after appropriate advice, with instructions to return immediately if there is any deterioration

LOCALIZED HEAD INJURY

In these injuries the damage is predominantly confined to a focal area of the head. Injuries of this type are relatively more common in children than in adults.

Effects

- Simple or compound depressed fractures are common
- Infection may occur with compound injuries
- Focal contusion or laceration of the brain may be present to a varying size or depth and may produce neurological signs or seizures
- Concussion may be absent

Management

- X-rays are always required, and should be performed as part of the admission including, where indicated, tangential views. CT is indicated in these focal injuries
- Admission for neurosurgical assessment is required in most cases
- Prevention of wound infection: all patients with compound injuries with head wounds should be placed on antibiotics (such as flucloxacillin or cephalothin for 24–48 h), and the wound covered by a head dressing. Prophylactic antibiotics are not indicated, however, for patients with internal compound fractures (base of skull) with CSF leaks. These patients should be observed closely, and if they develop a fever with no obvious focus, given empiric antibiotics (e.g. flucloxacillin and cefotaxime)

CARE OF THE UNCONSCIOUS PATIENT

- Maintain airways
- Observation for vital and basal neurological signs
- Temperature regulation
- Fluid and electrolyte balance
- Nasogastric aspiration to avoid inhalation of gastric contents (oro-gastric if fractured base of skull)

Anticipation of Complications

Early evaluation to assess the development of complications, such as compression and infection is essential. Observation for the complications associated with extracranial injury is also important. The patient who is not improving should be referred to the neurosurgeon.

Head Injury Instruction to Parents

For the next 24 h keep a careful watch over the patient who should be roused at least every 2 h. The child must be brought back to the emergency department immediately if you notice any of the following:

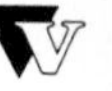

- The child becomes unconscious or more difficult to rouse
- The child becomes confused, irrational or delirious
- Convulsions or spasms of the face and limbs
- The child complains of persistent headache or neck stiffness occurs
- Vomiting occurs repeatedly
- Bleeding from the ear or recurrent watery discharge from the ear or nose

CSF SHUNT PROBLEMS

SUBACUTE SHUNT OBSTRUCTIONS

Aetiology

- *Upper end block.* The tube is too long or blocked by the choroid plexus
- *Lower end block.* The tube is too short or blocked by abdominal tissues
- *Disconnection*

Symptoms

- Headache

- Drowsiness
- Vomiting
- Fits
- The same as a previous episode

Signs

- Fontanelle tension
- Cranial percussion note
- Focal neurological signs
- Change in vital signs
- Deterioration in conscious state
- Recent increase in head circumference in infants

Specific Signs

- *Upper end block*. The pump depresses but does not refill
- *Lower end block*. The pump is difficult to depress. An X-ray of the chest or abdomen will give an indication of the length of the tube
- *Disconnection*. The signs depend on the site of the disconnection. Ventricular tube disconnection is unusual and has the same signs as upper end block. Pump disconnection produces local swelling. Disconnection along the course of the tubing may produce local swelling. X-rays may demonstrate a disconnection

Assessment

The neurosurgeon will want to know:

- The symptoms and signs including the state of the pump and shunt tubing
- The findings on plain X-ray, CT head scan or ultrasound
- The type of shunt: Pudenz or Holter, atrial or peritoneal

SHUNT INFECTION

These infections are often indolent, and should be suspected in any child with a shunt who is constitutionally unwell with fevers. There may be associated obstruction, with symptoms and signs as above.

CHAPTER 13

CARDIOVASCULAR CONDITIONS

Jim Wilkinson

WHEN TO INVESTIGATE A MURMUR

Approximately 70% of infants and 50% of normal schoolchildren have soft heart murmurs. In an asymptomatic child such murmurs most often have the characteristics of a *vibratory murmur* (Still's murmur), a *venous hum*, a *pulmonary flow murmur* or a *carotid bruit*. Such murmurs are identifiable on the basis of their characteristic timing, pitch, and behaviour with changes in posture. However, some practice is required to become confident in identifying these common innocent murmurs.

Where doubt exists about the nature of a murmur, it is appropriate to arrange an ECG and chest X-ray. If the X-ray or ECG are in any way abnormal, or if the patient has any symptoms which suggest a cardiac problem, a consultation with a paediatric cardiologist with a view to a possible echocardiogram should be arranged.

In the first 3 months of life distinction between organic and innocent murmurs can be particularly difficult. If in doubt the auscultation should be repeated at 3–6 months of age, by which time it is usually easier to achieve a firm diagnosis either way

HEART FAILURE

RECOGNITION

- The main symptoms in infants are dyspnoea on feeding or at rest, poor feeding and failure to thrive
- Physical signs include tachycardia, tachypnoea, intercostal and subcostal recession, Harrison's sulci, hepatomegaly, cardiomegaly and a gallop rhythm
- Cardiomegaly is almost always present on the chest X-ray; if not seen, other causes for the symptoms need to be explored
- A previously well child presenting with recent symptoms and manifestations of cardiac failure requires urgent echocardiography to exclude *pericardial effusion* and/or *tamponade*

MANAGEMENT

Diuretics

Frusemide: 1 mg/kg once or twice daily. This should be accompanied by a potassium sparing diuretic (e.g. *spironolactone*) or potassium supplements.

Digoxin

Digoxin: Formal digitilization is not necessary (except for patients with SVT). Maintenance dose is 10 μg/kg per day (usually given as 5 μg/kg 12 hourly). If rapid digitalization is considered necessary a loading dose of 40 μg/kg over 24 h may be given (in premature infants 20 μg/kg). The first dose should be one-half of the total digitalizing dose. Further doses (25% of total digitalizing dose) should be given after 6 and 12 h. Serum digoxin levels are useful in assessing adequacy of digitalization. A level of 1.5–2.5 ng/mL. is likely to be in the therapeutic range. Infants tolerate somewhat higher levels (up to 3.5 ng/mL).

Vasodilators

Vasolidators may be helpful (e.g. Captopril) and should be introduced with the patient in hospital, so that blood pressure may be monitored.

OTHER MEASURES

- *Oxygen* should be administered if hypoxia is thought to be related to pulmonary congestion or respiratory infection
- *Sodium bicarbonate.* Correction of severe acidosis may be required
- *Inotropic drugs* (e.g. dopamine, dobutamine) may be infused if severe cardiac failure is accompanied by poor peripheral perfusion. Dose: initially 5 μg/kg per min by intravenous infusion (dobutamine may be given into a peripheral line, dopamine requires a central line)
- *Prostaglandin E_1.* Infusion of prostaglandin should be considered in neonates presenting with manifestations of cardiac failure if it is probable on clinical grounds that they have a ductus-dependent defect, in which part or all of the systemic circulation is compromised as a result of a cardiac defect (e.g. hypoplastic left heart syndrome, critical aortic stenosis, aortic interruption, coarctation syndrome)
- *Positive pressure ventilation* should be considered if the infant is progressing to cardiorespiratory failure
- *Antibiotics* should be given if superimposed bacterial infection is present or suspected, especially in the sick neonate

NEONATAL CYANOSIS

Rapidly progressive cyanosis in the early newborn period may be due to a ductus-dependent cyanotic defect (e.g. pulmonary atresia), or to transposition of the great arteries.

INITIAL ASSESSMENT

- Chest X-ray
- Arterial blood gases
- Hyperoxic test
- ECG
- Blood group and cross-match

Hyperoxic Test

- Arterial P_{O_2} should be measured before and after administration of 100% oxygen by face mask, head box or endotracheal tube for 10 min. The sample should be taken from the right radial artery if possible (to avoid the possibility of desaturation related to right to left shunting through the ductus)
- Interpretation: P_aO_2 increasing to >150 mmHg suggests cyanosis is *not* due to structural heart disease; P_aO_2 remaining <150 mmHg suggests cyanosis may be due to structural heart disease. In most major cyanotic defects, P_aO_2 will remain <70 mmHg.

MANAGEMENT

- Initial management includes infusion of *prostaglandin* E_1 (10–20 ng/kg per min). Prostaglandin E_1 may cause apnoea, so **intubation for transport should be considered**
- Correction of acidosis if necessary.
- Oxygen may be administered, usually in a concentration of 30%
- Diagnosis can usually be made by echocardiography

CYANOTIC (HYPOXIC) ATTACKS

- Severe cyanotic attacks are a characteristic feature of Fallot's tetralogy, but may occasionally occur with other cyanotic lesions
- Episodes may be spontaneous, but are often precipitated by exertion, feeding or crying. They often occur first thing in the morning, and intercurrent infection and dehydration may play a part
- Attacks are manifested by increasing cyanosis and/or pallor, short-

MEDICINE

ness of breath and distress out of proportion to the precipitating situation. Loss of consciousness may occur in severe attacks

MANAGEMENT

- *First aid*. Try to stop the child crying. The child should be picked up, cradled and soothed, and nursed in the knee–chest position over the parent's shoulder. *Morphine* 0.2 mg/kg, i.m. may be helpful in severe cases
- *Oxygen* is of limited benefit, but may be given provided it does not provoke further distress in the child
- In extreme cases the infant may require intravenous fluid replacement, correction of acidosis, intubation and positive pressure ventilation
- *Beta-blocking drugs (propranolol)* may be used prophylactically to prevent spells in a child who has started to have attacks. This should only be used as a temporary measure while further investigation and surgery are planned

SUPRAVENTRICULAR TACHYCARDIA

CLINICAL FEATURES

- Pallor, dyspnoea and cardiac failure are the usual manifestations of an episode of supraventricular tachycardia (SVT) in infancy
- Pulse is very rapid (rate usually between 180 and 300 beats/min), of small volume and regular

DIAGNOSIS

- The ECG shows a regular narrow complex tachycardia
- If P waves can be seen these should be present with each complex. (In many cases P waves are not readily seen as they are hidden in the T waves)

MANAGEMENT

Early consultation is advised.

- '*Vagal*' *manoeuvres*. Place a polythene bag containing cold water with ice cubes over the upper face (forehead, eyes and nose) for 15–20 s. This will quite frequently lead to reversion of the tachycardia. Failing this, or other 'vagal' manoeuvres, adenosine should be considered

- *Adenosine* is highly effective in terminating SVT. The initial dose is 0.05 mg/kg, diluted in normal saline and given intravenously by rapid bolus injection, with continuous ECG monitoring. The effect wears off within 1 min, and further doses may be given at 2 min intervals, increasing the dose by 0.05 mg/kg for each dose up to a maximum dose of 0.25 mg/kg. The main side-effects in older children are flushing, agitation and a sensation of tightness in the chest, but these are brief and transient
- *Digoxin.* If adenosine is not available, and the infant's condition is stable and cardiac failure is absent, the next line of treatment is digitalization (see p. 176). The initial dose of digoxin should be given intravenously. The tachycardia will usually not revert for several hours with digoxin alone
- *Verapamil* may be given in children over the age of 1 year, but should be avoided in infants. The initial dose is 0.1 mg/kg given slowly intravenously (over 5–10 min), under continuous ECG monitoring. If no response, this may be repeated after 15–20 min. Intravenous calcium should be available if hypotension occurs. **Verapamil is contraindicated if the complexes are broad and/or if the rhythm is irregular**
- *DC cardioversion.* If the infant is severely symptomatic, has evidence of congestive failure or if drug therapy has failed to revert the tachycardia, DC cardioversion should be considered (1 J/kg shock – synchronized). **Verapamil and DC cardioversion are potentially dangerous, and should ideally only be given by (or under the supervision of) a paediatric cardiologist or intensivist**

MEDICINE

INFECTIVE ENDOCARDITIS

RISK GROUPS

- All children with structural congenital heart defects (except isolated atrial septal defect secundum)
- All children with *operated* heart defects (except repaired atrial septal defect secundum and patent ductus arteriosus)
- All children with acquired valve disease
- Children with endocardial pacemakers
- Patients with intravascular lines/shunts, etc.

The following patients are *not* at risk:

- Children with murmurs, if confirmed 'innocent'
- Children with non-structural problems (e.g. arrhythmia)

PRESENTATION

Infective endocarditis is usually caused by organisms of relatively low virulence. Onset of symptoms can be insidious, and often suggestive of an intercurrent viral illness. Fever, anorexia, general malaise and weight loss may persist over many weeks.

The classic physical signs of endocarditis (splenomegaly, splinter haemorrhages, petechiae, clubbing, etc.) are usually absent in children with endocarditis.

DIAGNOSIS

Any patient in the above risk groups presenting with such symptoms (especially if they persist for more than 7–10 days without other explanation), should be screened for evidence of infective endocarditis, including multiple blood cultures, full blood count, erythrocyte sedimentation rate or CRP, and urinalysis.

Echocardiography may demonstrate vegetations and is a helpful ancillary investigation, **although a negative echo does not exclude endocarditis.**

ENDOCARDITIS PROPHYLAXIS

Local anaesthesia (dental or ENT procedures):

- *Amoxycillin* 50 mg/kg, oral 1 h pre-operatively (max. 3 g)
- If penicillin sensitive or on penicillin recently:
    - *Clindamycin* 10 mg/kg, oral 1 h pre-operatively (max. 600 mg)
    - *Clindamycin* 5 mg/kg (max. 300 mg) 6 h later

General anaesthesia (dental or ENT procedures):

- *Amp/Amoxycillin* 50 mg/kg, i.v. at induction (max. 1 g) and *Amoxycillin* 25 mg/kg (max. 500 mg) oral/i.m./i.v. 6 h after
- If penicillin sensitive, either:
    - *Clindamycin* 10 mg/kg, orally, or by intravenous infusion over 30 min and *Clindamycin* 5 mg/kg, orally (max. 300 mg) 6 h later or:
    - *Vancomycin* 20 mg/kg, i.v. infused over 1 h pre-operatively (max. 1 g)

High-risk patients (prosthetic valve/previous endocarditis)
Also for *gastroenterologic or genitourinary procedures:*

- *Amp/Amoxycillin* 50 mg/kg, i.v. pre-operatively (at induction/max. 1 g) PLUS *Gentamicin* 1.5 mg/kg, i.v. at induction and *Amoxycillin* 25 mg/kg (max. 500 mg) oral, i.v./i.m. after 6 h

- If penicillin sensitive:
  Vancomycin 20 mg/kg, i.v. infused over 1 h pre-operatively (max. 1 g) PLUS *Gentamicin* 1.5 mg/kg, i.v. at induction

RHEUMATIC CARDITIS

Rheumatic carditis is associated with acute rheumatic fever and is now very uncommon in the developed world.

CLINICAL MANIFESTATIONS

Rheumatic fever follows an infection caused by group A β-haemolytic streptococcus.

Major Features

- Migratory *polyarthritis* mainly affecting large joints
- Evidence of *carditis* with one or more of the following: tachycardia at rest (e.g. while asleep); cardiac enlargement; the development of new murmurs, including an apical systolic murmur of mitral incompetence and/or diastolic murmurs at the apex (Carey-Coomb's murmur) or at the left sternal edge (aortic regurgitation); pericardial friction rub; cardiac failure
- A transient, demarcated skin rash on the trunk (*erythema marginatum*)
- The development of nodules over bony prominences (*'subcutaneous nodules'*)
- Choreiform limb movements – *Sydenham's chorea*, often appearing some weeks later than the other features

Minor Criteria

- Fever
- Arthralgia
- Previous history of rheumatic fever
- Raised erythrocyte sedimentation rate or C reactive protein
- Prolonged PR interval on ECG

All patients with suspected rheumatic fever should be tested for evidence of streptococcal antibodies (ASO titre, anti-DNAse titre). The diagnosis cannot usually be established unless evidence of recent streptococcal infection is demonstrable (positive throat culture or positive antibody titres). If such evidence is found, the presence of one major and two minor criteria, or two or more major criteria, is indicative of the presence of rheumatic fever (Jones' criteria).

MANAGEMENT

- Rest in bed
- *Aspirin* in full therapeutic doses (80–100 mg/kg per day in three to four doses to maintain serum salicylate levels of about 2 mmol/L)
- *Corticosteroids* may be administered in the presence of severe carditis (e.g. prednisolone 1–2 mg/kg per day). These usually reduce the duration of the acute episode, but probably do not affect the development of chronic valve disease
- During the initial illness streptococcal infection should be eliminated by appropriate *penicillin* therapy. Subsequently, long-term penicillin prophylaxis should be instituted to prevent recurrence and further cardiac damage

ENDOCRINE CONDITIONS

Garry Warne

SHORT STATURE

IS THE CHILD REALLY SHORT?

- Measure the child and, wherever possible, both biological parents. Plot all three heights on appropriate height centile charts, and compare the centiles (see Appendix 2). The child's height centile should approximate the mean of the parents' centiles
- Is the child short in relation to other children the same age (i.e. below the third centile)?
- Is the child unexpectedly short for his/her family?

IS THE CHILD GROWING SLOWLY?

- Ask for any previous height measurements and plot them on the centile chart
- If no previous measurements are available, ask to see the child again at 3 month intervals and, after 6 months, calculate the *height velocity* and check this against a growth velocity (GV) chart. GV can be reliably calculated from measurements taken over *not less than* 6–12 months
- In normal children GV tends to fluctuate, and only a *consistently* low GV will lead to a falling off in height centile
- The criterion for further investigation in a short child is a GV below the 25th centile

IF THE CHILD'S GROWTH IS SLOW, WHAT IS THE REASON?

Physiological

Constitutional delay in maturation

- This is a common (and often familial) normal variant
- Characteristically, growth slows at about age 2 years, producing a fall in height centile. Thereafter, growth is parallel to the third centile, but

the prepubertal decline in growth is exaggerated and the onset of the growth spurt is later than average
- Bone age is delayed (bone age = height age)
- Final height is likely to be in keeping with the height of other family members

Familial short stature

- Several adult family members are short
- Skeletal proportions and GV are normal
- Bone age is equivalent to the chronological age

Note: Some children from short families *also* have constitutional delay in maturation.

Organic

Organic causes of growth retardation are classified in Table 14.1.

Diagnosis

- Clues to the diagnosis may emerge from the history and the child's general appearance
- Measure skeletal proportions (span/height and upper/lower segment ratios). Span should be within a few centimetres of height at all ages. Lower segment should be >½ height beyond age 8 years
- Some serious medical conditions (chronic renal failure, coeliac disease, Crohn's disease) may present with slow growth as the only abnormal sign

Investigations

Initial

- Bone age

If GV <25th centile for bone age:
- Thyroid function tests (TFT), chromosomes in all girls (regardless of appearance)
- Haemoglobin, erythrocyte sedimentation rate (ESR; Crohn's), antigliadin antibodies, renal function, Ca/P/alkaline phosphatase
- Lateral skull X-ray
- Skeletal survey (if disproportionate)
- Growth hormone (GH) studies: (i) exercise (random serum GH values are meaningless); (ii) glucagon stimulation test (current definitive test)

Table 14.1 Organic causes of short stature

	Examples	*Clues to diagnosis*
Intrauterine	Russell-Silver syndrome	Birth length <third centile for gestational age
Skeletal	Bone dysplasia (e.g. achondroplasia)	Disproportion (short limbs)
	Rickets	
Nutritional	Protein–calorie malnutrition (no. 1 world-wide)	Weight centile <height centile
	Malabsorption (e.g. coeliac disease)	
	Chronic illness (e.g. renal failure, Crohn's)	
Iatrogenic	Corticosteroid therapy	Cushingoid features
	Spinal irradiation	Low upper/lower segment ratio
	Transfusion haemosiderosis (e.g. thalassaemia)	Pigmentation
Chromosomal	Turner, Down, Prader-Willi	Specific dysmorphic features
Other dysmorphic syndromes	Noonan, Cornelia de Lange, Rubinstein-Taybi	Specific dysmorphic features
Endocrine	Hypothyroidism, growth hormone deficiency, Cushing's disease	Height centile <weight centile (short and plump), associated examination findings
Inborn errors	Storage disorders (e.g. MPS, Gaucher's)	Facial features, organomegaly
	Organic/amino acidopathies (e.g. MMA, MSUD)	
Psychosocial	'Deprivational dwarfism'	Social history

MMA, methylmalonic acidaemia; MPS, mucopolysaccharidoses; MSUD, maple syrup urine disease.

MEDICINE

Growth Hormone Therapy

Recombinant human GH is government-controlled because it costs an average of A$20 000–30 000 a year per child. To qualify, children must meet certain criteria:

- Height <first centile
- GV <25th centile *for bone age*
- Bone age <13½ (girls) or <15½ (boys)
- Free of any condition known not to respond to GH (e.g. high-dose steroid therapy, thalassaemia) or that could be worsened by GH therapy (insulin-dependent diabetes mellitus (IDDM), Fanconi anaemia)

Good responses are seen in GH deficiency, Turner syndrome.

TALL STATURE

Aetiology

- Familial
- Precocious puberty
- Hyperthyroidism
- Syndromes: Marfan, Klinefelter, triple X, homocystinuria, Sotos
- Pituitary gigantism (juvenile acromegaly)

Treatment

- High-dose oestrogen is sometimes used in selected very tall girls to accelerate epiphyseal maturation and reduce final height. The ideal time to start is just after the appearance of the first pubertal changes
- Tall boys may be similarly treated with testosterone

HYPOTHYROIDISM

Hypothyroidism may be congenital or acquired.

CONGENITAL HYPOTHYROIDISM

- Incidence is 1 : 4500 births
- Most cases are detected by neonatal screening (high thyroid-stimulating hormone, TSH). Confirmation of the diagnosis on whole blood TFT is essential
- Technetium scanning shows that most cases have either absent or

ectopic (sublingual) thyroid. Enzyme deficiencies associated with goitre are found in about 10%

- *Thyroxine therapy (3–5 μg/kg per day) must be started as early as possible* – before 2 weeks

Clinical Features

- Jaundice
- Large fontanelles
- Coarse features
- Dry skin
- Supra-orbital oedema
- Umbilical hernia
- Harsh cry
- Slow feeding
- Distal femoral epiphysis not ossified

ACQUIRED HYPOTHYROIDISM

- Acquired hypothyroidism is called *primary* when the thyroid gland itself is abnormal (ectopic thyroid dysgenesis, autoimmune chronic lymphocytic thyroiditis, dyshormonogenesis) and *secondary* when the abnormality is a deficiency in pituitary TSH
- Helpful investigations include: serum TSH, thyroid auto-antibodies, technetium thyroid scan

Clinical Features

- Growth retardation
- Constipation
- Cold intolerance
- Goitre
- Dry cool skin
- Prolonged ankle jerk relaxation time

Referral to a paediatric endocrine clinic is important for the management of hypothyroidism.

HYPERTHYROIDISM

- Hyperthyroidism is almost always due to Graves' disease. Six times as many girls are affected as boys, most commonly during puberty
- A family history of thyroid disease (hyper- or hypothyroidism) is common. Family members may also have one of the following: IDDM,

vitiligo, pernicious anaemia, Addison's disease or premature gonadal failure

Clinical Features

- Goitre (nearly all)
- Weight loss; heat intolerance; tiredness
- Warm sweaty hands; tremor; tachycardia
- Irritability; restlessness
- Proximal muscle weakness and wasting; accelerated ankle jerk relaxation time
- Lid lag; exophthalmos
- Accelerated growth

Investigations

TFT, TSH receptor antibodies, bone age (usually advanced).

Management

- Antithyroid drugs (carbimazole, propylthiouracil), interrupted every 2–3 years until remission occurs
- Subtotal thyroidectomy is recommended if the disease is still active by age 19–20, or the patient is unable to take antithyroid drugs
- The use of radioactive iodine in children and adolescents is controversial and we do not advocate it

DELAYED PUBERTY

Delayed puberty is defined as the absence of pubertal changes: over 14 years for girls and over 15 years for boys (see Appendix 2 for pubertal stages charts/diagrams).

Aetiology

With normal or low serum gonadotrophins

- Constitutional delay (usually familial) is the most common cause. It is associated with slow growth and a delayed bone age
- Chronic illness/poor nutrition (e.g. cystic fibrosis, thalassaemia, juvenile chronic arthritis, Crohn's)
- Endocrine causes: hypopituitarism (gonadotrophin, and possibly GH and other hormonal deficiencies), Kallmann syndrome (isolated gona-

dotrophin deficiency with anosmia), hypothyroidism and hyperprolactinaemia (consider prolactinoma)

With elevated serum gonadotrophins

This signifies *primary gonadal failure*, which may be due to:
- A genetic abnormality associated with gonadal dysgenesis (Turner, Klinefelter, Noonan syndromes)
- Anorchia
- Gonadal destruction secondary to vascular damage, irradiation, infection, torsion or autoimmune disease

MEDICINE

Investigations

- Serum follicle-stimulating hormone (FSH), luteinizing hormone (LH), testosterone or oestradiol; serum prolactin; other pituitary function tests (e.g. GH studies), as indicated by growth
- Full blood examination, ESR
- Urea, creatinine, serum proteins
- TFT
- Chromosomes
- Bone age

Treatment

Referral should be made to a paediatric endocrinologist who may use oxandrolone or testosterone in boys, and oestradiol in girls. GH therapy may be offered to girls with Turner's syndrome.

PRECOCIOUS PUBERTY

Precocious puberty is defined as under 8 years in girls and under 9.5 years in boys.

For pubertal staging, refer to Appendix 2.

Aetiology

Gonadotrophin-dependent ('Central' or 'True')

- True precocious puberty is more common in girls than boys, and girls are *less* likely to have an underlying pathological cause than boys

- *Girls* with this disorder have accelerated growth, development of both pubic hair and breasts, and a pale, shell-pink-coloured vaginal mucosa with increased mucus secretion
- *Boys* with true precocious puberty have enlargement of both testes, as well as accelerated linear and genital growth
- The commonest pathological cause is *hypothalamic hamartoma*
- Practically all intracranial pathologies (malformation, trauma, tumour, infection, haemorrhage) are associated with an increased prevalence of precocious puberty

Investigations are designed to demonstrate the premature activity in the hypothalamo-pituitary–gonadal axis, and to exclude intracranial pathology.

Gonadotrophin-independent (or 'Pseudo')

- Congenital adrenal hyperplasia
- Adrenal, testicular or ovarian neoplasms
- Tumours that secrete non-pituitary gonadotrophin such as chorionic gonadotrophin (hCG)
- McCune-Albright syndrome
- Familial male precocious puberty

Investigation

- Serum FSH, LH
- Gonadal steroid (testosterone or oestradiol)
- 24 h urinary FSH, LH (integrated value)
- Bone age
- MRI head scan, if increased FSH, LH

Treatment

Referral should be made to a paediatric endocrinologist, who may use medroxyprogesterone acetate, cyproterone acetate or a luteinizing hormone releasing hormone superagonist. Not all cases require treatment.

CONDITIONS RESEMBLING PRECOCIOUS PUBERTY

Premature Thelarche

Isolated breast development is common in girls under 2 years of age (8–10%) and can be expected to regress spontaneously in most cases. Simple observation is sufficient.

Premature Adrenarche

- The isolated appearance of pubic hair (usually in a girl) under the age of 8 years may occur as a variant of normal, but may also signify *non-classical congenital adrenal hyperplasia*. Careful inspection of the genitalia for clitoral enlargement is important
- Appropriate investigations are bone age, basal serum dehydroepiandrosterone sulfate (DHEA-S), androstenedione, testosterone and 17-hydroxyprogesterone (17-OHP). The measurement of 17-OHP at 30 and 60 min after intramuscular Synacthen (synthetic adrenocorticotrophic hormone) is recommended to diagnose mild forms of congenital adrenal hyperplasia
- Referral to a paediatric endocrinologist is recommended

PUBERTAL GYNAECOMASTIA

- In true gynaecomastia there will be a palpable disc of breast tissue; this is to be distinguished from adiposity of the breast area
- Breast development occurs transiently in many boys mid-way through puberty and is physiological
- If associated with testicular volumes <6 mL, Klinefelter's syndrome must be excluded by a chromosomal analysis
- Adrenal and gonadal tumours rarely cause gynaecomastia
- Many drugs, notably cimetidine, digoxin, spironolactone and even intramuscular testosterone can induce breast development, as can heavy marijuana use
- Prepubertal gynaecomastia also occurs, but in most cases no cause can be found

Treatment

There is no medicinal treatment. Refer boys with significant breast enlargement to a plastic or general surgeon for subareolar mastectomy.

OBESITY

- *Nutritional obesity* is associated with growth acceleration and advancement of bone age
- *Endocrine obesity* is associated with growth retardation and a delay in bone age

Table 14.2 Causes of obesity

	Clinical features	*Screening investigation*
Cushing's disease	Growth retardation, typical facial changes, hypertension, hirsutism, bruising	24 h urine free cortisol
Hypothyroidism	Growth retardation, tiredness, constipation, dry skin	TFT
GH deficiency	Growth retardation	GH studies
Prader Willi syndrome	Neonatal hypotonia, growth retardation, developmental delay, typical face, hypogonadism	Chromosomes Specific DNA test

AMBIGUOUS GENITALIA

An underlying endocrine or genetic cause should be sought in:
- Any infant with ambiguous genitalia
- Boys with perineal hypospadias
- Boys with any combination of the following: micropenis, hypospadias, short stature, dysmorphic features, undescended testis
- Girls with inguinal herniae containing gonads

Note: Clitoral enlargement of any degree is abnormal.

Aetiology (in Order of Frequency)

- Gonadal dysgenesis
- Congenital adrenal hyperplasia
- Androgen insensitivity syndrome
- Testosterone biosynthetic defects

Investigations

- Pelvic ultrasound
- Serum 17-hydroxy progesterone, 24 h urine steroid profile
- Chromosomes
- Electrolytes, urea, blood glucose

Management

- Refer urgently to an experienced paediatric endocrinologist or surgeon
- Inform the parents about the problem and show them the genitalia; say that the infant appears otherwise healthy, and that the true sex will be ascertained within a few days
- Offer emotional support (refer to social worker)
- Transfer the baby to tertiary referral centre without delay
- Avoid offering unsubstantiated opinions about the sex of the baby
- Call a meeting of all nursery staff and discuss policy about communication with the parents about the baby. Keep detailed notes about communication with the parents

15

CHAPTER 15

DISORDERS OF GLUCOSE METABOLISM

Jennifer Batch and George Werther

HYPOGLYCAEMIA

DEFINITION

Blood glucose <2.5 mmol/L (beyond the neonatal period). If hypoglycaemia is suspected on the basis of typical symptoms and a reflectance meter measurement, **it should be confirmed on a venous sample with a true blood glucose measured in the laboratory.**

PRESENTATION

- Altered conscious state
- Drowsiness
- Abnormal behaviour
- Seizures

RELEVANT HISTORY

- Birthweight
- Family history of neonatal deaths
- Previous episodes
- Intercurrent illness
- Relationship of episode to meal
- Duration of fasting
- Drug ingestion, including alcohol

SPECIFIC EXAMINATION FEATURES

- Growth parameters (weight and length/height): overweight may suggest *hyperinsulinism;* underweight may suggest *ketotic hypoglycaemia*
- Midline defects (e.g. cleft lip, micropenis) may suggest *hypopituitarism*

- Jaundice (e.g. *galactosaemia*)
- Cataracts (e.g. *galactosaemia*)
- Hepatomegaly (e.g. *glycogen storage disease, galactosaemia*)
- Muscle bulk, power and tone (e.g. *glycogen storage disease*)
- Unusual odours (e.g. ketones or other odours suggesting *metabolic disease*)

CAUSES OF HYPOGLYCAEMIA

Neonatal: Transient

- *Inadequate substrate or enzyme function* (prematurity, intrauterine growth retardation)
- *Hyperinsulinism* (infants of diabetic mothers, Beckwith-Wiedemann syndrome)

Neonatal, Infantile, Childhood: Persistent or Recurrent

Disorders of hepatic glucose production

- Ketotic hypoglycaemia (accelerated starvation, see below)
- Defects in hepatic glycogenolysis, e.g. type I glycogen storage disease
- Defects in hepatic gluconeogenesis, e.g. fructose-1, 6-diphosphatase deficiency
- Galactosaemia
- Hereditary fructose intolerance

Disorders involving production of alternative fuels

- Defects in fatty acid oxidation (e.g. medium chain acyl coenzyme A dehydrogenase deficiency)
- Defects in ketogenesis

Hormonal abnormalities

- Hyperinsulinism
- Deficiency of counter-regulatory hormones: growth hormone deficiency; cortisol deficiency (primary or secondary to adrenocorticotrophic hormone deficiency)

Miscellaneous

- Inborn errors of amino acid metabolism
- Drugs (alcohol, propranolol, salicylates)
- Severe liver disease (fulminant hepatitis, Reye syndrome)
- Sepsis in newborn

The two most common causes of hypoglycaemia beyond the neonatal period are:

- *Hyperinsulinism* in the first 2 years. This usually results in persistent, severe hypoglycaemia and may lead to permanent brain damage, as the brain depends on glucose in the first 2–3 years of life.
- *Ketotic hypoglycaemia* (accelerated starvation) beyond the first 2 years. This is the most likely cause of hypoglycaemia in children over 2 years of age. These children are often small for age and were small for gestational age. Poor oral intake or vomiting in the 24 h before the hypoglycaemic episode is common. An early morning seizure in a child should suggest the diagnosis. The cause is unclear, and this entity may simply be one end of the normal spectrum. Natural history is for spontaneous remission by 8–10 years.

INVESTIGATION

Before intravenous glucose is given (and often before the true blood glucose is available), blood and urinary samples *must* be obtained as these are essential for diagnosis.

- *Venous blood*
  - True blood glucose
  - Lactate (may be elevated in glycogen storage disease and gluconeogenic defects)
  - Ketones (absent in hyperinsulinism, may be low in fat oxidation defects)
  - Free fatty acids (elevated fatty acid/ketone ratio in fat oxidation defects)
  - Insulin and C-peptide (both elevated in endogenous hyperinsulinism; must be hypoglycaemic at the time)
  - Cortisol and growth hormone (should be elevated with hypoglycaemia; if not may be deficient)
  - Amino acids (if sufficient blood available; may be useful for diagnosis of amino acid metabolic defects)
- *Arterial or capillary acid–base*
- *Urine — test for presence of ketones* (20 mL should also be reserved at 4°C for possible subsequent metabolic analysis)

Ketonuria excludes hyperinsulinaemia. If the cause of hypoglycaemia is not apparent, hospital admission may need to be planned for further investigation including prolonged fast.

MANAGEMENT

One mL/kg of 50% dextrose or 2 mL/kg of 25% dextrose given intravenously over 2–3 min. **Care should be taken to monitor recovery of blood glucose and thereby avoid administration of excessive amounts of hyperosmolar dextrose.** *Note:* Document time to recovery. If conscious state remains impaired, continue 10% dextrose at 0.1 mL/kg per min (may occur in children with fat oxidation disorders).

DIABETES MELLITUS

DIAGNOSIS

- Random blood glucose >11.0 mmol/L *or*
- Fasting blood glucose >7.7 mmol/L *and* typical symptoms (polydipsia, polyuria)

Glycosuria and ketonuria are also usually seen in newly diagnosed Type I diabetes. *Note:* Oral glucose tolerance tests have no place in the diagnosis of Type I diabetes in childhood and adolescence.

TRANSIENT HYPERGLYCAEMIA

Transient hyperglycaemia and glycosuria may be seen in children in association with intercurrent illnesses. The risk of subsequently developing diabetes mellitus is small (approximately 3%), but may be greater if the child has associated *islet cell antibodies* (a risk marker for the development of diabetes). Consider measuring islet cell antibodies if hyperglycaemia is seen in the absence of a severe illness or other stress.

PRESENTATION OF NEWLY DIAGNOSED DIABETES

Diabetic Ketoacidosis

Assessment

- Degree of dehydration (*Note:* this is often overestimated):
  - *Mild* (3%) – not detectable clinically;

- *Moderate* (6%) – reduced skin turgor, poor capillary return, Kussmaul respiration
- *Severe* (10%) – poor perfusion, tachycardia, reduced blood pressure

- Conscious state
- Evidence of associated infection

Investigations

Blood

- True blood glucose
- Electrolytes, urea, creatinine (should be done on venous blood to avoid haemolysis and thus spurious elevation of potassium level)
- Capillary or arterial acid–base assessment
- Glycosylated haemoglobin
- Islet cell antibodies and insulin antibodies (optional)

Note: **serum sodium must be adjusted in the presence of hyperglycaemia.**

To adjust serum Na^+, add 1.6 mmol/L of sodium for each 5.5 mmol/L of glucose above 5.5 mmol/L.

Urine

- Test for ketonuria and glycosuria
- Test for proteinuria, pyuria and nitrites (may indicate infection)

Other

Consider blood culture, chest X-ray or other tests for infection if clinically appropriate.

Resuscitation/rehydration

- *Hypoperfusion/shock.* Give 10 mL/kg of plasma expander (Haemaccel or 5% albumin) or normal saline stat. Repeated boluses of 10 mL/kg should be given until perfusion is re- established
- *Dehydration but perfusion adequate.* Aim to give *deficit + maintenance and rehydrate over 48 h* (remember to calculate maintenance for 2 days) *Deficit* = % dehydration × bodyweight. *Maintenance* depends on bodyweight (see p. 347).

The fluid should be given evenly over 48 h (see Table 15.1 for easy reference). After the first 24–36 h when the patient is well and able to tolerate fluids, intravenous fluids may be withdrawn and rehydration completed orally.

Table 15.1 Intravenous fluid rates in diabetic ketoacidosis (mL/h)*

Body-weight (kg)	*Degree of dehydration*		*Body-weight (kg)*	*Degree of dehydration*	
	3%	*6%*		*3%*	*6%*
5	24	27	38	101	125
7	33	38	40	104	129
8	38	43	42	107	133
10	48	54	44	110	137
12	53	60	46	113	141
14	58	67	48	116	146
16	64	74	50	119	150
18	70	80	52	122	154
20	75	87	54	124	158
22	78	91	56	127	162
24	80	95	58	130	167
26	83	100	60	133	171
28	86	104	62	136	175
30	89	108	64	139	179
32	92	112	66	142	183
34	95	116	68	145	187
36	98	120	70	148	191

*Includes deficit and maintenance fluid needs for 48 h. Patients with greater degrees of dehydration should initially be resuscitated until perfusion is adequate. Further fluid management should be discussed with a paediatric diabetes or intensive care unit.

MEDICINE

Type of fluid to be given

- *Normal saline* should be given for the first 12 h, as this is an isotonic fluid and will help prevent sudden changes in plasma osmolality
- When the blood sugar falls to 12–15 mmol/L and the acidosis is improving, change to *0.45% normal saline with 5% dextrose*
- If blood sugar falls to 12–15 mmol/L in the first 12 h, give *normal saline with 5% dextrose* to complete a full 12 h of normal saline therapy

Potassium replacement

- Should commence when insulin infusion begins
- If bodyweight <30 kg, give KCl 40 mmol/L
- If bodyweight >30 kg, give KCl 60 mmol/L

Check serum K^+ levels 2 h after starting the resuscitation and 2–4 hourly thereafter.

Bicarbonate (HCO_3)

- Not routinely required (acidosis usually resolves with rehydration)
- If acidosis persists or worsens, consider inadequate fluid resuscitation or infection
- If initial pH <7.0 may give bicarbonate after discussion with consultant

Formula for bicarbonate

HCO_3 (mmol/L) = 0.3 × bodyweight × base deficit

Give half of this amount over 30 min by slow infusion with cardiac monitoring, then reassess acid–base status.

Insulin infusion

- Commence insulin infusion and potassium replacement when the patient is in the ward
- To prepare the insulin infusion, add 50 units of rapid acting insulin (e.g. Actrapid or Humulin R) to 49.5 mL normal saline. This makes a concentration of insulin 1 unit in 1 mL of fluid. The insulin infusion may be run as a sideline with the rehydrating fluid via a three-way tap, provided a volumetric or syringe pump is used. **Clearly label the insulin infusion**
- Run the infusion at 0.1 units/kg per h in newly diagnosed children and where blood glucose is >15 mmol/L. If blood glucose <15 mmol/L, may reduce the insulin infusion to 0.05 units/kg per h
- Adjust the insulin infusion rate and/or the dextrose infusion to keep the blood glucose level between 10 and 12 mmol/L. An adequate insulin dose is required to clear the ketonaemia and reverse the acidosis
- Stop the insulin infusion when the patient is metabolically stable (blood glucose level <10 mmol/L, pH >7.3 and HCO_3 >15) and ready/able to eat

- Change from intravenous to subcutaneous insulin just before a mealtime. Do not stop the insulin infusion until 30 min after the first subcutaneous injection of insulin

Monitoring

Clinical:

- Hourly observations for 24 h, including neurological
- Nil by mouth (12–24 h, small amounts of ice to suck only)
- Strict fluid balance
- 4 hourly temperature measurement

Note: **Complaint of a headache may be a warning sign of incipient cerebral oedema.**

Biochemical:

- Hourly blood glucose while on intravenous insulin (reflectance meter is adequate)
- 2–4 hourly total CO_2 or capillary acid–base
- 2–4 hourly electrolytes

Cerebral oedema

Cerebral oedema is an uncommon but extremely serious complication of the treatment of diabetic ketoacidosis commencing 6–12 h after onset of treatment. This condition is usually fatal. If the patient survives there may be profound neurological impairment.

Risk factors

- Age <5 years
- Severe initial acidosis (pH <7.0)
- History of chronic poor control
- Excessive fluid rehydration
- Hyponatraemia or hypernatraemia (when sodium levels adjusted) at presentation (may need to rehydrate more slowly, i.e. over 72 h)
- *Negative sodium trend during resuscitation.* With appropriate resuscitation the serum Na^+ should remain stable or rise slightly as blood glucose falls. **If the adjusted serum Na^+ falls during resuscitation, this may be a sign of excess fluid administration and may be associated with the development of cerebral oedema**

MEDICINE

Early signs

- Negative sodium trend (as above)
- Headache
- Behaviour change (e.g. sudden irritability, depression of conscious state)
- Incontinence
- Thermal instability

Late signs

- Bradycardia
- Elevated blood pressure
- Depressed respiration

Treatment of cerebral oedema

- Mannitol 12.5% 2–4 mL/kg (0.25–0.5 g/kg), i.v. stat. Repeat in 15–20 min if necessary
- Fluid restrict
- Nurse head up
- Transfer to a paediatric Intensive Care Unit
- Support ventilation with intubation and intermittent positive-pressure ventilation if necessary

Note: Cerebral oedema is a clinical diagnosis and treatment should be given without waiting for investigations such as CT scans.

Prevention of cerebral oedema

- **Do not overestimate degree of dehydration**
- Correct fluid and electrolyte disturbance slowly
- Monitor closely and alter fluid regimen if negative sodium trend develops
- Have 12.5% mannitol available at all times

Hypoglycaemia

- May also occur with treatment for diabetic ketoacidosis
- Treat with 25% dextrose 2 mL/kg infused over 3 min
- Continue insulin infusion, but adjust/add dextrose to normal saline as necessary

Hyperglycaemia and Ketonuria Without Dehydration

If newly diagnosed patients are not vomiting or acidotic, they may be stabilized with oral fluids and subcutaneous insulin. Assessment and investigations are as outlined in the section on Diabetic ketoacidosis (see p. 197).

- Give quick-acting insulin 0.25 units/kg, stat. unless within 2 h of a meal.
- Give quick-acting insulin 0.25 units/kg before each meal (07.30, 11.30 and 17.30 h)
- Give intermediate-acting insulin 0.25 units/kg at 17.30 h, but *not* if this is the first dose. Instead give 0.25 units/kg short-acting insulin at 17.30 and 24.00 h (followed by snack).

Note: If patient is <5 years of age, may give insulin doses as 0.125 units/kg instead of 0.25 units/kg as young children may be very sensitive to initial doses of insulin.

- Allow child to eat normal diet according to appetite excluding sugars and foods high in refined carbohydrate
  Meals at 08.00, 12.00 and 18.00 h
  Snacks at 10.30, 15.30 and 20.00 h
  Diet will later be adjusted by dietitian according to patient's needs and appetite
- Change to twice daily insulin (mixture of short and intermediate acting) when ketonuria cleared and blood glucose controlled. Approximately 1 unit/kg per day is given on day 1, modified on the basis of the previous day's requirements
  - Give 25% of total daily dose as short acting, half before breakfast and half before evening meal
  - Give 75% as intermediate-acting insulin, two-thirds before breakfast and one-third before evening meal

Note: Some patients (particularly adolescents) may be transferred to the basal bolus regimen consisting of pre-meal short-acting insulin (three doses) and evening intermediate-acting insulin rather than twice daily insulin.

PRESCRIBING INSULIN

Note: All insulin doses should be clearly written on insulin order sheet. The number of units should either stand alone or have 'units' written after it. Using the abbreviation 'u' may lead to a serious drug dose error (e.g. Actrapid 6u read as Actrapid 60 units).

MEDICINE

MANAGEMENT OF INTERCURRENT ILLNESS

Intercurrent illness usually results in insulin resistance and often extra insulin is required. Even if oral carbohydrate intake is low, there is a mandatory need for insulin to suppress excessive endogenous glucose production and ketonaemia. Therefore, whatever the circumstances, **insulin should never be omitted.**

- The illness (e.g. gastroenteritis, tonsillitis) should be treated on its own merits
- Give carbohydrate as simple sugar containing food or fluids

Hyperglycaemia

Increase daily insulin dose by 10% (give extra intermediate-acting insulin). If ketonuria is present, it may be necessary to give additional increments of short-acting insulin (10–20% of total daily dose) every 2–4 h until ketonuria has cleared. Give carbohydrate as simple sugar containing fluids.

Vomiting

Must assess blood glucose and urinary ketones and be aware of possible development of dehydration and ketoacidosis

Low Blood Glucose

Reduce the insulin dose to two-thirds of usual dose. Give carbohydrate as simple sugar containing fluids. Check blood glucose hourly, and give extra short-acting insulin if necessary.

MANAGEMENT OF PATIENTS WITH DIABETES HAVING SURGERY

The main aims are to prevent hypoglycaemia before, during and after surgery and to provide sufficient insulin to prevent development of ketoacidosis.

Factors that must be considered are:
- Time of surgery
- Duration of surgery
- Urgency of surgery

Minor elective morning surgery:
- Admit child on previous evening
- Aim for patient to be first on operating list
- Normal food and insulin until midnight on night before surgery

- At 06.00 h perform blood glucose. If blood glucose <10 mmol/L give lemonade or sugar containing clear fluid 5–10 mL/kg (max. = 200 mL) and inform anaesthetist
- Monitor blood glucose every 2 h and immediately before surgery. If blood glucose <6 mmol/L insert intravenous line and give intravenous glucose
- Give insulin dose = 1/10th of total daily insulin dose (short and intermediate acting) at usual time
- Intravenous line with glucose will be inserted in the operating theatre (if not required pre-operatively)
- Postoperatively perform regular blood glucose every 2–4 h, adjust intravenous glucose infusion as necessary and give extra insulin 0.25 units/kg every 4–6 hours to keep glucose between 5 and 10 mmol/L
- When tolerating oral fluids stop intravenous infusion and resume normal insulin regimen

Minor elective afternoon surgery:

- Normal food and insulin until midnight on night before surgery
- Give light breakfast at the usual time
- Give insulin dose = 1/10th of total daily insulin dose (short and intermediate acting) at usual time
- Monitor blood glucose every 2 h. (Commence intravenous glucose if blood glucose <6 mmol/L, otherwise may leave intravenous until theatre)
- Give additional insulin at same dose at 12.00 h
- Postoperatively adopt same regimen as above

Minor surgery/short anaesthetic:

- Intravenous glucose may not be necessary providing that oral intake can be resumed soon after surgery and providing the pre- operative blood glucose concentration does not fall <6 mmol/L. If any doubt, it is safer to follow the routines above

Emergency and major surgery:

- Urgent clinical and biochemical assessment as for diabetic ketoacidosis
- Rehydrate and start intravenous insulin as required
- Maintain intravenous 0.45% normal saline with 5% dextrose and insulin infusion at 0.05–0.1 units/kg per h pre- and postoperatively until patient able to resume oral feeding

GLYCOSYLATED HAEMOGLOBIN (HBA_1C)

Performed at 3 monthly intervals and provides a measure of long-term diabetes control. Contact individual laboratories for interpretation of results.

COMPLICATIONS SCREENING PROGRAMME

Many paediatric and adolescent diabetes centres around the world have programmes for early detection of possible long-term complications of diabetes. These programmes include screening for:

- Nephropathy (microalbuminuria)
- Retinopathy (ophthalmological assessment + fundal photography)
- Neuropathy (peripheral and autonomic)
- Hyperlipidaemia
- Thyroid dysfunction

CHAPTER 16

METABOLIC CONDITIONS

Jim McGill

The major obstacle in the diagnosis of an inborn error of metabolism is the failure of the clinician to consider them in the differential diagnosis. **Metabolic disorders should be considered in any child presenting with unexplained hypoglycaemia, acidosis, recurrent vomiting, impaired consciousness or seizures.** A history of *consanguinity*, *unexplained stillbirths* or *neonatal or early childhood deaths* are important clues for metabolic disorders.

DIAGNOSIS

The possibility of an inborn error of metabolism needs to be considered before therapy is commenced. **The diagnosis often depends on appropriate samples being collected at the time of presentation.**

In suspected cases, collect samples for the following tests.

BLOOD

Acid–base, ammonia (on ice), amino acids, lactate, ketones, fatty acids, glucose, electrolytes, liver function tests, galactoscreen, full blood examination, white cell count/differential.

Freeze plasma from additional 5–10 mL heparinized blood.

Note: 'Dextrostix' are unreliable if hypoglycaemia is suspected.

URINE

Ward test for glucose, reducing substances, pH and ketones. Save 10–20 mL (minimum 2 mL) for urine amino acids and organic acids (especially if anion gap increased).
Note: Reducing substances may be *negative* in galactosaemia.

CSF

Freeze 0.5–1 mL CSF immediately (preferably on dry ice) for future testing as indicated by blood/urine tests (e.g. lactate, amino acids).

INITIAL MANAGEMENT

- In most instances the aim of treatment is to create an *anabolic state*
- In the seriously ill child this is achieved by intravenous glucose, usually as 15–20% dextrose with maintenance Na, K and Cl. Fluid volume should be the normal maintenance amount (see p. 347) plus correction of any dehydration
- Aim to keep blood glucose in 6–10 mmol/L range. An insulin infusion may be necessary to facilitate glucose utilization
- Less ill (conscious) patients able to tolerate oral fluids can be managed with oral or nasogastric high caloric drinks, such as polyjoule or polycose. Concentrations recommended are 15% for 0–12 months; 20% for 1–6 years and 30% for >6 years

For symptomatic *hyperammonaemia*, sodium benzoate should be started with a loading dose of 250 mg/kg followed by a constant infusion of 250 mg/kg per day. In some patients *haemofiltration*, *haemodialysis* or *peritoneal dialysis* may be necessary to eliminate the metabolic toxin. Some inborn errors of metabolism are responsive to pharmacological doses of vitamins. A *vitamin cocktail* can be given in an emergency if there is likely to be a significant delay in results from diagnostic tests (Table 16.1).

URGENT AUTOPSY

Where a child/infant has died and a metabolic disorder is suspected, urgent autopsy should be performed as soon as possible after death (maximum of 2 h).

Table 16.1 Vitamin therapy for metabolic disorders

Disorder	*Vitamin*	*Dose (mg)*
MSUD, PDH	Thiamine (B_1)	50–100
Glutaric aciduria II	Riboflavin (B_2)	20–50
Homocystinuria	Pyridoxine (B_6)	100–200
MMA, TCII deficiency	Cobalamin (B_{12})	1
Biotinidase and multiple carboxylase deficiencies	Biotin	100

MSUD, maple syrup urine disease; MMA, methylmalonic acidaemia; PDH, pyruvate dehydrogenase deficiency; TC II, Transcobalamin II.

MEDICINE

Table 16.2 Biochemical profile of major inborn errors of metabolism

Classification	*Metabolic acidosis*	*Ketosis*	*Lactic acidosis*	*Hyper-ammonaemia*	*Hypo-glycaemia*	*Most common diagnosis*
Aminoacidopathies	–	+ + +	–	–	±	MSUD
Organic acidopathies	+ + +	+ + +	+	+ +	–	MMA, PA, IVA
Primary lactic acidosis	+ + +	+ + +	+ + +	–	±	PDH, PC, RC
Urea cycle defects	–	–	–	+ + +	–	OTC, citrullinaemia, arginosuccinic aciduria
Unusual defects	–	–	–	–	–	Peroxisomopathies, sulfite oxidase deficiency, RC, NKH
Hepatic involvement (hepatomegaly/abnormal LFT/ hypoglycaemia)	+ + +	+ + +	+ + +	±	+ + +	Galactosaemia, tyrosinaemia, gluconeogenesis defects, GSD

MSUD, maple syrup urine disease; MMA, methylmalonic acidaemia; PA, propionic acidaemia; IVA, isovaleric acidaemia; PDH, pyruvate dehydrogenase deficiency; PC, pyruvate carboxylase deficiency; RC, respiratory chain defects; OTC, ornithine transcarbamylase deficiency; NKH, non-ketotic hyperglycinaemia; GSD, glycogen storage diseases.

SAMPLES NEEDED

- *Blood:* freeze plasma from 5 to 10 mL heparinized blood
- *Urine:* freeze 10–20 mL
- *CSF:* freeze 0.5–2.0 mL
- *Liver and muscle:* (i) 2 × 0.5 cm cubes of each wrapped in aluminium foil and snap frozen in dry ice. (ii) Small sample of each into glutaraldehyde for electron microscopy
- *Skin:* small piece 3–4 mm diameter into tissue culture or viral transport medium. Keep in normal refrigerator (4°C) – *do not freeze*

All tissue samples can be collected through right upper quadrant incision obtaining muscle from rectus.

BIOCHEMISTRY

A guide to the likely diagnosis can be obtained by comparing the biochemical profile with Table 16.2. This may aid in specific investigations.

CHAPTER 17

RHEUMATOLOGIC CONDITIONS

Roger Allen

Musculoskeletal signs and symptoms are common in children and adolescents, and a broad spectrum of conditions needs to be considered. As the clinical features and laboratory findings may be relatively nonspecific, it is important to look for disease patterns when evaluating the presenting complaint and conducting systems review.

This chapter is in two basic parts: (i) an approach to diagnosis by history, examination and investigation, and (ii) a brief outline of some of the more common rheumatologic conditions.

EVALUATION OF ARTHRITIS/ARTHRALGIA

HISTORY

- Nature of onset: acute or insidious. **Acute-onset monoarticular arthritis associated with fever is septic until proven otherwise**
- Timing of symptoms during day: as general guide *early morning stiffness = inflammatory; post-activity pain = mechanical*
- Any intercurrent infections: respiratory, enteric or skin? *Postviral infections are probably the commonest cause of transient arthritis*
- Where does the child, or parent, consider to be the most symptomatic site — joint, muscle, adjacent bone or a more diffuse area?
- Extra-articular symptoms: ensure a thorough systems review and keep the three 'major sleepers' in mind: systemic lupus erythematosus, acute lymphoblastic leukaemia and inflammatory bowel disease
- To what extent have normal physical activities/interests been interrupted?
- Assess the 'functional milieu' of the patient (e.g. school progress, family and peer relationships, potential stress experiences)
- Family history: other inflammatory arthritis particularly the spondyloarthropathies, autoimmune disorders, pain syndromes (e.g. fibromyalgia or other potential pain models)

EXAMINATION

- *Examine all joints* (not only the site of the presenting complaint)
- Aim to *localize the site of maximal discomfort* (e.g. is it the joint capsule, adjacent bone or muscle belly, tendon or ligament attachments?)
- Examine for signs of systemic diseases with an articular component and/or extra-articular features of juvenile chronic arthritis (JCA)

Musculoskeletal assessment should include:

- Joint – signs of inflammation, range of movement, deformity
- Entheses – bone attachment sites of ligaments/tendons (e.g. Achilles)
- Tendon sheaths of fingers and toes (e.g. dactylitis in psoriasis)
- Gait – antalgic (pain) or limp, Trendelenberg's sign
- Weakness (e.g. inability to toe or crouch walk)
- Patellar tracking pattern – does the patella move vertically on walking?
- Shoe sole and heel wear pattern
- Leg length measurement
- Spinal flexion, including Schober test (measurement of lumbosacral range – should increase by at least 6 cm on maximal flexion; starting range is between lumbosacral junction and a point 10 cm above)

INVESTIGATIONS

Often Useful

- *Full blood examination*, *erythrocyte sedimentation rate* (ESR) and/or *C-reactive protein*
- *Synovial fluid culture* – only if sepsis considered
- *Antinuclear antibody (ANA)* – beware of over-interpretation as up to 20% of normal children may have a low positive ANA

Occasionally Useful

- *Specific bacterial/viral studies* (e.g. ASOT, antiDNase B, Yersinia, parvovirus) if the clinical picture is suggestive
- *Rheumatoid factor;* in polyarticular patients, older children or if the pattern of disease appears unusual
- *HLA B27* – in an apparent spondyloarthropathy (remember almost 9% of the Caucasian population are positive)
- *Imaging:* plain X-ray, bone scan, ultrasound. Early in an arthritis, plain films give no more information than a careful examination. They may

be useful in difficult sites such as the hip, or if there is a long history of arthritis

- *'Diagnostic' aspirate:* worthwhile if sepsis or haemarthrosis is considered *but* will not necessarily differentiate between other inflammatory arthritides

Not Useful

Serum uric acid

CAUSES OF ARTHRITIS/ARTHRALGIA IN CHILDHOOD

JUVENILE CHRONIC (RHEUMATOID) ARTHRITIS (JCA)

Table 17.1 Medication therapy for juvenile chronic arthritis

Common drugs used	*Dosage (mg/kg per day)*
Non-steroidal anti-inflammatory drugs (NSAID)	
Naproxen	10–15
Diclofenac	2–3
Ibuprofen	30–40
Aspirin	60–100
Slow-acting antirheumatic drugs (SAARD)	
Sulfasalazine	30–40
Hydroxychloroquine	5–6
Methotrexate	0.3 or 10 mg/m^2 per week*
Auranofin	0.15
Penicillamine	10–15
Gold (intramuscular)	1 mg/kg per week
Corticosteroids	
Oral: may initially require 0.5–1.0 mg/kg day, but if long-term aim for alternate day <0.5 mg/kg or if necessary daily 0.1–0.2 mg/kg	
Intra-articular: triamcinolone acetonide – dose relates to joint size (e.g. knee 20–40 mg, ankle 7.5–10 mg)	

*See Nomogram, p. 453

Assessment

- *Age at onset:* <16 years
- *Minimum duration of arthritis:* 6 weeks (some criteria suggest 3 months)

Remember: most acute non-septic arthritis is not JCA

Disease Subtypes

- Pauciarticular: affects four or fewer joints
    - young, often ANA positive female
    - older, often B27 positive male
- Polyarticular: affects five or more joints; sero (Rh factor) positive or negative
- Systemic: joints plus fever, rash, lymphadenopathy, etc.

Useful to look for: enthesitis (suggestive of a spondyloarthropathy), nail pits/scalp rash (indicative of psoriasis), Still's rash (faint urticarial-like erythema) – mostly when febrile, uveitis (especially pauci-JCA patient) by slit-lamp.

Management

Management depends on the clinical picture of disease severity and subtype.

Medication

Apart from some features of systemic onset disease (e.g. severe pleuropericarditis) **corticosteroids should not constitute first-line therapy for children with arthritis.**

Physical therapy

Physical therapy is essential to maintain joint range and function. *Splinting* should be considered where appropriate.

HENOCH-SCHOENLEIN PURPURA (HSP)

Clinical Features

- Evolving crops of palpable purpura – predominantly buttocks and legs
- Abdominal pain (occasionally melaena)
- Large joint migratory arthritis (variable duration and severity)

- Nephritis
- Other (e.g. oedema dorsum of feet and hands, acute scrotal swelling and 'bruising')

Investigations

- Full blood examination (mainly to exclude thrombocytopenia)
- Urinalysis: haematuria/proteinuria
- Renal function: urea/creatinine, urinary protein estimation

Management

- Supportive: bed rest and analgesia
- *Corticosteroids:* may reduce duration of abdominal pain, but uncertain if significantly affect other features
- Other: rarely more severe renal impairment may warrant immunosuppression or plasmaphaeresis and antihypertensive therapy (requiring nephrological supervision, see p. 133); surgical intervention if appendicitis or intussusception (see p. 232)

IRRITABLE HIP (TRANSIENT SYNOVITIS)

See p. 247.

SEPTIC ARTHRITIS

See p. 248.

KAWASAKI DISEASE (MUCOCUTANEOUS LYMPH NODE SYNDROME)

This is an increasingly recognized cause of vasculitis, particularly in young children and infants. Its particular importance is because of the risk of coronary artery aneurysms and thrombosis.

Clinical Features

The diagnosis is one of exclusion (e.g. scarlet fever, measles, drug reaction) and is based on five of six criteria, but *incomplete forms* may occur so that lack of all criteria should not negate the diagnosis.

- Prolonged fever for 5 or more days
- Bilateral non-exudative conjunctivitis

MEDICINE

- Mucositis: strawberry tongue, dry cracked lips, oropharyngeal erythema
- Rash: polymorphous truncal rash, perineal rash
- Cervical lymphadenopathy >1.5 cm diameter
- Peripheral changes: palmar–plantar erythema, indurated hands and feet; digital desquamation

Other relatively common features include: history of diarrhoea; marked irritability; uveitis; sterile pyuria; pneumonitis; hydrops of the gall-bladder.

The clinical course is in three relatively distinct phases:

- *Acute* (week 1): fever, rash, mucosal symptoms, etc.
- *Subacute* (weeks 2–3): thrombocytosis, desquamation, coronary artery dilatation
- *Chronic* (week 4+): coronary (and peripheral) artery aneurysms, arthritis, nail changes (Beau's lines)

Investigations

- Haematology: white cell count, platelet count and ESR are usually elevated acutely
- Cardiac: chest X-ray; ECG (S-T, T wave changes of ischaemia/infarction); 2-D echocardiogram (left ventricular function, coronary arteries, pericardial fluid)

Management

- Intravenous *γ-globulin* 2 g/kg (as single infusion)
- *Aspirin:* initial dose 100 mg/kg per day until afebrile, then 5–10 mg/kg per day until platelet count normalizes and aneurysm risk resolved (usually 4–8 weeks)
- *Dipyridamole* is added if there is giant aneurysm formation

POSTINFECTIOUS ARTHRITIS

Acute rheumatic fever

See p. 181.

Post-streptococcal reactive arthritis

- Symmetrical non-migratory poly- or pauciarticular arthritis
- Carditis may occur and may form part of a spectrum with acute rheumatic fever
- Arthritis responds slowly to salicylates
- Consider penicillin prophylaxis if carditis is present

Postenteric reactive arthritis (Reiter's syndrome)

- Mainly *Salmonella*, *Shigella* and *Yersinia* (also reported with *Campylobacter* and *Giardia*)
- Clinically similar to the spondyloarthropathies; therefore: predominantly lower limb, including sacro-iliitis; enthesitis common; positive family history (especially if HLA B27 positive)
- Associated features: acute anterior uveitis; sterile pyuria
- Treatment: NSAID – indomethacin is often the most effective

Postviral arthritis

- Many viral illnesses are associated with arthritis
- Uncertain in most situations whether primary (infective) or secondary (reactive) event, for example Epstein-Barr; rubella; adenovirus; varicella (beware septic arthritis secondary to infected skin lesion); parvovirus B19, hepatitis B
- A transient arthritis often follows a non-specific 'viral' illness, the confirmation of which may be difficult and unnecessary
- Treatment: NSAID probably shorten duration

NON-INFLAMMATORY CAUSES OF JOINT PAIN

Benign Nocturnal Limb Pain ('Growing Pains')

- Recurrent pain mainly involving knee, calf and shin
- *No* signs or symptoms of inflammation either on examination or history
- Investigations (if done) are normal
- Management is analgesia (usually paracetamol) and reassurance; rubbing often helps

Benign Hypermobility

- Typical sites: hyperextension of fingers parallel to forearm; apposition of thumb to anterior forearm; hyperextension of elbows and/or knees $>10°$; excessive dorsiflexion of ankles; hip flexion allowing palms to be placed flat on ground
- Pain occurs typically in afternoon or post-exercise
- May have features of patellofemoral dysfunction
- May have 'bland' transient joint effusions

Reflex Sympathetic Dystrophy

This condition is more common in paediatrics than is generally realized.

Clinical features

- Diffuse pain exacerbated by touch (hyperaesthesia)
- Diffuse swelling beyond region of joint
- Ruddy or suffused colour change
- Cool to touch
- May follow relatively trivial trauma

Investigation

- Bone scan often abnormal – increased or decreased uptake
- Plain X-ray – osteopenia in prolonged cases
- Acute phase markers normal

Management

- Requires skilful physical therapy and pain management:
- Avoidance of immobilization
- Consideration of psychiatric assessment
- Possible sympathetic nerve blocks

CHAPTER 18

GYNAECOLOGIC CONDITIONS

Sonia Grover

PREPUBESCENT PROBLEMS

VULVOVAGINITIS

This is the commonest gynaecologic problem in childhood, usually occurring in girls aged between 2 and 8 years. The vaginal skin in childhood is thin and atrophic. Overgrowth of mixed bowel flora occurs in this environment and the resultant discharge can be irritant to the vulval area, which is also atrophic.

Presentation

- An offensive vaginal discharge
- Erythema/irritation of the labia and perineal skin
- Itch and dysuria may also be present

Management

Investigations are usually *not* required. Management consists of:

- Explanation and reassurance to parents
- Vinegar (1/2 cup white vinegar in a shallow bath) and/or use of simple barrier, soothing cream to labial area (e.g. zinc–castor oil, nappy rash cream)
- Toileting/hygiene advice: avoid potential irritants such as soaps and bubble bath

Rarely, if the problem persists, further action may be required. The natural history is for recurrences to occur up until the age when oestrogenization begins.

- If a heavy discharge persists – take swabs from the perineum in case of an overgrowth of *one organism* (e.g. group A Streptococcus) and treat with appropriate antibiotics (usual culture findings are mixed coliforms)
- Do *not* take vaginal swabs as it is painful and distressing. If swabs for culture are required introital area swabs will suffice

- If itch/irritation is the main complaint – consider *pinworms*
- *Foreign body* is a potential cause for a persistent, unresolving discharge. An examination under anaesthesia with vaginoscopy is required to exclude this
- Keep the possibility of *sexual abuse* in mind

Thrush is uncommon in this age group unless there has been significant antibiotic use. (Thrush thrives in an *oestrogenized* environment, not in the atrophic setting.) *Vaginal pessaries should* never *be prescribed to this age group.*

LABIAL ADHESIONS

Labial adhesions are seen most frequently during *infancy* when the child is still in nappies. The adhesion is not congenital but acquired from secondary adherence after nappy rash causes ulceration of the apposing surfaces of the labia minora. They are easily separated by lateral traction or a thermometer in infants and readherence is prevented by application of Vaseline and treatment of the nappy rash.

If labial separation is unacceptable to parents, an alternative approach is to apply oestrogen cream to the area. Two to three weeks of treatment is usually required to be effective.

Labial adhesions may also occur in girls between 2 and 8 years, often in combination with vulvovaginitis. Labial adhesions in older children *do not* need to be divided. (Division of the adhesions with lateral traction is usually possible but is frequently distressing for the older child and the parents.) As long as the child is able to void, and the vulvovaginitis is managed as described above, reassurance can be given. Parents should be told that the labia will separate when oestrogenization occurs as the child grows, combined with general physical activities.

MENSTRUAL PROBLEMS

DYSMENORRHOEA

Clinical Features

- Cramping lower abdominal pain, low back pain and pain radiating to the anterior aspects of the thighs with menses (may begin a few days before menstruation)
- Associated symptoms such as *nausea, vomiting, change in bowel actions* (usually softer bowel actions or diarrhoea, but occasionally constipation), *headaches* and *general lethargy* may occur. These symptoms should be looked for as they support the diagnosis of a

prostaglandin-induced dysmenorrhoea. Occasionally these symptoms, occurring in an intermittent pattern, may begin a few months prior to menarche
- Stress will often precipitate more severe episodes of dysmenorrhoea
- Vaginal examination is *not* performed if the young woman is not sexually active. Occasionally in young women who are using tampons a vaginal examination may be possible but alternatives such as a pelvic ultrasound examination should provide all the required information (e.g. obstructive congenital anomalies, ovarian cysts)

Management

- General measures: assess stresses/pressures, encourage exercise
- *Antiprostaglandins* (e.g. mefenamic acid, naproxen, ibuprofen) ideally should be commenced *prior to* the onset of symptoms. Failure to respond to one type of antiprostaglandin warrants trial of an alternative one
- If the menstrual cycle is too irregular for prophylactic use of antiprostaglandins, the menstrual cycle may need to be regulated with hormonal treatment. The *oral contraceptive pill* can also be used for dysmenorrhoea. This may be the first-line treatment in a sexually active teenager
- Non-responsive or worsening dysmenorrhoea will require investigation. Pelvic ultrasound can usually identify an obstructive congenital anomaly and detect significant *endometriosis* (that is, an endometrioma)

Diagnostic laparoscopy may identify mild endometriosis. However, the value of treating this with specific hormonal therapy or operative laser/diathermy is unclear from both the short-term and long-term perspective. Therefore, this operative investigation should be withheld until optimal management with antiprostaglandin therapy has been tried and failed.

AMENORRHOEA

Primary

(See Delayed Puberty, p. 188).

Secondary

Consider the following diagnoses:
- Pregnancy

- Weight loss/anorexia nervosa
- Strenuous exercise
- Stress (exams, social – family, travel)
- Polycystic ovaries: associated problems of hirsutism and obesity are usually present. These patients often have irregular, infrequent periods rather than amenorrhoea. Investigations can help confirm/support the diagnosis, but are *not* essential (e.g. follicle-stimulating hormone, luteinizing hormone, sex hormone binding globulin, pelvic ultrasound).

Amenorrhoea itself does not need treatment but associated problems may require intervention (e.g. obesity – dietary/nutritional, exercise; hirsutism – oral contraceptive pill, which causes an increase in sex hormone binding globulin with subsequent fall in free androgens). Using hormonal treatment to cause withdrawal bleeds has the advantage of making periods lighter and more regular rather than infrequent and heavy.

METROSTAXIS (SEVERE HEAVY LOSS)

Check Hb and clotting profile; exclude pregnancy. Metrostaxis in the young woman having her first or second period usually requires *oestrogen* therapy (Fig. 18.1a). As with older women, the young woman who has been menstruating for some time will usually respond to *progestogen* therapy (Fig. 18.1b).

Ongoing Management

Treatment should be continued for at least 3–6 months before considering a trial without hormonal therapy. Alternatives are:

- Cyclical progesterones (norethisterone 5 mg daily or b.d. for 14 or 21 days/month)
- Oral contraceptive pill

Either of these approaches would also be appropriate for the management of the adolescent with *menorrhagia*.

PELVIC PAIN: GYNAECOLOGICAL CAUSES

MIDCYCLE PAIN (MITTELSCHMERZ)

This occurs midcycle; therefore, it can often be diagnosed on history.

OVARIAN CYSTS

Most ovarian cysts detected on scan will be *normal follicles* and reassur-

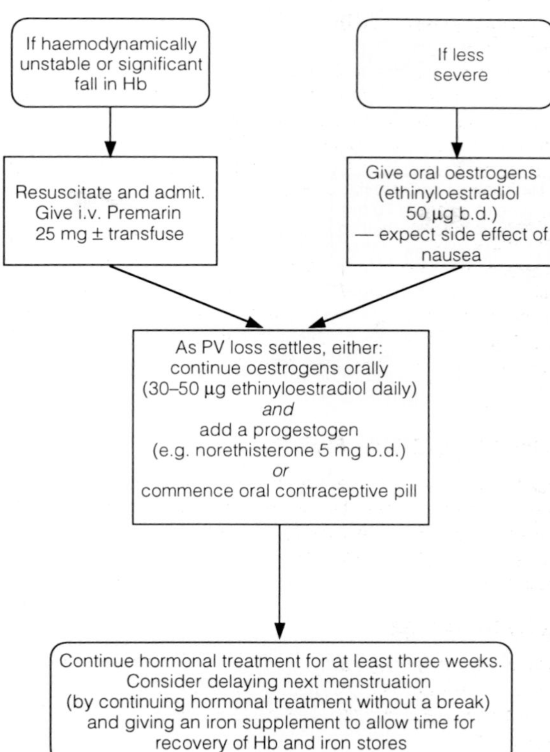

Figure 18.1a Heavy loss at first or second period

ance that these are physiological and represent healthy functioning ovaries is important. Presume all cysts <6 cm are physiological unless specific features are present to suggest otherwise. Repeating a scan 6 weeks later to prove resolution of cysts <6 cm can prevent operative intervention

Torsion of the ovary usually occurs in the presence of an ovarian cyst. The history is of sudden onset of severe pain with associated nausea, vomiting and dizziness. A diagnostic laparoscopy is the best way of

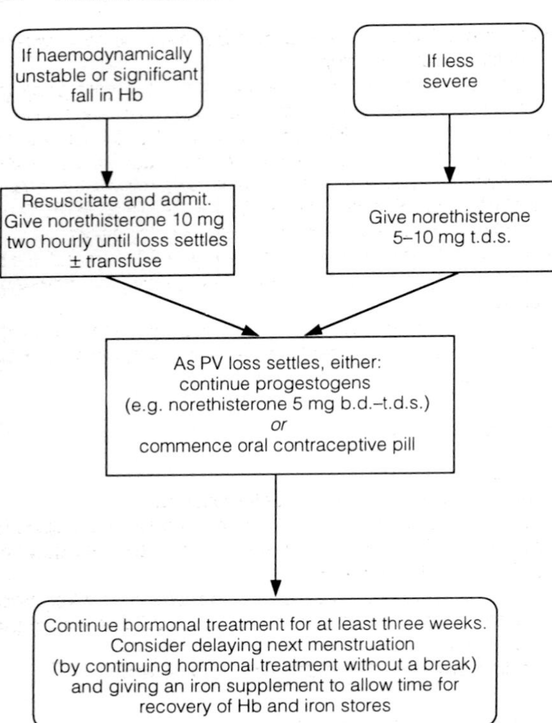

Figure 18.1b Heavy loss in the young woman who has been menstruating for some time

excluding this condition, although if an immediate ultrasound can be performed and the ovaries are normal the diagnosis is most unlikely.

PELVIC INFLAMMATORY DISEASE (PID)

- Only occurs in women who have been sexually active
- A history of dyspareunia, discharge and fever may be associated with the pelvic pain.

- Chlamydial PID may cause endometritis with intermenstrual bleeding, menorrhagia or metrostaxis
- As these young women are sexually active it is appropriate that *cervical* swabs be taken, including specific swabs for chlamydia
- *Management:* admit for intravenous antibiotics if febrile; otherwise oral antibiotics (e.g. metronidazole, amoxycillin and doxycycline). *Note:* If gonococcal disease is a significant risk in the community, appropriate antibiotics are ceftriaxone 250 mg, i.m. stat plus doxycycline (for 14 days) *or* amoxycillin–clavulanate plus doxycycline (14 days)
- In the sexually active teenager Papanicolaou (PAP) smears should be taken annually commencing approximately 6 months after intercourse began
- Discuss contraception. If PID is suspected it generally implies that condoms are not being used. Discuss benefits of condoms for protection from STD

ECTOPIC PREGNANCY

- Sexually active teenager
- A recent 'period' does not exclude this diagnosis
- Use of contraception does not exclude this diagnosis. Suspicion is increased if IUD is used (unlikely in a teenager), and decreased with oral contraceptive pill use
- Perform pregnancy test and organize pelvic ultrasound unless clinical situation (shock) necessitates immediate resuscitation and surgical intervention
- Contraception and PAP smear need to be discussed

CONGENITAL OBSTRUCTED ANOMALIES

- May cause acute onset pain or progressively increasing dysmenorrhoea (if unilateral obstruction) or progressively increasing pelvic pain without menstruation (if complete obstruction)
- Pelvic mass may be palpable
- Pelvic ultrasound or other imaging techniques will help clarify anatomy
- Associated renal agenesis on side of the obstructed genital tract may occur

BREAST PROBLEMS

- Asymmetrical development of the breast bud may lead to the presentation with a 'breast lump'. Reassure during time of breast growth and development. Growth that is initially asymmetric may correct itself

- Persistent unequal breast size can cause considerable embarrassment and distress to the teenager and referral to a specialist (usually a plastic surgeon with an interest in breast surgery) may be appropriate. Eventually, surgical correction may be required but this would not be undertaken until growth has ceased

CONTRACEPTION: BEST OPTIONS FOR YOUNG WOMEN

CONDOMS

Condoms offer the advantage of protection from STD as well as fairly good contraception.

ORAL CONTRACEPTIVE PILL (OCP)

Contraindications

- History of thromboembolic disease
- Liver disease
- Oestrogen-dependent tumours

Short-term Side-effects

- Nausea
- Breakthrough bleeding: should resolve with continuing usage
- Migraines

Types

- Sequential pills (e.g. Triquilar, Triphasil): generally first choice
- Constant dose (e.g. Microgynon 30ED, Nordette): if erratic, heavy periods, premenstrual moodiness or irregular life-style routines (slightly greater leeway in time of taking pills)
- Higher oestrogen content: if using anticonvulsants or if persistent breakthrough bleeding

Intrauterine contraceptive devices and *diaphragms* are generally not appropriate for young women. The *progesterone-only pill* is also generally not appropriate as it needs to be taken at the same time every day to be effective, and is less reliable than the combination OCP.

EMERGENCY CONTRACEPTION: MORNING-AFTER PILL

- Can be used up to 72 h after unprotected intercourse

- Contraindications are as for OCP
- Give two 'pill' tablets immediately and another two pills 12 h later. 'Pill' tablets should be any OCP containing 50 μg ethinyl oestradiol (e.g. Nordiol, Microgynon 50)
- As nausea and vomiting may occur, give an oral anti-emetic (e.g. metoclopramide) 1/2 hour before the 'pill' tablets

This treatment is effective (>90%), but does not provide continuing contraception. Discuss and plan ongoing contraception and PAP smears, and plan follow-up to ensure emergency treatment has worked.

19

CHAPTER 19

COMMON SURGICAL CONDITIONS

John Hutson

INGUINOSCROTAL CONDITIONS

The underlying pathological basis of an inguinal hernia, an encysted hydrocele of the cord and a scrotal hydrocele is persistence of the patent processus vaginalis after completion of testicular descent.

INGUINAL HERNIA

The opening of the processus vaginalis is large enough to allow the protrusion of bowel through the inguinal canal and sometimes down to the scrotum. The younger the child, the greater is the danger that the bowel will become strangulated. **Inguinal hernias always need surgery because of the ever present danger of bowel strangulation and compression of the testicular vessels.** The operation is short and children beyond the neonatal period are managed as day patients.

Reducible Inguinal Hernia

- Birth to 6 weeks: surgical consultation on the day of diagnosis, surgery on the next convenient list (preferably within 2 days)
- Six weeks to 6 months: urgent surgical outpatient appointment with surgery within 2 weeks
- Over 6 months: surgical outpatient appointment should be within 2 weeks and surgery within 2 months. This is normally done as a day case

Irreducible Inguinal Hernia

These should be referred to a surgeon as soon as the diagnosis is made (Fig. 19.1a). Normally, the surgeon is able to reduce the hernia manually and surgery is performed the following day. The child is admitted overnight and discharged the day after surgery.

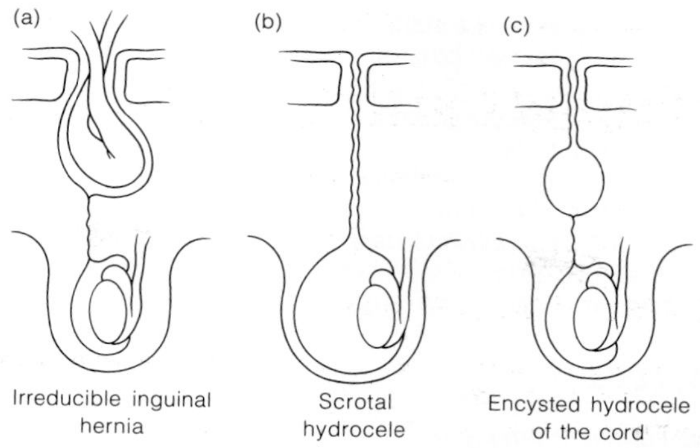

Figure 19.1 Inguinoscrotal conditions

SCROTAL HYDROCELE, ENCYSTED HYDROCELE OF THE CORD

In both these conditions, the opening of the processus vaginalis is narrow and may close of its own accord in children up to 18 months to 2 years (Fig. 19.1b, c). Important clinical signs are:

- A brilliantly transilluminable swelling
- A narrow cord above the swelling
- The swelling does not empty on squeezing

If any of these features are *not* present, the swelling may be an irreducible hernia.

If hydroceles persist beyond 2 years, surgery is recommended and inguinal herniotomy (i.e. division of the patent processus vaginalis) is performed at a convenient time, usually as a day case.

UNDESCENDED TESTES

When the testis cannot be brought to the bottom of the scrotum, it is 'undescended'. Assessment of the undescended testis is easiest between 3 and 6 months of life (avoiding confusion with retractile testis) and early referral to a surgeon is important. Experienced surgeons will perform an orchidopexy at about 6 months to 2 years as a day case.

THE ACUTE SCROTUM

A child with a painful, tender and often red scrotum should be

seen by a surgeon as a matter of urgency. It is usually impossible to differentiate the two common following causes without surgical exploration:

- *Torsion of the testicular appendage*
- *Torsion of the testis*

A testis lying horizontally in the scrotum indicates an anatomical predisposition to torsion. In a boy with recurrent brief episodes of testicular pain, consider the possibility of intermittent testicular torsion. *Epididymo-orchitis* is a rare disease in prepubertal boys who do not have urinary tract infections. Mumps orchitis is not seen before puberty.

THE PENIS

THE FORESKIN/PREPUCE

The foreskin is normally adherent to the glans at birth and remains so for a variable amount of time. Usually it is fully retractable by 4 years of age, but partial adherence is still normal up to 10 years. *There is no need to retract foreskins in preschool children.*

SMEGMA DEPOSITS

These present as yellow/white firm masses beneath the prepuce in young boys with non-retractable foreskins (Fig. 19.2a). It is a normal variant and requires no treatment.

BALANITIS

This is infection under the foreskin with redness, inflammation, swelling and sometimes a white exudate (Fig. 19.2b). Immediate treatment with local penile toilet (i.e. soak in an antiseptic solution), local antiseptic ointment (e.g. neomycin eye ointment) beneath the foreskin and oral antibiotics (e.g. cotrimoxazole) is usually sufficient. If the whole penis is red and swollen to the pubis, hospital admission and intravenous antibiotics (e.g. amoxycillin and gentamicin) may be required.

PHIMOSIS

This is scarring of the preputial opening causing:

- Urinary obstruction
- Ballooning of the foreskin on micturition

It is often the end result of recurrent episodes of balanitis (Fig. 19.2c). It usually requires circumcision if severe, although mild cases respond to

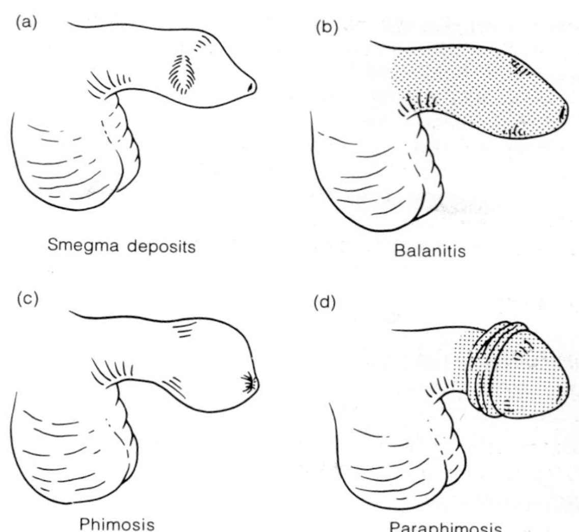

Figure 19.2 Conditions of the penis

topical 0.05% betamethasone valerate cream applied three to four times daily for 10 days.

PARAPHIMOSIS

In this acutely painful condition, the retracted foreskin is trapped behind the glans and forms an oedematous ring of foreskin proximal to the exposed and swollen glans penis (Fig. 19.2d). A surgeon should be consulted immediately if it cannot be reduced manually.

CIRCUMCISION

The indications for circumcision are phimosis and recurrent balanitis. Hypospadias is an absolute contraindication.

It is important to stress to parents that circumcision is not required for cleanliness and that these days less than a quarter of Australian male children are circumcised. It is an unnecessary operation with definite complications of surgery and anaesthesia.

UMBILICAL HERNIA

Umbilical hernia – the protrusion of the umbilicus – is a common finding in newborn children. In most it will resolve spontaneously and not require surgery. If it persists beyond 2 years of age, day surgical repair is recommended because the risk of strangulation increases with age.

ACUTE ABDOMINAL PAIN

Abdominal pain is a common symptom in children. *Appendicitis* needs to be distinguished from the other common causes: *viral infection, urinary tract infection* and *constipation*.

In the younger child, and especially in those less than 4 years of age, the diagnosis can be difficult. It is important to refer a child who complains of persistent abdominal pain, even if this is associated with vomiting or diarrhoea (i.e. do not assume it is gastroenteritis). If the child will not allow abdominal examination, one should suspect peritonitis.

INTUSSUSCEPTION

In a 3 month to 2 year old infant who presents with intermittent pallor, lethargy, vomiting and abdominal colic, the diagnosis of intussusception should be considered. These are the early symptoms and should be acted upon, rather than awaiting the 'classical' red currant jelly stool, which is a feature of advanced disease. The abdominal mass is central beneath rectus abdominus and is often difficult to feel.

A child with suspected intussusception requires urgent surgical assessment and a contrast enema for diagnosis and/or treatment. If a hydrostatic pressure 80–100 mmHg fails to reduce the intussusception, emergency surgery is indicated. Contrast enema should not be performed in the presence of peritonitis, significant dehydration or established bowel obstruction. Early diagnosis is the key to easy and successful treatment.

VOMITING IN INFANCY

MALROTATION AND VOLVULUS

It is important to determine whether the vomiting is bile stained or not. **Green vomiting is an indication for urgent surgical consultation to exclude the anatomical variant of intestinal malrotation and**

its associated lethal complication of midgut volvulus. Initially, there may be no other symptoms or signs of abdominal disease. Abdominal distension is not present and should not be waited for. The twisted intestine may become gangrenous within 6 h after the onset of bile-stained vomiting.

PYLORIC STENOSIS

In infants with non-bile-stained vomiting, *pyloric stenosis* needs to be distinguished from *feeding problems*, *gastro-oesophageal reflux* and *infection* (e.g. urinary tract infection, meningitis).

Pyloric stenosis should be suspected if the vomiting is projectile, persists despite correction of feeding difficulties and/or the use of anti-gastro-oesophageal reflux measures or is associated with failure to thrive.

Examination

- Look for gastric peristalsis during test feeding, and feel for the pyloric tumour, either during test feeding or after vomiting
- Passage of a nasogastric tube and drainage of the stomach is sometimes required to aid palpation of the tumour
- The child should be referred to a paediatric surgeon on the basis of *symptoms*, as the demonstration of signs can be difficult

Investigations

Biochemistry

Metabolic alkalosis; chloride usually <100 mmol/L, sodium usually <130 mmol/L (cf. gastro-oesophageal reflux – electrolytes usually normal); serum potassium may be normal despite significant losses.

Ultrasound

Required only if diagnosis is unclear after consultation with a paediatric surgeon.

RECTAL BLEEDING

This is a common symptom and does not normally imply a sinister cause. It is usually associated with *constipation* and is caused by a superficial, acute anal fissure which may not be visible. The constipation

SURGERY

should be treated with laxatives with the expectation that the rectal bleeding will resolve.

- An *intestinal polyp* is associated with more persistent rectal bleeding and is not necessarily associated with constipation. The polyp may resolve spontaneously
- A large volume of rectal bleeding requires further investigation to exclude the possibility of a *Meckel's diverticulum*

SURGICAL CONDITIONS OF THE NEONATE

IMPORTANT WARNING SIGNS

- **Excessive drooling of frothy secretions from the mouth may suggest oesophageal atresia**
- **Bile (green) stained vomiting is always abnormal**
- **Malrotation may be present with minimal bile stained vomiting at any age**. Admission to a paediatric hospital is essential
- **Delayed passage of meconium** (beyond 24 h) **is abnormal** and may indicate Hirschsprung's disease
- **Inguinal hernias need urgent attention to avoid strangulation**

'RARE AND DANGEROUS' CONDITIONS

Ambiguous Genitalia

Genitalia which are frankly ambiguous need urgent consultation with an experienced paediatric endocrinologist or surgeon on the first day of life (see p. 192).

An enlarged clitoris in an apparent female is also abnormal and needs immediate referral.

Hypospadias may overlap with ambiguous genitalia and needs careful initial assessment as someone already has assumed the gender should be male. If one or both testes are undescended and/or the scrotum is bifid, the baby should be treated as having ambiguous genitalia until proven otherwise by immediate referral for further investigation.

Oesophageal Atresia

Excessive drooling or frothy, mucousy secretions from the mouth suggests inability to swallow in a newborn. Test for oesophageal atresia by passing a 10 gauge catheter (which will not curl up) gently through the mouth: in atresia the catheter stops at about 10 cm from the gums, while in a normal baby it will pass to 20–25 cm and return acid on litmus testing. Proven oesophageal atresia needs urgent referral and transfer to a neonatal surgical unit. First aid includes nil orally, intravenous fluids, and frequent (10–15 minutely) oropharyngeal suction to keep the airways clear (thereby preventing contamination of the lungs).

Diaphragmatic Hernia

Respiratory distress in a newborn with a scaphoid abdomen suggests diaphragmatic hernia. Cardiac displacement and an X-ray of chest and abdomen showing bowel loops in the chest (left more commonly) confirms the diagnosis. Urgent referral and transfer by the neonatal emergency transport service is needed. First aid includes intravenous fluids, nil orally, nasogastric tube to prevent gaseous distension, and respiratory support with oxygen. If a baby with suspected or diagnosed diaphragmatic hernia needs mechanical ventilation, then intubate the trachea. **Bag and mask ventilation may exacerbate the respiratory distress by distending the bowel.**

Exomphalos/Gastroschisis

These anterior abdominal wall defects put the child at great risk of heat and water loss from the exposed surface of the sac (exomphalos) or bowel (gastroschisis). First aid is needed urgently prior to transfer: intravenous fluids, nil orally, nasogastric tube (to prevent gaseous distension) and wrapping the sac or exposed bowel in plastic kitchen wrap or aluminium foil to prevent evaporative cooling. The baby should be kept in an incubator while awaiting the neonatal transport service.

Babies of excessive size and body weight (>4 kg) who have exomphalos should be suspected of having *Beckwith-Wiedemann syndrome*, with excessive production of insulin. Blood glucose testing and intravenous 10% dextrose can avoid fitting, mental retardation or death caused by unrecognized neonatal hypoglycaemia.

Sacrococcygeal Teratoma

Any lump over the coccyx of the baby should be assumed to be a teratoma until proven otherwise, and needs immediate referral at birth.

Malrotation with Volvulus

Volvulus or twisting of the bowel is a potentially fatal complication of congenital malrotation, where the gut is abnormally positioned and inadequately fixed in the abdominal cavity. A well baby (or older child) may suddenly vomit bile-stained fluid without other symptoms (as would be seen with sepsis). Immediate referral for a barium meal to exclude midgut volvulus is required, as the twisted bowel will become infarcted in 6–12 h.

CHAPTER 20

ORTHOPAEDIC CONDITIONS

Kerr Graham and Peter Barnett

NEONATAL ORTHOPAEDIC CONDITIONS

DEVELOPMENTAL DYSPLASIA OF THE HIP

Previously known as *congenital dislocation of the hip*; however, not all cases are present at birth, and the hips are not necessarily dislocated. Risk factors are breech delivery, Caesarean section, family history, congenital foot abnormality, other congenital anomaly, first born, female sex.

Diagnosis

General screening

All neonates should have a clinical examination for instability: the Ortolani and Barlow tests.

Selective screening

Infants in high-risk groups and those with an abnormal routine clinical screening examination should have an *ultrasound* examination of their hips.

- As clinical diagnosis can be difficult and ultrasound has diagnostic limitations, repeated examination of children during the first year of life is important
- X-rays are helpful after 3 months

Management

The earlier the diagnosis the easier the management.

- Most neonates can be successfully treated by abduction bracing with a Pavlik harness
- Operative treatments including open reduction may be required with later diagnosis

CLUB FOOT (CONGENITAL TALIPES EQUINOVARUS)

Most infants with abnormal looking feet are said to have 'talipes'. However, the majority have postural problems such as talipes calcaneovalgus (excessive dorsiflexion and eversion), metatarsus varus (adduction of the forefoot) or postural talipes equinovarus (see Fig. 20.1). These deformities are usually mild and mobile, i.e. they correct easily and fully with the pressure of one finger. They resolve spontaneously with no treatment.

The true club foot deformity is more severe and is often stiff. The foot is in equinus, with the hindfoot in varus and the forefoot supinated.

Management

- All require manipulation and casting
- Soft tissue surgery for many
- Bone surgery for a few

ANGULAR DEFORMITIES IN CHILDREN

Many children are seen with normal angular or torsional variants. It can be difficult to distinguish physiological variation from pathological conditions. The range of 'normality' is very wide but what parents accept is much narrower. The physiological variations in normal children can result in as much anxiety as the pathological disorders.

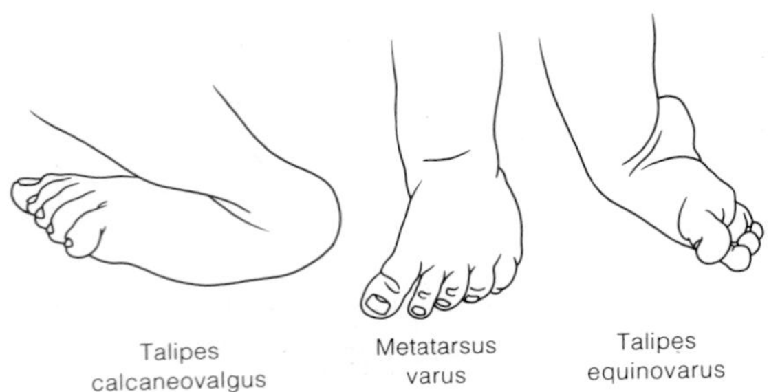

Figure 20.1 Congenital foot deformities

INTOEING

Table 20.1 Intoeing in childhood

	Metatarsus varus	*Internal tibial torsion*	*Medial femoral torsion*
Synonyms	Metatarsus adductus		Inset hips
Age at presentation	Birth	Toddler	Child
Site of problem	Foot	Tibia	Femur
Examination	Sole of foot bean-shaped	Thigh–foot angle is inwards	Arc of hip rotation favours internal rotation
Management	Observe or cast	Observe and reassure	Observe, rarely surgery
When to refer if not resolved	3 months after presentation	6 months after presentation	8 years after presentation

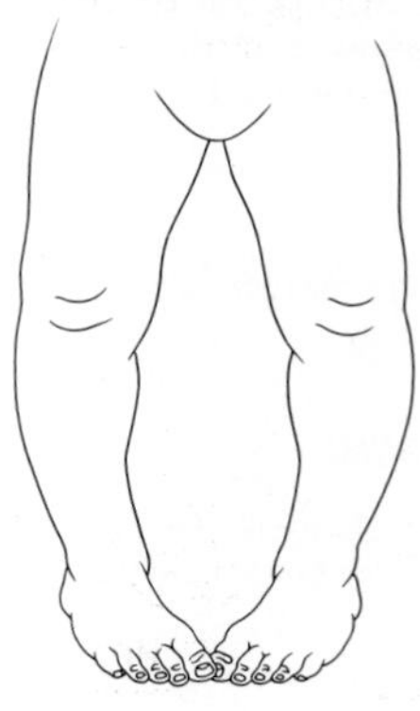

Figure 20.2 Internal tibial torsion

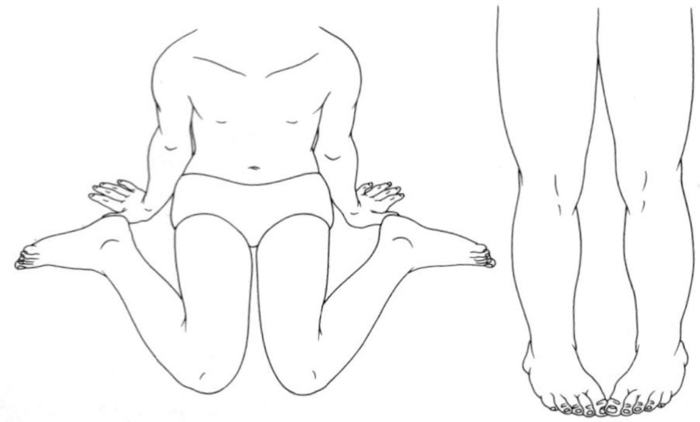

Figure 20.3 Medial femoral torsion

OUT-TOEING

Infants and toddlers have restricted internal rotation at the hip because of an external rotation contracture, not retroversion of the femur.

Infants

- Present with 'Charlie Chaplin' posture between 3 and 12 months
- Child weight bears and walks normally
- Resolution occurs with no treatment

Children

- May be due to neurologic disorder
- Surgery may be necessary

BOW LEGS (GENU VARUM)

The vast majority are physiological. Rare causes include skeletal dysplasias, rickets and Blount's disease (tibia vara)

Presentation

- Toddlers are usually bowed until 3 years of age

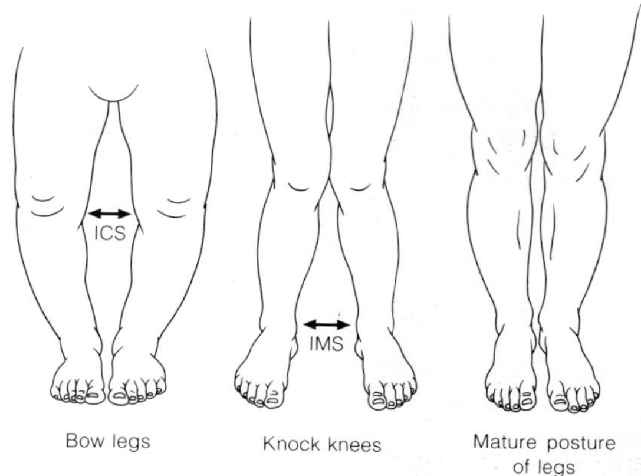

Figure 20.4 Postural variance of lower limbs

- Physiological bowing is symmetrical, not excessive and improves with time

Management

- Monitor intercondylar separation (ICS; see Fig. 20.4)
- Refer on when ICS >6 cm, not improving or asymmetric

KNOCK KNEES (GENU VALGUM)

Again, the vast majority are physiological. Rare caures are rickets and trauma

Presentation

- Children are usually knock kneed from 3 to 8 years
- Physiological knock knee is symmetrical, not excessive and improves with time

Management

- Monitor the intermalleolar separation (IMS; see Fig. 20.4)
- Refer if IMS >8 cm

Note: Most children with bow legs or knock knees are normal with only <1% having an underlying problem.

FLAT FEET (PES PLANO VALGUS)

This condition is painless and asymptomatic. *Note:* **If painful or stiff, referral is needed.**

Causes

- Physiological (vast majority): all newborns have flat feet due to fat which fills the medial longitudinal arch; 80% of children develop a medial arch by their sixth birthday
- Tarsal coalition (in older children and adolescents only)

Management

- No treatment required unless painful or stiff
- Unaffected by orthotics or exercises
- Majority resolve spontaneously

TRAUMA

Injuries are the leading cause of mortality and morbidity in children. The management of fractures and dislocations is an integral part of the overall management of the traumatized patient. Common fractures in children involve the wrist, elbow, clavicle, distal tibia and fibula and femur. Each has distinct management strategies but common themes run through.

ASSESSMENT

Patients presenting with a suspected fracture or dislocation require a full evaluation of the fracture, and damage to other structures needs to be excluded.

An accurate history of the mechanism of injury will determine which structures may potentially be damaged.

Examination

- Closed or open wound (the latter will require operative intervention)
- Deformity or swelling (*Note;* Acute swelling in children usually indicates a fracture)

- Neurological status distal to the injury
- Peripheral pulses – if the blood flow to the limb is compromised urgent orthopaedic referral is needed

Management

- Affected limb should be splinted by a board or plaster slab prior to X-ray
- Analgesia (usually parenteral) is required (e.g. pethidine 1 mg/kg i.m.)
- X-ray should be obtained examining the joint above and below the suspected fracture site. An anteroposterior and lateral view should be obtained
- If the angle between the shaft of the bone and the fractured fragment is >15–20° manipulation of the fracture needs to occur prior to the placement of a plaster. Forearm fractures in children 6 years or older can usually be manipulated using a local anaesthetic block (e.g. Bier's Block)
- If the fracture involves both cortices of the bone then a plaster involving the joint above and below should be placed (e.g. above elbow for forearm fracture)
- A simple undisplaced greenstick or buckle fracture can be treated in a short cast

Home Treatment After a Full Plaster

- Elevate the limb above heart level for the next 24–48 h
- A sling should only be worn after this period and the hand should not be below the elbow while in the sling
- Crutches should only be used by children over 6–7 years
- Written plaster instructions should be explained and given to parents

Follow-up

For patients who have had a manipulation of fracture or a fracture involving both cortices of the bone, a repeat X-ray should be obtained in 1 week to ensure the correct position is maintained. Plaster should remain in place for 3–6 weeks depending on the degree of injury. Following removal of the cast the bone is still at risk of re-fracture for the next 8–12 weeks and therefore contact sports are not recommended during this period.

SPECIFIC INJURIES

Supracondylar Fractures

Undisplaced fracture can be treated in a collar and cuff for 3–4 weeks. All displaced fractures need to be evaluated urgently by an orthopaedic surgeon and most will need a manipulation under general anaesthesia.

Forearm Fractures

Make sure the thumb is free and that the plaster only goes up to the knuckle line (MPJ).

Femur Fractures

Isolated femur fractures in young children rarely cause hypotension; however, in adolescents and patients with potential multi-trauma an intravenous line should be inserted. Analgesia can be achieved by femoral nerve block (see p. 27).

Clavicle Fractures

These almost always are treated in a simple sling for 3 weeks with follow-up by the local doctor.

Note: **Consider child abuse in infants with fractures.**

Ankle Injury

True sprains or soft tissue injuries are more common in adolescents. Younger children with open growth plates are more likely to sustain a growth plate injury or fracture and should be treated in a plaster cast.

Clinical Assessment

- Mechanism of injury – usually caused by an inversion injury to the ankle
- Was the patient able to bear weight immediately after the injury?
- Where is the swelling most prominent?
- What is the point of maximal tenderness?

Investigation

X-rays are required if:
- Deformity is present
- Maximal tenderness occurs over the tibia or fibula

- Patient is unable to weight bear

Note: If the patient is tender over the growth plate of the tibia or fibula and the X-rays are normal, the patient has a Salter Harris 1 epiphyseal injury and should be treated in a below-knee plaster. If there is a large amount of swelling a plaster slab should be used first, and a full plaster placed after the swelling has gone down.

If the X-rays are normal or none of the above conditions apply then treatment will depend on the severity of symptoms.

Management: Mild–moderate sprain

- ***R***est – non-weight bearing should occur for a few days to 2–3 weeks
- ***I***ce – should be applied every 2–3 h for 15 min during the first 48 h; then heat can be applied
- ***C***ompression – should be accomplished either with a firm bandage or a plaster slab
- ***E***levation – the limb should be elevated on a few pillows whenever possible to allow the swelling to subside

Management: Severe sprain

Treat like a fracture:

- Below-knee plaster (or if swelling is severe, a plaster slab followed by a full plaster) for 2–4 weeks
- Non-weight bearing for the first week
- Gradual rehabilitation should occur after several days of rest. This includes gentle weight bearing and ankle exercises to strengthen the damaged ankle ligaments (initially plantar- and dorsiflexion exercises as soon as possible; later toe raises and inversion/eversion exercises when the pain has subsided)
- Running and sport should not be undertaken for 1–2 weeks after the injury. In a competitive athlete, physiotherapy or sports medicine referral is appropriate

Pulled Elbow

Clinical features

- Age: usually 1–3 years
- Mechanism of injury is usually another person pulling the child's arm forcefully. There may be a crack or popping sound at the time. Occasionally, it may occur after a fall

- Arm is held pronated and slightly flexed (i.e. limp by their side as if they are ignoring it)
- Child is not distressed and is not using the apparently lifeless limb
- Palpation from the clavicle to the wrist does not demonstrate any swelling or tenderness
- Supination of the arm causes pain

Investigations

If typical of a pulled elbow no investigations are necessary.

Management

- Hold the child's hand as if to shake it and with your other hand encircle the elbow with the thumb over the annular ligament of the radius
- Gently apply traction and supinate the hand. Then flex the forearm at the elbow all the way to the shoulder. You should feel a pop as the radial head is relocated
- The child should be moving the arm normally within 10–15 min

Note: If the history is not typical or *there is swelling* or *your attempts fail,* then an X-ray of the elbow should be obtained to exclude a radial head fracture.

LIMP IN CHILDHOOD

Limp is a common presenting complaint in childhood (see Table 20.2).

Table 20. 2 Differential diagnosis of limp in childhood

Acute	*Subacute*	*Chronic*
Fracture	Juvenile rheumatoid arthritis	Cerebral palsy
Irritable hip	Tumour/leukaemia	Developmental dysplasia of the hips
Septic arthritis	Acute on chronic SCFE	Perthes' disease
Osteomyelitis		Chronic SCFE

SCFE, slipped capital femoral epiphysis.

Clinical assessment

- Is the limp acute, subacute or chronic?
- Is there associated pain and/or fever?
- Are there other constitutional symptoms?
- Have there been previous episodes of pain or limp?
- What position is the leg held in (e.g. flexed and externally rotated)?
- Does joint movement or bony pressure cause pain?
- Is there limitation of movement?

Investigations

- Full blood examination (FBE), differential, erythrocyte sedimentation rate (ESR); and possibly C-reactive protein
- Plain X-ray of joint or affected limb
- Ultrasound of hip if painful (looking for fluid in the joint)
- Bone scan (after orthopaedic consultation)

Management

This will depend on the underlying problem:

- Slipped capital femoral epiphysis (SCFE), tumours, Perthes' disease or developmental dysplasia of the hip should be referred immediately to an orthopaedic surgeon
- Toddlers' fractures may be occult and not seen on X-ray. If the child is afebrile then observation is appropriate
- Bone scan should be arranged for worsening or changing symptoms

IRRITABLE HIP (TRANSIENT SYNOVITIS)

This is a common condition which presents with a painful hip and difficulty walking in a child who is constitutionally well. This condition needs to be distinguished from others in Table 20.2. Although it is the commonest reason for limp in the preschooler, irritable hip is a diagnosis of exclusion.

Clinical features

- Usually 3–8 years old
- Recent viral illness (last 1–2 weeks)
- Absence of trauma
- Usually able to walk but with pain
- Severity of the symptoms may vary with time

- Temperature is usually <38°C and the patient appears well
- Mild–moderate decrease in range of motion due to pain, particularly internal rotation

Note: The less movement in the joint, the more likely the cause is infective.

Investigations

- As for limp (ultrasound usually demonstrates an effusion)
- X-rays and FBE are normal with an ESR of <20

Note: The history, symptoms and signs of an irritable hip overlap with septic arthritis which is a serious condition requiring urgent treatment. **If there is any suspicion of bone or joint sepsis, orthopaedic consultation is required and admission to hospital should be arranged.**

Management

Rest in bed and simple analgesics are the treatment of choice. The more the child can rest the quicker the recovery. Patients may have a relapse if they increase their activity too quickly. Occasionally, these patients need to be admitted to hospital for bed rest and traction.

ACUTE BONE AND JOINT SEPSIS (SEPTIC ARTHRITIS [SA] AND OSTEOMYELITIS [OM])

This can affect any joint or bone but most commonly involves the lower limbs. **SA is an orthopaedic emergency with drainage and antibiotics essential to prevent long-term morbidity.**

Clinical features

- Acute onset of limp/non-weight bearing/non-movement of limb (may be delayed in OM)
- Pain localized to joint or metaphysis of bone
- Irritability and poor feeding in infants
- Temperature usually >38.5°C
- Joint held in neutral position
- Pain on all movements with decreased range of movement (severe in SA)

Investigations

- As for limp
- ESR usually >20–30
- White cell count (WCC) raised in SA, usually raised in OM
- Bone scan may be indicated if the diagnosis is not clear

Management

- Admission to hospital, keep nil orally
- Intravenous antibiotics (covering *Staphylococcus aureus*, *Haemophilus influenzae* and Gram-negative organisms in neonates)
- Urgent orthopaedic referral, and possibly surgery

PERTHES' DISEASE

This is a specific hip disease of childhood. Affected children have a generalized disorder of growth with a tendency to low birthweight and delayed bone age. The pathology is avascular necrosis of the capital femoral epiphysis followed by a sequence of changes including resorption of necrotic bone, reossification and remodelling. This sequence of events is seen radiologically as density of the capital epiphysis, patchy osteolysis, new bone formation and remodelling with a variable degree of femoral head deformity.

Clinical features

- Age range: 2–12 years but the majority present between 4 and 8 years
- Sex ratio: five males to one female, 20% bilateral
- Symptoms: pain and limp, usually for at least a week
- Signs: restriction of hip motion

Investigations

- X-ray
- Bone scan useful in the early stages before the signs are clear on X-ray

Management Principles

- Resting the hip in the early irritable phase
- Regaining motion if the hip is stiff
- *Containing* the hip by bracing or surgery in selected patients

SLIPPED CAPITAL FEMORAL EPIPHYSIS (SCFE)

Can occur acutely or chronically. Early detection will prevent later morbidity.

Clinical features

- Age: late childhood to early adolescence
- Usually >90th percentile for weight
- Pain in hip or *knee*
- Limp
- Hip appears externally rotated and shortened
- Decreased hip movement, particularly internal rotation

Note: Can be bilateral

Investigation

X-ray of pelvis and *frog leg lateral* of affected hip.

Management

- Patient should not weight bear if the diagnosis is entertained
- Needs urgent orthopaedic referral and surgery to prevent further slipping

SCOLIOSIS

Definitions

- Scoliosis is a curvature in the spine when viewed from the frontal (coronal) plane
- A *structural* scoliosis is when the curvature has an element of rotation and may progress with growth
- A *non-structural* scoliosis may be secondary to a problem outside the spine, such as unequal leg lengths

Detection

The most common type of scoliosis is *adolescent scoliosis*, affecting girls in 90% of cases. Because abnormal spinal curvatures start small and may progress with time and growth, efforts have been made to detect the condition at an early stage by school screening programmes. This is usually done by the *forward bend test*, in which the examiner observes the spine from behind as the subject bends forwards. Flexion of the spine usually demonstrates the deformity much more clearly because of the asymmetry of the ribs and chest wall.

Very small curves are relatively common and it can be difficult to decide when an X-ray is required, which curves are likely to progress and which require brace treatment or surgery. The risk of curve progression is related to the age at presentation and the size and cause of the curve.

Ten per cent of normal teenagers have a curve of 5° or more, but 0 only 2% have curves >10°.

Management

All children with scoliosis should be referred to a paediatric orthopaedic surgeon.

- <20° – observe
- 20–40° – brace
- >40° – surgery

CHAPTER 21

EAR, NOSE AND THROAT CONDITIONS

Robert Berkowitz and John Vorrath

OTITIS MEDIA

See also p. 66. This term covers a spectrum of conditions, which are characterized by the presence of fluid in the middle ear, diagnosed on either tympanic membrane appearance or immobility (as documented by either pneumatic otoscopy or tympanometry). Clinically, otitis media presents as either: *acute suppurative otitis media* (ASOM) or *otitis media with effusion* (OME).

ACUTE SUPPURATIVE OTITIS MEDIA

A middle ear effusion *plus* features of inflammation which are either localized (ear pain) or generalized (fever, irritability) where there is no other cause to explain these generalized features of inflammation. *The degree of redness of the tympanic membrane is unhelpful in deciding whether or not inflammation is present.*

The causative organism is usually either *Streptococcus pneumoniae*, non-typable *Haemophilus influenzae* or *Moraxella catarrhalis*. A proportion of cases are viral; however, it is difficult to distinguish these clinically.

Management

Initial Management

Amoxycillin 40 mg/kg per day in three divided doses is recommended. Most episodes of ASOM respond well to amoxycillin. When ASOM is associated with acute tympanic membrane perforation, drainage of the middle ear is often incomplete as the perforation heals rapidly, and therefore antibiotics still need to be given. There is no benefit in adding topical antibiotics.

Follow-up

The inflammation and middle ear effusion need to be followed up separately.

Review in 48 h if there is no resolution of the features of *inflammation*. Possible explanations include:

- Failure to take the medication (either the antibiotics not given or being vomited)
- Inappropriate antibiotic (the amoxycillin may need to be changed to the more broad-spectrum amoxycillin with clavulanic acid)
- Wrong diagnosis
- The antibiotic itself is responsible for the child remaining unwell
- A suppurative complication of ASOM has developed (e.g. mastoiditis)

If appropriate medical treatment has been unsuccessful, acute drainage of the ear (myringotomy) with or without insertion of a tympanostomy tube should be considered.

Follow-up of the *middle ear effusion* should be based on a knowledge of the expected persistence of fluid following an ASOM. Following an ASOM there is persistent middle ear effusion in 70% of cases at 2 weeks, 40% at 1 month, 20% at 2 months and 10% at 3 months. Follow-up in the first few weeks following an ASOM is therefore unnecessary.

OTITIS MEDIA WITH EFFUSION

This presents as a middle ear effusion *without* features of inflammation.

Management

Medical

Antibiotics may be of value as bacteria can be cultured in approximately 20% of cases of OME. Where OME is associated with recurrent ASOM, prophylactic antibiotics may be of benefit to prevent further episodes of ASOM and therefore allow the middle ear effusion to resolve spontaneously. However, this must be balanced against the risk of inducing resistant organisms.

No other medications are of practical benefit and the use of eustachian tube auto-inflation is of limited value.

Surgical

Insertion of tympanostomy tubes does not cure the underlying eustachian tube dysfunction responsible for OME, but only temporarily removes the symptoms. If OME is symptomatic and is likely to be present for a significant period of time, insertion of tympanostomy tubes should be considered. Adenoidectomy may be beneficial in addition (by removing a reservoir of infection from the nasopharynx), but adds significant morbidity to an otherwise very minor procedure. The prerequisites for tympanostomy tubes are:

- Middle ear effusion present for at least 3 months. This is important because 90% of effusions will resolve within the first 3 months and early treatment is therefore unnecessary
- There should be no expectation of early resolution of the middle ear effusion. For example, OME and ASOM are often related to upper respiratory tract infections and are therefore more common over the winter months. Where OME has been present for 3 months by the end of winter, it may be appropriate to delay inserting tubes in the expectation that there may be resolution with the onset of warmer weather
- Symptoms must be present—either recurrent ASOM or functionally significant hearing loss (e.g. speech delay, behavioural disturbance or poor school performance)

The benefits of temporary alleviation of symptoms of OME by the insertion of tympanostomy tubes need to be balanced against the disadvantages:

- Tubes usually remain *in situ* for only 6–9 months (although longer-stay tubes are available) and the reinsertion rate of tubes is approximately 25%
- Tympanic membrane perforation rate of approximately 1% per year that the tube is *in situ*
- Otorrhoea occurs in up to 25% of cases, often associated with an upper respiratory tract infection. It may also occur due to external contamination (e.g. swimming or bathing without ear protection). A discharging ear should be treated by ear toilet and topical antibiotics. An oral antibiotic may also be of benefit in younger children, but not in children older than 3 years of age as the infective organism is likely to be *Pseudomonas* and therefore not sensitive to the oral antibiotics commonly used. Discharge refractory to medical treatment can be managed by 3% hydrogen peroxide ear washes; however, the possibility of an underlying immunodeficiency or cholesteatoma should be considered

OTITIS EXTERNA

Clinical features

Inflammation of the ear canal (which includes the tympanic membrane) and pre-auricular tenderness, with tympanic membrane mobility on pneumatic otoscopy (which rules out otitis media).

Management

Regular ear toilet and topical antibiotics. Where the ear canal is very oedematous, an ear wick should be inserted and moistened frequently with topical antibiotics to maintain patency of the ear canal.

Hospital admission for administration of (anti-*Pseudomonas*) intravenous antibiotics may be necessary when ear pain is severe and not relieved by regular analgesics, or where cellulitis has extended beyond the ear canal.

ACUTE TONSILLITIS

Aetiology

Acute tonsillitis is usually due to group A β-haemolytic streptococcal infection, but viral causes such as infectious mononucleosis and adenovirus also need to be considered (see also p. 65).

Clinical features

Acute tonsillitis is characterized by fever, sore throat, tonsillar inflammation, cervical lymphadenitis and the absence of cough or other symptoms suggestive of a respiratory tract infection.

Management

Penicillin must be administered for a full 10 day course to prevent early recurrences. Frequent recurrences of acute tonsillitis can be treated by either low-dose prophylactic penicillin or adenotonsillectomy.

OBSTRUCTIVE ADENOTONSILLAR HYPERTROPHY

Pathophysiology

Upper airways obstruction occurs where there is an imbalance between the neuromuscular control, which supports the airways, and the negative inspiratory pressure, which tends to collapse the airways. The site of obstruction is generally in the oropharynx at the level of the tonsil, and tonsillectomy therefore is beneficial in relieving upper airways obstruction. Removal of the adenoids improves the nasal airways and thereby decreases the negative pressure generated during inspiration.

Indications for Surgery

Involution of the adenoids and tonsils will occur with time, and be accompanied by resolution of obstructive symptoms. With this in mind, the indications for surgical management depend on the severity of the symptoms, which can be classified as follows:

- *Snoring alone:* this does not require surgical management
- *Laboured respiration and restlessness at night or chronic mouth breathing by day.* If the adenoids alone are enlarged then adenoidectomy (which is associated with much less morbidity than adenotonsillectomy) is sufficient, but if the tonsils are also enlarged then adenotonsillectomy is required
- *Obstructive sleep apnoea* (OSA): this usually requires adeno-tonsillectomy unless there is no significant lymphoid tissue enlargement (as may be the case in children with neuromuscular disorders or craniofacial anomalies). Complications of OSA include failure to thrive, significant hypoxia, and cor pulmonale

PERIORBITAL AND ORBITAL CELLULITIS

Periorbital cellulitis is commonly due to acute sinusitis, particularly involving the ethmoid sinus (see also p. 261). Antibiotics should cover the organisms causing acute sinusitis (same as for ASOM, see above) and acute-on-chronic sinusitis (*Staphylococcus aureus*, anaerobes). No specific radiological imaging is required.

Periorbital cellulitis may progress to *orbital cellulitis*, which is characterized by chemosis proptosis, ophthalmoplegia, decreased visual acuity and systemic symptoms. If features of orbital cellulitis are present, a CT scan is required to determine whether or not the sinusitis is complicated by abscess formation, particularly a subperiosteal abscess, which requires surgical drainage usually by an external ethmoidectomy approach. If no abscess is present, treatment is by intravenous antibiotics alone; however, CT scanning may need to be repeated if there is progression of symptoms and signs or if there is failure of improvement with medical treatment.

EPISTAXIS

This is usually due to bleeding from anterior nasoseptal vessels. Acute bleeding usually settles with local pressure, but occasionally the application of a cotton wool pledget soaked with a topical decongestant is necessary.

Recurrent bleeding can be treated by the application of an antibiotic ointment if there is significant nasal crusting present or by cautery if enlarged blood vessels are seen. Nasal cautery can be performed as an office procedure following the application of a topical anaesthetic/decongestant, for example Cophenylcaine spray (lignocaine and phenylephrine), using a silver nitrate stick. Only one side should be cauterized at a time, and local trauma to the nose should be avoided for 2 weeks to allow healing to occur without further bleeding.

Epistaxis is very unlikely to be due to a nasal tumour or a previously undiagnosed coagulopathy, but further evaluation may be necessary if there are suggestive symptoms or signs present.

TRAUMA

NASAL TRAUMA

Treatment is required for either cosmesis or septal haematoma.

Cosmesis

A nasal deformity due to a displaced nasal fracture should be reduced within 7–10 days of injury. The presence of a bony deformity due to a nasal fracture is best determined at about 5 days following the injury once the soft tissue swelling has resolved. The decision to reduce the nasal fracture is based on clinical grounds and radiology is unhelpful.

Septal Haematoma

This can occur following nasal trauma whether or not a fracture is present, and invariably leads to septal abscess formation with cartilage destruction and nasal collapse. A septal haematoma presents with a bulge of the septum and can be confirmed by palpation with an instrument (e.g. wax curette) following the application of topical anaesthetic. Treatment involves incision and drainage, nasal packing to prevent recurrence, and anti-staphylococcal antibiotics.

ORAL/OROPHARYNGEAL TRAUMA

Although these injuries are often trivial, hospital admission and further evaluation may be required in the following situations:

- Child unable to feed
- Upper airways obstruction
- Significant laceration requiring debridement and/or closure

- Significant retropharyngeal injury. Involvement of the retropharynx may not be obvious by oral examination particularly for injuries through the soft palate. The retropharynx is ideally examined by flexible nasopharyngoscopy. In addition, a lateral cervical spine X-ray is required to rule out the presence of gas in the soft tissues, presence of a foreign body and any associated cervical spine injury. Widening of the retropharynx may also be demonstrated, but this may be misleading unless the radiological features are confirmed by nasopharyngoscopy. A significant retropharyngeal injury requires intravenous antibiotics and a period of nasogastric feeding
- Suspicion of injury to the internal carotid artery. The internal carotid artery lies posterolateral to the tonsil. An injury to this region may be associated with injury to the internal carotid artery whether the trauma is blunt or sharp. While internal carotid artery injuries are rare, they are usually due to blunt trauma which causes intimal disruption and progressive thrombosis presenting with neurological signs over a period of about 24 h. Where an internal carotid artery injury is suspected, the patient should be admitted for observation and consideration given to angiography

AURAL TRAUMA

Trauma to the *external auditory canal* is usually associated with bleeding but is an insignificant injury and requires no treatment.

The *tympanic membrane* can be perforated by direct trauma or a pressure wave (e.g. a slap across the ear, diving). Acute tympanic membrane perforations usually heal within weeks and do not require acute intervention. Topical antibiotics, however, are recommended for water-related injuries. Direct trauma may rarely cause ossicular disruption, facial paralysis or inner ear damage (with complete deafness and vertigo).

FOREIGN BODIES

The first attempt at foreign body removal is always the easiest and should be performed by an experienced clinician with appropriate instruments and good illumination. Failure of initial removal may lead to the need for an otherwise unnecessary general anaesthetic.

EAR

Foreign bodies in the external auditory canal are best removed by a hook-shaped instrument, which is passed behind the foreign body and is then used to pull it out. Grasping instruments, such as forceps, should not be used as they invariably lead to the foreign body being displaced further medially. Suction may occasionally be useful.

NOSE

The technique for the removal of nasal foreign bodies is the same as for foreign bodies in the external auditory canal. A topical anaesthetic (e.g. Cophenylcaine) should, however, be applied prior to attempted removal.

The risk of inhalation of a nasal foreign body is minimal and therefore acute removal should be deferred until appropriate personnel and equipment are available.

FISH BONE IN PHARYNX

A fish bone usually lodges in the tonsil or base of tongue and therefore can be relatively easily seen on oral examination and then removed following the prior application of topical anaesthetic. If the fish bone is not seen on oral examination, a more thorough examination by nasopharyngoscopy is required. Fish bones rarely reach the oesophagus and therefore oesophageal evaluation is unnecessary.

Where a fish bone is not found despite a suggestive history, the child should be reviewed until symptoms resolve. Although fish bones are radiolucent radiology may be helpful to detect the presence of complications when symptoms have persisted.

OESOPHAGUS

- The vast majority of swallowed foreign bodies pass without difficulty
- If a foreign body becomes lodged in the oesophagus, it usually does so in the upper oesophagus, at the level of the cricopharyngeus. Lower oesophageal foreign bodies suggest the presence of underlying oesophageal pathology (e.g. stricture)
- The likelihood of impaction is dependent on the size and shape of the foreign body. Objects larger than 20 mm are more likely to impact
- Broken plastic toys are particularly dangerous, as they often impact, yet their radiolucency may lead to a delay in diagnosis, and they may present with respiratory symptoms some time after ingestion
- If a swallowed object reaches the stomach it will almost always pass without incident. Two types of object, however, may cause problems: (i) long thin objects (e.g. hair pins, locker keys) may impact at the

duodenojejunal flexure, and (ii) button batteries, if held up at any point in the alimentary canal, may release alkali, causing local necrosis and perforation

- X-rays should be taken if there are symptoms suggestive of oesophageal lodging (e.g. drooling, dysphagia), or if long thin objects or button batteries have been swallowed. X-rays should include the neck, chest and abdomen. Oesophageal foreign bodies impact in the coronal plane, whereas tracheal lodgement occurs in the sagittal plan. Radiolucent foreign bodies may be imaged by barium swallow
- If an object is impacted in the oesophagus, arrangements should be made for endoscopic removal

CHAPTER 22

EYE CONDITIONS

James Elder

IMPORTANT PRINCIPLES

- *Always test and record vision as the first part of any eye examination.* In infants note following and other visual behaviour and listen to parents' impression about their child's vision
- *A child with a squint is never too young to be seen.* Transient malalignment of the eyes is common up to 6 months of age. A child with a constant squint at any age or any transient squint after 6 months of age should be referred to an ophthalmologist promptly. True squints in general never get better by themselves
- *Never pad a discharging eye*
- *Always pad an eye into which local anaesthetic has been instilled*
- *Do not use local steroid drops unless corneal ulceration has been excluded* by fluorescein staining. Then only use them for short periods (2 days or less) before consulting an ophthalmologist
- *X-ray the orbit (anteroposterior and lateral) if an intraocular foreign body is suspected* from the history, even though the eye may appear normal
- In cases of photophobia or watery eyes in the first year of life, when there is no significant discharge, *consider the possibility of congenital glaucoma*
- All children with a *white red reflex or white masses in the retina must be referred immediately* to an ophthalmologist to exclude retinoblastoma

TRAUMA

FOREIGN BODIES

If a foreign body or corneal ulcer is suspected instil one drop of local anaesthetic to ease the pain and facilitate examination. Suitable local anaesthetics are Ophthaine 1%, amethocaine 0.5 or 1% or benoxinate 0.4%. **Do not use local anaesthetics for the continuing treatment of ocular pain under any circumstance.**

Conjunctival

These are common and are often found on the posterior surface of the upper lid; therefore, *eversion of the lid is essential.* Most foreign bodies are easily removed with a moist cotton wool swab. If they are embedded or difficult to remove, refer the patient to the duty ophthalmologist.

Corneal

If not readily removed with a moistened cotton wool swab, refer to the duty ophthalmologist. Beware of an iris naevus and iris prolapse through a perforating injury of the cornea mimicking a corneal foreign body.

Intraocular

These are generally high velocity fragments. Suspect if the history involves an explosion, striking metal on metal or any other situation involving high-speed objects (e.g. power tools, lawn mower). If the history is at all suggestive, even in the absence of local signs, *X-ray of the orbit* (anteroposterior and lateral) is necessary. If an intraocular foreign body is demonstrated, immediate referral to the duty ophthalmologist is mandatory.

EYELID INJURIES

All eyelid lacerations except the most minor should be repaired as an inpatient procedure. Suspect canalicular injury in all lacerations involving the medial aspect of the eyelids and refer to the duty ophthalmologist. All lacerations involving the lid margin should be referred to the duty ophthalmologist.

HYPHEMA (BLOOD IN THE ANTERIOR CHAMBER)

This generally requires admission to hospital. All cases require ophthalmic referral as there is a potential for secondary haemorrhage and loss of vision.

FRACTURE OF THE ORBITAL BONES

A blow-out fracture through the wall of the orbit is suspected if one or more of the following three cardinal signs are present:

- Restricted movement of the eye, particularly in a vertical plane, with double vision
- Infra-orbital nerve anaesthesia

- Enophthalmos. This may be difficult to assess initially because of lid haematoma

Diagnosis is most often clinical. Plain X-rays and CT scan are used to demonstrate fracture of orbital wall and entrapped orbital tissue (classical sign is tear-drop 'polyp' hanging from the roof of the maxillary antrum). Refer to the duty ophthalmologist.

PENETRATING INJURY

This should always be considered in patients with lacerations involving the eyelids, particularly after motor car accidents. Suspect if the pupil is distorted or iris is prolapsing through the cornea, or pigmented tissue is seen over the sclera. If suspected protect the eye with a cone or shield that places no pressure on the eyelids or eye and admit. Prevent vomiting with anti-emetic. Refer to duty ophthalmologist immediately.

CHEMICAL BURNS

Irrigate the eye with saline or water copiously for 15 min. Instillation of local anaesthetic will facilitate this. Intravenous solution administered by a giving set is the practical method of irrigation. Refer all chemical burns to the duty ophthalmologist. Most alkali burns will require admission.

THERMAL BURNS

The ocular surface is rarely involved. Check for ulceration with fluorescein staining. Butesin picrate ointment is suitable for use on lid burns. Secondary lid swelling may result in corneal exposure and ocular lubricants are then required.

THE ACUTE RED EYE

Common causes of the acute red eye are conjunctivitis, corneal ulceration, corneal or conjunctival foreign body (see above) and iritis.

CONJUNCTIVITIS

Aetiology

- Bacterial — generally pus present
- Viral — generally watery discharge
- Allergic — history of atopy and 'itchy eyes'

Neonatal Conjunctivitis (Ophthalmia Neonatorum)

Neisseria gonorrhoeae

Acute severe, purulent discharge associated with marked conjunctival and lid oedema (clinical appearance is of 'pus under pressure'). Occurs within a few days of birth. This is an ocular emergency because of the risk of corneal perforation.

- *Diagnosis.* Urgent Gram stain (for Gram-negative intracellular diplococci) and culture
- *Treatment.* In uncomplicated cases (i.e. without evidence of sepsis), a single intramuscular dose of ceftriaxone 50 mg/kg (maximum 125 mg) is sufficient. If complicated by sepsis or pre-septal cellulitis, admit and give intravenous ceftriaxone. In all cases local measures such as ocular lavage and topical antibiotics (chloramphenicol or neomycin) may be of help.
- Investigate and treat mother and partner

Chlamydia

Causes about 30% of sticky eyes in neonatal period. Fails to respond to routine topical antibiotics. Untreated, there is a risk of pneumonitis.

- *Diagnosis.* Giemsa stain of conjunctival scraping for intranuclear inclusions. Also antibodies in tears and immunofluorescent stains of conjunctival scrapes. Consult ophthalmologist for advice on specimen collection
- *Treatment.* Oral erythromycin and eye toilet.
- Investigate and treat mother and partner

Other bacteria

Generally caused by *Staphylococcus*, *Streptococcus* or diphtheroids. Culture and treat with neomycin or chloramphenicol eye drops. Rapid clinical response anticipated.

Chemical

Purulent discharge with lid oedema seen within 24 h of instillation of silver nitrate prophylaxis. *Treatment:* frequent lavage and topical neomycin.

Conjunctivitis in Older Children

Management depends on aetiology.

Bacterial

Chloramphenicol eye drops 2 hourly by day and ointment at night.

Viral

Usually clears spontaneously. If it is unclear whether infection is viral or bacterial, neomycin eye drops may be given.

Herpes simplex conjunctivitis

Suspect if have lid vesicles. Check for corneal ulceration and treat with 4 hourly acyclovir ointment. Refer to the duty ophthalmologist.

Allergic

In mild cases, use astringent (phenylephrine 0.125% or naphazoline 0.1%); in moderate cases, use topical antihistamine (antazoline 0.5%). In severe cases, refer to the duty ophthalmologist. Topical steroid or sodium cromoglycate should be given under the supervision of an ophthalmologist.

CORNEAL ULCERATION

Aetiology

- Trauma (with or without a foreign body)
- Herpes simplex (dendritic ulcer)

Diagnosis

- Symptoms: pain, photophobia, lacrimation and blepharospasm
- Fluorescein stain after instillation of local anaesthetic

Treatment

- Traumatic: *chloramphenicol* ointment (1%) and pad. Review in 24 h; if not healed in 48 h refer to ophthalmologist. If healed, continue chloramphenicol ointment b.d. for 1 week
- Herpes simplex: *acyclovir* eye ointment (1 cm inside lower conjunctival sac five times a day for 14 days) and refer to next eye clinic

IRITIS

Rare in children. Symptoms as for corneal ulcer. Pupil small and does not react well to light. Refer to the duty ophthalmologist. Consider iritis in children with juvenile chronic arthritis (JCA) in whom iritis is generally painless.

PRE-SEPTAL (PERIORBITAL) AND ORBITAL CELLULITIS

Both conditions present with erythematous, swollen lids in a febrile, unwell child. In pre-septal cellulitis the lid swelling frequently prevents eye opening. The lids must be separated (a Desmarre's lid retractor may be used) to exclude proptosis and limitation of eye movement. These are important signs of orbital cellulitis, which is associated with sinusitis. Proptosis may be so severe that it prevents lid closure and corneal exposure may result. Bilateral orbital (or pre-septal) cellulitis may be associated with cavernous sinus thrombosis.

TREATMENT

All cases require admission (under General Paediatrics) and intravenous antibiotics (flucloxacillin and penicillin *or* a third-generation cephalosporin if very young or uncertain Hib immunization status).

Refer all cases of suspected orbital cellulitis to ophthalmology and ENT surgeon. **These children require urgent CT scan** to identify orbital collection of pus and sinus pathology. Orbital abscess requires urgent drainage by ENT surgeon. Delay in diagnosis of orbital cellulitis may result in permanent loss of vision.

STRABISMUS OR SQUINT (TURNED EYE)

Refer all children with squint or suspected squint to the eye clinic. This will allow amblyopia to be detected early, and perhaps prevented, and will enable any underlying pathology such as retinoblastoma or cataract to be detected. A child does not 'grow out of' a squint. However, babies in the first few months of life may have an intermittent squint, especially when feeding. If the parents report a squint, the child should be referred to the eye clinic. All children with a first-degree relative with a squint should be seen by an ophthalmologist at about 3–3 1/2 years of age even if there is no squint as they may have a refractive error alone.

A pseudo-strabismus (pseudo-squint) is due to a broad nasal bridge, and/or epicanthic folds. This results in the appearance of a squint, but

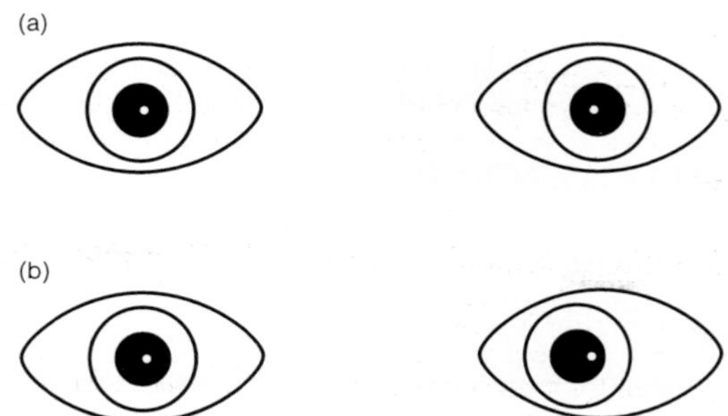

Figure 22.1 Corneal light reflex. Shine a light at the child's eyes and observe the reflection. (a) Eyes are straight and the corneal light reflex is symmetrical. (Note that it is displaced slightly to the nasal side of centre in each eye.) (b) Left convergent strabismus. Reflection from deviated eye is displaced laterally.

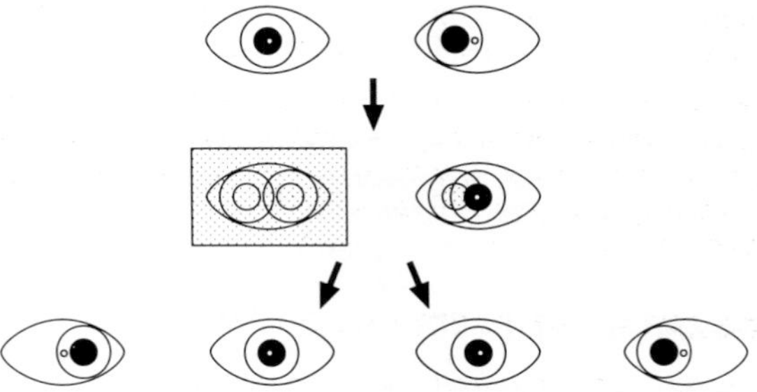

Figure 22.2 The cover test. The child's attention is attracted with a toy. The eye which appears not to be deviating is covered. The uncovered eye is then observed for movement. If there is a convergent squint, the eye will move outwards (top and middle). The uncovered eye should also be observed when the cover is removed from the fellow eye. In alternating squint there will be no movement of the uncovered eye and the previously covered eye will now be deviated (bottom left). In non-alternating or constant squint (vision is usually reduced in deviating eye) there will be a rapid return to the original situation (bottom right). If no movement is detected, the test should be repeated but cover the other eye first.

corneal light reflexes are central and there is no movement on cover testing (see Figs 22.1,2). Only make the diagnosis of pseudostrabismus if absolutely certain. Refer doubtful cases to the eye clinic.

BLOCKED NASOLACRIMAL DUCT

This is a common cause of discharge which persists after the first 2 weeks of life. It presents with a watery eye and mucopurulent discharge. The discharge is worse upon waking and the conjunctiva is not inflamed.

It usually resolves spontaneously, due to opening of the lower end of the tear duct. If infection is troublesome, topical neomycin eye drops may be given (avoid repeated courses of chloramphenicol). Massage over the tear sac after each feed. If discharge and watering have not settled by 12 months of age, refer to an eye clinic for possible probing.

CONGENITAL GLAUCOMA

PRESENTING FEATURES

- Hazy cornea
- Enlarged cornea
- Watery eyes
- Photophobia

This is a rare condition, but early recognition is vital as prompt surgery offers a chance of cure and preservation of vision. All infants with suspected glaucoma require examination under anaesthesia to measure corneal diameter, optic disc cupping and intraocular pressure.

CONGENITAL CATARACTS

Congenital cataracts are rare, but early detection and removal with subsequent optical correction (contact lenses or spectacles) offers a good chance of visual preservation. **All newborn infants should have their red reflexes examined prior to discharge from hospital.** Check the red reflexes and fundi in any infant with poor visual performance (fixation and following). Nystagmus is a late sign of congenital cataracts. Any child suspected to have congenital cataract must be referred to the eye clinic urgently. Unilateral cataract will often present as a squint.

BURNS

Julian Keogh
In collaboration with Russell Taylor

AIMS OF TREATMENT

- Prevent and treat burn shock
- Prevent infection
- Obtain early skin cover
- Prevent hypertrophic scar formation
- Restore function and correct cosmetic defects

ASSESSMENT

AGE

The younger the child, the more likely is shock to occur for a given extent of burn.

ESTIMATION OF THE SURFACE AREA BURNED

The usual adult formula (rule of nines) is not applicable to children, because the proportions contributed by the head and limbs vary at different ages. The burned areas should be plotted accurately on the body chart, and the area calculated with the aid of the Lund-Browder chart (see p. 271). The extent of the burn is only rarely underestimated, but overestimation is common and frequently leads to excessive fluid administration.

ASSESSMENT OF THE DEPTH OF BURN

In most burns, there are varying grades of injury (see Table 23.1).

Table 23.1 Assessment of burn depth

Depth of burn	*Degree*	*Cause*	*Surface/colour*	*Pain sensation*	*Treatment*
Superficial (partial loss of skin)	1st degree	Sun, flash; minor scald	Dry, minor blisters, erythema	Painful	Expose
	2nd degree	Scald	Moist, reddened with broken blisters	Painful	Non-adherent dressing
	Deep 2nd degree	Scald, minor flame contact	Moist white slough, red mottled	Painless	Graft otherwise scarring
Deep (complete loss of skin)	3rd degree	Flame, severe scald or contact	Dry, charred whitish	Painless	Graft

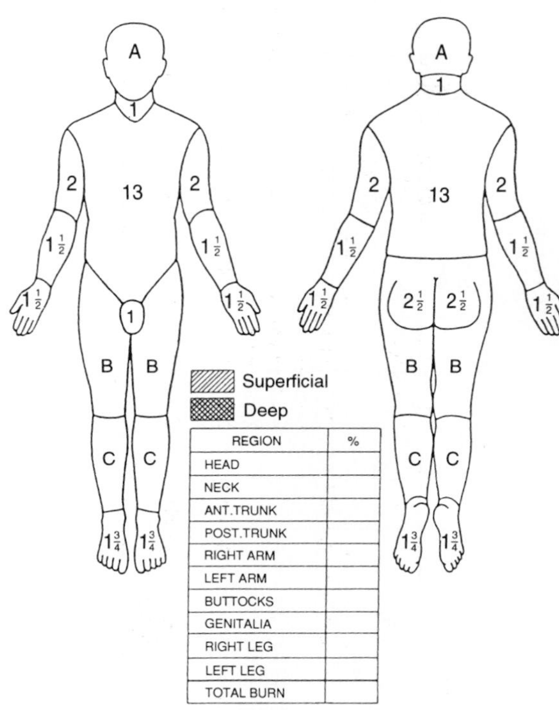

Relative percentage of areas affected by growth

Age (years)	0	1	5	10	15	Adult
A – $\frac{1}{2}$ of head	$9\frac{1}{2}$	$8\frac{1}{2}$	$6\frac{1}{2}$	$5\frac{1}{2}$	$4\frac{1}{2}$	$3\frac{1}{2}$
B – $\frac{1}{2}$ of one thigh	$2\frac{3}{4}$	$3\frac{1}{4}$	4	$4\frac{1}{4}$	$4\frac{1}{2}$	$4\frac{3}{4}$
C – $\frac{1}{2}$ of one leg	$2\frac{1}{2}$	$2\frac{1}{2}$	$2\frac{3}{4}$	3	$3\frac{1}{4}$	$3\frac{1}{2}$

Figure 23.1 Lund–Browder chart

Figure 23.2 Resuscitation of burnt child during first 24 hours

BURNS SURFACE AREA (BSA)............................% TIME IV COMMENCED............................24 HR CLOCK
TIME OF BURN............................24 HR CLOCK DATE............................
WEIGHT IN KG............................

A. BURN RESUSCITATION * 3 × kg × % = ...mL	**1st 24 HOURS (volume)**	**1st 8 HOURS (volume)**	**2nd 8 HOURS (volume)**	**3rd 8 HOURS (volume)**
TYPE OF INFUSION ** **1. 5% Normal Serum Albumin Solution (NSAS)** *** **2. Remainder as Hartmann's Solution** 50% of each type solution is used concurrently	________ mL ________ mL	1/2 of 24 hr vol. ________ mL ________ mL	1/4 of 24 hr vol. ________ mL ________ mL	1/4 of 24 hr vol. ________ mL ________ mL
B. MAINTENANCE FLUID **See oral fluids Information below** 1/2 N saline in 5% dextrose (estimated volume on body wt in kg)	________ mL	1/3 of 24 hr vol. ________ mL	1/3 of 24 hr vol. ________ mL	1/3 of 24 hr vol. ________ mL
TOTAL A & B BURN RESUSCITATION + MAINTENANCE FLUID				

URINARY OUTPUT EXPECTED 0.75 mL/kg/hr = ________ **mL**

ORAL FLUIDS: Most children with burn injury tolerate oral fluids. Initially all children may be offered small amounts of milk and if tolerated the quantity is increased at hourly intervals. Usually after a few hours the patients is receiving most maintenance fluid by mouth, except for those patients with very severe burns.
IF ORAL FLUIDS NOT TOLERATED SEE (B) ABOVE.

NOTES: * In less severe burns 2 mL × kg × 1% in the first 24 hours may be sufficient.
** Normal Serum Albumin Solution (NSAS) is interspersed and not given as one bolus.
*** If no Hartmann's available use normal saline.

2nd 24 HOURS: After the initial 24 hours of fluid replacement, the type of fluid replacement will depend on urinary output, serum electrolytes and haemoglobin. The volume

MANAGEMENT

FIRST AID

Instantly remove clothing or smother flame and apply cold water.

In a minor burn, continue cold water application in a bowl or by compress for up to 30 min. In a major burn, bathe for 20 min while awaiting transport to hospital. Cover to guard against hypothermia or cold injury. Never use ice or ice slush.

Major burns are covered in a special foam transport dressing (if available) or plastic cling wrap, with a blanket for warmth. These patients should be given intravenous fluid, oxygen and morphine, if necessary, before admission to hospital.

MINOR BURNS

Superficial burns of less than 5% of the body surface are suitable for outpatient treatment, unless they occur on the face, neck, hands, feet or perineum. Infants under the age of 12 months are at risk and are more likely to require admission.

Initial Management

- Blisters should be left intact
- Gently cleanse and remove loose skin
- Dress with tulle gras and an absorbent dressing (polyurethane, e.g. Opsite, Tegaderm; or combination polyurethane and absorbent backing, e.g. Mellolin)
- Immobilize with a crepe bandage, plaster slab or sling, if indicated

Subsequent Management

- Leave the initial dressing for 5–8 days. If the dressing is soaked by exudate, redress as necessary without disturbing the adherent tulle
- Consider grafting to the residual areas if healing is not complete by the end of the second week. Graft deep 2nd degree burns by 5–10 days
- Pain, fever and soiled or offensive dressings indicate that the dressing should be changed earlier than anticipated

MAJOR BURNS

Superficial burns to greater than 5% of the body surface area, and deep burns, require admission to hospital. **Transfer should be considered in any child with burns to greater than 10% of body surface area.** Older children with more extensive superficial burns, such as sunburn, may be managed as outpatients (see Fig. 23.1).

General

- A brief history should document the time, causative agent and circumstances of the burn, the therapy already given and the child's general health
- Carefully estimate and chart the extent and depth of the burn
- Weigh the patient if possible—otherwise estimate weight
- Insert an intravenous line in patients with burns greater than 10%. If a central venous line is needed, a specialist burn centre should be involved. Plan intravenous therapy (see below) and commence treatment with Hartmann's solution (lactated Ringers)
- Draw blood for baseline laboratory studies including haemoglobin and haematocrit, serum electrolytes and, in severe burns, blood-grouping and cross-matching
- Insert a urethral catheter for hourly urine volume in all patients with burns greater than 15%
- Analgesia or sedation should be administered as necessary (see p. 393)
- Prevent infection. Care should be taken in ward management to guard against cross-infection. Antibiotics are not prescribed routinely
- Observations of general condition, pulse, respiration rate, temperature, BP and fluid balance (including hourly urine output estimations) are necessary
- **With severe burns to the face, consider early endotracheal intubation. As the face swells, airways obstruction may occur, making intubation very difficult**

Fluid Resuscitation

See Fig. 23.2.

Fluid volume

Three millilitres per kilogram bodyweight per 1% burn surface area (BSA) for the first 24 h. In less severe burns 2 mL/kg bodyweight per 1% BSA may be sufficient.

SURGERY

Type of fluid

Colloid (5% normal serum albumin or substitutes) should constitute one-quarter (in burns greater than 20%), one-third (in burns greater than 30%) or one-half (in burns greater than 40%) resuscitation fluid. The remainder is given as Hartmann's solution in 5% dextrose.

Fluid Maintenance

Type of fluid

Use 1/2 isotonic saline in 5% dextrose to provide extra sodium.

Rate of infusion

In first 24 h:

- First 8 h: one-half resuscitation fluid plus one-third maintenance fluid
- Second 8 h: one-quarter resuscitation fluid plus one-third maintenance fluid
- Third 8 h: one-quarter resuscitation fluid plus one-third maintenance fluid

The 24 h period commences from the time of burning, not from the time of admission. Adjustments are made according to the hourly urine output, which is the best guide to the adequacy of fluid replacement. Expected flow is 0.75 mL/kg per h in children; in the infant and toddler, a urine output of up to 1.0 mL/kg per h is required. Specific gravity of the urine is recorded, as is osmolality of urine and serum if renal function is poor.

Repeated haemoglobin, haematocrit and electrolyte estimations are made. Restlessness may indicate inadequate fluid replacement.

Second 24 h and onwards:

Replacement fluid: approximately one-half volume for first 24 h; maintenance fluid as before. Total volume is given at an even rate over 24 h, and the volume and type of fluid given are adjusted according to urine flow and electrolyte estimations, and decreased as shock diminishes over the succeeding days. Diuresis occurs 2–3 days post-burn.

Oral fluids

Most children will tolerate small amounts of milk (30–60 mL/h) after 4–8 h. If this is tolerated, increase the quantity 4 hourly. In minor burns oral fluids may be commenced earlier. If gastric dilatation associated with vomiting occurs, a nasogastric tube should be inserted.

After 48 h, the majority of fluid intake is usually oral. Children who refuse to drink, or who have burns to the face and mouth may require tube feeding.

Blood

Whole blood is not required initially except in severe, deep burns, and then usually only 24 h post-burn, when the haemoglobin concentration is falling.

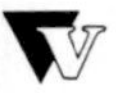

Local Wound Care

Minimal debridement of loose skin is performed initially and then management continues by exposed or closed methods.

Escharotomies should be considered if the peripheral circulation to a limb is jeopardized, but before commencing this procedure contact with a paediatric burns unit is desirable.

Respiratory difficulties require particular attention; intensive care or escharotomy to the trunk may be required.

Exposure

- Indications: for burns on face, perineum, or one surface of the trunk
- Treatment: allow eschar to form if superficial, or apply topical silver sulfadiazine cream. A daily bath is given with warm water and mild soap, followed by application of antibiotic cream

Closed

- Indications: for small children and burns on extremities. Except for burns to the face or perineum, nearly all children are ultimately nursed with closed dressings
- Treatment: an antiseptic tulle gras and gauze for superficial burns, or topical silver sulfadiazine cream and Melolin for deep burns. Fingers and toes are separated with non-adherent tulle and wrapped together (not separately). A daily bath is given with warm water and mild soap, before the dressing

Antibiotics

These are usually only given for proven infection and on the basis of sensitivity tests. On admission, swabs should be taken of the burn area, nose, throat and rectum, and the burn area should be re-swabbed twice weekly. In major burns, multiple 3 mm punch biopsy specimens are the most reliable method of detecting infection. If septicaemia is suspected clinically, blood culture should be performed and antibiotics such as gentamicin and flucloxacillin are commenced.

Nutrition

All children with burns should receive a high-calorie diet containing adequate protein, and vitamin and iron supplements. In severe burns there is a marked increase in metabolic rate, and gastric tube feeding with a complete fluid diet (e.g. Isocal, Osmolite) should be instituted early and adjusted to maintain or increase bodyweight. Involvement of a dietitian is recommended.

Room Temperature

It is desirable that this is in the range of 22–26°C. If a child is partly exposed and nursed in a cool environment, metabolic requirements will increase.

Special Therapy

Physiotherapy and occupational therapy should be commenced early, and continue throughout the course of burn care. Splints and pressure dressings are necessary to control hypertrophic scar formation. The play therapist also has an important role.

Social rehabilitation is important, as many burned children come from disadvantaged homes. **Maltreated children constitute approximately 6% of admissions to the burns unit.** Psychological and psychiatric consultation is often required, and the hospital teacher should liaise with the child's school teachers.

Follow-up

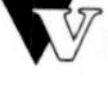

Healed burns and grafts are kept soft with emollient. Pressure therapy and splintage supervision is continued by physiotherapist and occupational therapist. Parents and children need continuing support, and further operations are sometimes necessary to correct contractures and relieve cosmetic defects.

CHAPTER 24

DENTAL CONDITIONS

James Lucas

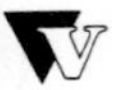

TOOTHACHE AND INFECTION

Patients presenting with toothache or dental abscess and who have severe pain, elevated temperature, obvious facial swelling and/or associated lymph node involvement will require treatment with antibiotics such as penicillin (drug of first choice) and may need admission. A dental consultation should be made immediately for all such patients

Children with intermittent toothache only after eating may be given analgesia and referred to a dentist (unless they are medically compromised, e.g. patients of haematology, cardiology, etc.). This does not apply to the severe spontaneous pain at night which is indicative of pulpitis, periodontitis or early abscess

LOCAL BLEEDING FROM THE MOUTH

- *Always wear gloves*
- If possible irrigate the patient's mouth with cold water or saline, or remove with gauze or tweezers any loose, broken down or excess clots
- Identify the source of bleeding, such as a soft tissue laceration or a tooth socket (bone)
- A bleeding tooth socket is usually due to extraction of a tooth with untreated infection (more rarely a haematological disorder)

SOFT TISSUE LACERATION

All soft tissue lacerations should be assessed for:
- Displacement from bony base (i.e. degloving injury)
- Requirement for repositioning and suturing

BLEEDING TOOTH SOCKET

- Compress alveolus between finger and thumb firmly. Topical Thrombin may be placed on the pack

- If the child is co-operative, place a gauze pad over the socket. Have the child bite on it for 20 min and change when soaked. If the child is not co-operative, a parent should hold the gauze in place. Never pack anything into the socket
- Sedation is frequently necessary. This should be given immediately if indicated
- Antibiotics should be given if infection is present, as indicated by a history of preceding pain or abscess formation. *Penicillin* is the drug of first choice
- The on-call dentist should be contacted for further management or if bleeding continues

TRAUMA TO TEETH AND JAWS

Treatment should be commenced as early as possible if complications such as disturbed jaw growth, malformation or malposition of permanent teeth, tooth loss or pulp death with abscess formation are to be prevented.

SUSPECTED FRACTURES OF THE MANDIBLE AND MAXILLA

- Tetanus prophylaxis (see p. 61) and antibiotics should always be given for a compound fracture opening into the mouth or skin. Penicillin is the drug of choice initially
- A dentist and/or maxillofacial surgeon should be involved in the management of these children from the time of presentation

DENTO-ALVEOLAR INJURIES

- Tooth fracture can occur to the primary or permanent dentition. This may involve the crown or root of the tooth with or without associated alveolar bone fracture
- Assessment is required to establish the extent of the fracture and possible pulp involvement. It is important to determine what has happened to the tooth fragments
- Assess tetanus prophylaxis (see p. 61) and the need for antibiotics
- Dental consultation is necessary for all injuries to teeth, soft tissue and alveolar bone

TOOTH DISPLACEMENT

- This may be palatal or labial, intrusion or total dislodgement, or extrusion with fracture of the labial and/or lingual alveolar bone. Before dental consultation, assess the following and order orthopantomograph (OPG) if possible:

Table 24.1 Eruption times of normal dentition

Primary or deciduous teeth (total 20)

	Central incisors	Lateral incisors	Cuspids	First molars	Second molars
Age (months)	6–12	8–10	16–20	12–16	20–30

There is wide variation in eruption times, particularly of the deciduous teeth. At 1 year an infant has six to eight teeth, at 18 months 12 teeth, and at 2½–3 years 20 teeth. *Should there be no teeth erupted by 12 months, dental consultation should be sought.*

Permanent teeth (total 32)

	Central incisors	Lateral incisors	Cuspids	First bicuspid	Second bicuspid	First molars	Second molars	Third molars
Age (years)	6–9	7–10	10–12	10–12	11–12	6–7	11–13	17–21

The first permanent teeth to erupt are the lower first molars and central incisors.

- Degree of fracture and/or amount of displacement
- Occlusion (whether bite is distorted)
- Mucosal lacerations

Displaced Primary Teeth

- If a primary tooth is avulsed (knocked out) do not reimplant it
- The on-call dentist should be made aware of the degree of displacement, tooth fracture and soft tissue or mucosal laceration, and called to assess other injuries of the primary teeth
- Appropriate treatment will then be either extraction or stabilization of soft tissues

Displaced or Avulsed Permanent Incisor Teeth

- *Ideally, the tooth should be reimplanted in the socket immediately.* Handle the tooth gently by the crown only, not by the root surface
- If it is not possible to reimplant, keep the tooth stored in milk, saliva or plastic wrap until the on-call dentist arrives. If the tooth is replaced within 30 min there is a high chance of success
- Order appropriate radiographs: OPG, lateral cephalogram and chest X-ray if the tooth is missing (to make sure it has not been inhaled)
- Once the tooth has been reimplanted, a temporary splint may be constructed from aluminium foil moulded around the tooth

Splinting and stabilization of the teeth will be required, as well as treatment of associated soft tissue lacerations. Appropriate dental follow-up should be arranged.

OTHER DENTAL PROBLEMS

The following problems may present as emergencies, but are generally not so:

- Lost filling (unless associated with significant pain)
- Broken denture or orthodontic plate
- Loose band or wire of fixed orthodontic appliance. Tuck wire out of the way with haemostat. The sharp end can be covered with chewing gum or blue tac
- Loose artificial crown
- Superficially chipped tooth
- Minor laceration not requiring suturing. Give mouth rinses with warm saline and chlorhexidine gluconate 0.2% (Chlorhex, Savacol)

These patients may be advised to ring their own dentist for an appointment at the earliest opportunity.

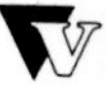

25

CHAPTER 25

COMMON DEVELOPMENTAL AND BEHAVIOUR PROBLEMS

Frederick Jarman

In collaboration with Bronwyn Parry-Fielder

Behavioural and developmental problems are best understood in a transactional framework, where symptoms and signs are the result of the interaction between inborn biological attributes of the child and factors within the environment.

INFANT 'COLIC'

Colic is defined as primary excessive crying in young infants of undetermined cause. The crying develops during the early weeks of life and may persist until the baby is 3 or 4 months of age. Crying often lasts for several hours, worse in the late afternoon and evening, and is associated with the baby drawing up his/her knees as if in pain and passing flatus. However, there is no evidence that colic is associated with abdominal pain or that it represents anything more than the upper limit of crying seen in all young infants over the early months of life. Wessel's definition of 'paroxyms of irritability, fussing or crying lasting for more than 3 hours per day for 3 or more days per week for 3 or more weeks' identifies a group of infants who cry more than 90% of other babies their age.

Colic should be distinguished from:
- Otitis media, raised intracranial pressure, corneal abrasion, intestinal obstruction, urinary tract infection via history, examination and urine examination
- Cow milk intolerance (rare without vomiting, abdominal distension, skin rashes)
- Lactose intolerance (frothy stools, abdominal distension)
- Gastro-oesophageal reflux with oesophagitis (rare without vomiting)

MANAGEMENT

- Reassurance that the infant is not sick or in pain and that some babies cry more than others in early infancy because of an intrinsic sensitivity and/or environmental overload
- Regular supportive contact with parents; monitor for maternal depression
- Reduce environmental overstimulation: noise, light, excessive handling
- Adherence to routines
- Demand feeding: semi-upright posture, comfortable chair
- Carrying in an infant *snuggly*, pacifier, baby massage, gentle rocking and patting
- Medication is rarely indicated
- **Random changes of feed/formula are not advised,** nor are trials on antireflux therapy unless reflux is strongly suspected on clinical grounds or confirmed on oesophagoscopy/pH monitoring

SLEEP PROBLEMS

ASSESSMENT

Most new babies do not establish nocturnal sleeping patterns until 3 months of age or sleep through the night until 6 months. Up to one-third of Australian children continue to wake once or more per night until 3–4 years of age. In the majority of cases these 'abnormal' sleep rhythms are learned behaviours, from children never having learned how to drop off to sleep on their own or get back to sleep without their parents' help when they wake through the night as part of the normal cycling of sleep. If parents and children are not unduly distressed by this behaviour there is no reason to intervene.

Medical causes of sleep disturbance are rare and can be ruled out on history, examination and limited laboratory investigation before a behavioural programme is commenced. Consider *otitis media with effusion, upper airways obstruction causing obstructive sleep apnoea, gastro-oesophageal reflux, nocturnal seizures and raised intracranial pressure* as conditions that might cause night-time 'arousals'. Psychosocial stresses, such as family conflict, parental separation, moving house or other major disruptions to routine can also trigger sleep problems. However, serious psychological problems in children with sleep disturbance are uncommon.

MANAGEMENT

Ask parents to keep a 24 h diary of the child's sleep patterns for several days prior to any intervention.

Behavioural techniques are best reserved for infants over 6 months of age.

For *settling problems at bedtime:*
- Note the time and duration of daytime naps and set a temporarily later bedtime
- Adhere to a strict pre-bedtime routine, so that the child moves through the same sequence in the same order each night
- *Take the child into the bedroom awake*
- Use a night light and a fur toy for toddlers and preschoolers, and a door gate across the doorway for children old enough to be in a bed
- Leave the room within a few minutes; prolonged parental presence in the bedroom exacerbates separation difficulties
- Return the child to their bedroom if they come out, and use a door gate to block their escape if this becomes a persistent problem
- Use 'controlled crying' for persistent crying after leaving the bedroom (see below)

For *frequent waking through the night* various behavioural techniques can be used. The most commonly used involves *controlled crying.* Respond to the child's crying at progressively lengthening intervals until they drop back to sleep, e.g. leave the child to cry for 2 min and then go into the bedroom, soothe the child and leave the room. Wait 4 min before going back in the second time, 6 min before going back in the third time, 8 min before going back in the fourth time, etc. until the child cries him/herself back to sleep.

Other techniques found to be useful include *camping out* (which involves one parent sleeping in the child's room on a camp stretcher next to the child's bed/cot and progressively moving further and further away from the child), and *scheduled waking* (which involves the parent actively waking the child on two occasions during the night, about 30 min before an expected spontaneous arousal). Two weeks are usually required for either of these strategies.

Whatever behavioural technique is used **it is important that spontaneous arousals not be reinforced by feeding, or the use of pacifiers or excessive parental attention through the night.**

Sedative medication given nightly for 1–2 weeks (*trimeprazine* 1–2 mg/kg per dose, *chloral hydrate* 25–50 mg/kg per dose) can be used as a supplement to the behavioural techniques listed above, but only in babies over 12 months of age.

Parasomnias, such as *night terrors, sleep walking* and *sleep talking* are not true night-time arousals because they occur in deep stage 4 sleep. Night terrors, the most disturbing of these disorders, are characterized by the child suddenly screaming and thrashing about in the early part of the night and occasionally running around the house in a state of high agitation. The child is usually inconsolable and has no memory for the event afterwards. The parasomnias cluster in two age ranges: 2–3 year olds and 6–9 year olds. They are self-limiting over a period of weeks to months and usually require no active treatment other than to usher the child back to bed and sit with them until the agitated state has settled. Persistent problems may be treated with scheduled waking or *imipramine* (0.5–2 mg/kg per night for 6–8 weeks).

TEMPER TANTRUMS

A normal developmental task of toddlers is to assert their independence and test parental limits. The 'terrible twos' and the resultant tantrums that herald this developmental stage actually start in most children at 15–18 months and often persist until 3–4 years of age. Tantrums are best ignored, providing both parents persist with this strategy and follow the guidelines below:

- Stay calm
- Look away
- Move away
- Say nothing
- Go into another room and busy yourself with something else (lock the door if necessary)
- Persistently ignore until the tantrum stops
- Praise appropriate behaviour as soon as it occurs

Note: Ignoring a behaviour that has previously attracted attention will result in its escalation over the first few days before the behaviour starts to decline.

OPPOSITIONAL BEHAVIOUR

Resistant and oppositional behaviour is universal in all young children from time to time, and is rarely an indicator of individual or family psychopathology. Surveys indicate that over 75% of parents of 2–4 year olds report their children to be stubborn and disobedient on a frequent basis. Most oppositional behaviour in school-age children and adolescents is also developmentally normal, providing it is not associated with violent or antisocial behaviour or serious school difficulties. Diagnostic interviews with the child and family are necessary to exclude serious pathology that might warrant referral for psychotherapy. Standardized child behaviour checklists completed by parents and teachers help quantify the severity of the behaviour disturbance objectively.

In most instances, general supportive counselling and behaviour modification is highly effective in working with parents of younger children:

- *Praise and reward the child's 'good' behaviour.* When children are being difficult they rarely receive much attention for good behaviour. To redress this balance parents can be encouraged to *'catch the child being good'* as often as possible. Verbal praise works best if it is immediate and specific, and if the parents 'praise the behaviour not the child'
- Special behaviour can be acknowledged with concrete rewards, given after the fact, not offered as a bribe beforehand. Green marks with a texta pen or stamps on the back of the child's hand work well for toddlers. Over age 2 years, good boy or good girl sticker charts attached to the refrigerator door are very powerful visual reinforcers of positive behaviour. Lucky dips or points/poker chips which can be cashed in later for an agreed-upon set of rewards are effective for older children. Rewards and punishments should be kept separate, lest the difficult child quickly slide into debt!
- *Prioritize the child's difficult behaviour.* Parents need to save their energy for the behaviours that matter most, and punishments lose their effectiveness if overused. Parents should nominate and agree on four or five high-priority behaviours that they will tackle actively in the first instance; everything else by definition becomes a lesser priority behaviour
- *Ignore lesser priority difficult behaviours.* Many irritating behaviours are exacerbated by the parental attention they attract. Breaking eye contact, staying calm and walking away will lessen these behaviours if all family members are consistent and parents can persist with this for at least several days
- *Provide immediate disciplinary consequences for high-priority difficult behaviour.* Consequences work best if they are applied immediately for high-priority behaviours, such as non-compliance, oppositionalism and physical aggression. Parents should work towards staying calm, avoiding threats and applying consequences immediately without second chances
- *Time out* is the preferred disciplinary consequence for children over 18 months of age. *Time out* can be applied in a playpen, a chair in the

corner, the bedroom, the back steps, or if away from home, against a fence or in the car. The child should stay in time out for a maximum of 1 min per year of age; if they leave time out without permission they should be returned and the time started again
- *Withdrawing privileges* is effective for children over 6 years old. Withdrawals work best if they are enacted as soon as possible after the offending behaviour occurs, and if the punishment is not too protracted. Punishments do not have to cause suffering to be effective

Refining the way parents handle young children is often all that is necessary to bring many non-compliant behaviours under control. These techniques can be applied sequentially by the doctor over three to four 30 min sessions.

BREATH HOLDING

Breath holding has a peak incidence in the toddler years, occurring in 5% of all children (see also Table 12.3, p. 169). Both cyanotic and acyanotic (pallid) events have been described, the former being much more common. Cyanotic spells are inevitably triggered by the child encountering frustration, becoming distressed and crying intensely. The child then holds his/her breath at the end of expiration and becomes centrally cyanosed, often losing consciousness in the process. Occasionally, loss of consciousness is followed by a generalized seizure. Consciousness is usually regained within 15–30 s. Discrimination from a primary seizure disorder is made on the basis of the breath holding child becoming cyanosed *before* losing consciousness, with the prodrome as described above.

Acyanotic 'breath holding' attacks are vasovagal spells (simple faints) which occur in response to fear or pain. Crying is minimal, with the child suddenly becoming apnoeic and losing consciousness. The child is pale and bradycardic during such episodes.

MANAGEMENT

- Reassurance that breath-holding spells are harmless and require no active treatment
- Avoid reinforcing the tantruming behaviour through excessive parental anxiety or attention (see Temper Tantrums, p. 285)
- Coma position until the child regains consciousness spontaneously

DEVELOPMENT

HEAD BANGING

Head banging is a common distressing behaviour manifest by young children, occurring in 5–15% of normal infants and toddlers. Head banging typically occurs up to 60–80 times/min and lasts for several minutes to 1 h or more per episode. The child almost always appears undistressed; in fact the association between head banging and other repetitive behaviours in children (e.g. body rocking, thumb sucking) has led most experts to view this activity as one of self-soothing. The child almost never sustains significant injury as a result of head banging, although mild bruising and abrasions are common. In developmentally delayed, autistic or severely emotionally deprived children head banging may occur with such force to warrant the use of helmets and/or psychotropic medication (e.g. thioridazine).

MANAGEMENT

- Reassure parents that head banging is a normal self-limiting behaviour in most children and will not cause brain damage
- Avoid reinforcing the behaviour through excessive parental attention and/or punishment
- Distraction or active ignoring are the 'treatments' of choice while awaiting for spontaneous resolution, which almost always occurs by age 3 years

EATING/FEEDING PROBLEMS

Through the second and third year of life the normal growth rate of children decreases dramatically as does the relative requirement for most nutrients (see p. 362). The average monthly weight gain in children between 6 and 12 months of age is 500 g, compared with 183 g for children between 12 and 24 months and 166 g for children between 2 and 3 years. Most parents are concerned about the apparent poor weight gain and food intake of their toddlers, despite being reassured that their child is growing at a normal rate for age. This concern arises at the very time toddlers are asserting their independence and coming to a rapid understanding about the power not eating has on their relationships. If a child is physically healthy and active, most mealtime problems are behaviour problems not medical problems.

The correlates of poor eating behaviour in toddlers include variable mealtimes, grazing between meals, excessive juice and/or milk intake, excessive parental attention to eating, and the 'food is love' association, whereby food and the act of eating take on a significance far beyond a simple nutritional one.

MANAGEMENT

The *management* of poor eating behaviour is as follows:

- Rule out physical causes of poor eating such as reflux oesophagitis, milk allergy, lactose intolerance, pharyngeal incoordination and neurological disorders
- Monitor the child's growth velocity on standardized charts
- Help the parents adopt reasonable expectations about the child's eating behaviour and support them in their anxiety about the child not eating. Help the parents to 'back off'!
- Establish clear mealtime routines and insist that the child sit with the family at mealtimes
- Restrict milk and/or juice intake
- Limit 'between meal' grazing
- Encourage independent feeding with finger foods
- Ignore poor eating behaviour
- Do not prepare special meals or pander to 'exotic' tastes
- Praise and reward appropriate eating behaviour

PHYSICAL AGGRESSION

Physical aggression is a common reaction to frustration in young children and is often modelled on similar behaviour within the family or social environment. The origins of serious aggressive behaviour are multifaceted and are usually the result of a complex series of interactions between the following:

- Child factors: temperament, brain injury, low IQ, learning difficulties, chronic illness, psychopathology
- Family factors: poor modelling, inadequate monitoring, parenting incompetence, poverty, parental criminality, parental psychopathology, physical/sexual abuse
- Social factors: socio-cultural norms, media influences, school failure, socio-economic disadvantage, lack of vocational opportunities

The doctor should explore these issues with the child and family and develop a formulation about probable contributing factors. At a practical level the doctor can work with parents on fine tuning the way they handle such behaviours (see Oppositional Behaviour, p. 285). Providing clear consistent disciplinary limits will assist the child in developing better self-control. Smacking used as a punishment models physical violence and sends an ambiguous message to children about the appropriateness of hitting another person, and should therefore be avoided. Time out or withdrawal of privileges as described above are the consequences of choice for aggressive behaviour for children under 10 years of age.

Referral for psychotherapy is indicated if aggression is:
- Repeated
- Severe
- Causes injury
- Is associated with lack of remorse, other delinquent/antisocial behaviours or family psychopathology

STEALING

Isolated minor theft is surprisingly common in school-aged Australian children, and while not acceptable, is usually not an indication of serious pathology. Isolated theft is often associated with one or more of the following characteristics:
- Typical school-age risk-taking behaviour
- Low self-esteem in a child searching for peer acceptance
- A reaction to recent family or psychosocial stress
- A cry for help and attention, with a subconscious desire to be caught

Stealing may also be associated with the same child, family and social factors seen in children with other conduct/antisocial behaviours (see Physical Aggression, p. 289)

MANAGEMENT

- Insist that the child return the stolen goods and/or personally apologise to the person(s) from whom they were stolen
- Child to pay in part for stolen items through deduction in pocket money or by working off debt
- Punishment may include withdrawal of privileges, such as grounding or restriction of TV
- Referral for psychotherapy if stealing is recurrent, associated with lack of remorse or other antisocial/delinquent behaviours

ATTENTION-DEFICIT HYPERACTIVITY DISORDER

Attention-deficit hyperactivity disorder (ADHD) is a disorder characterized by *developmentally inappropriate* degrees of inattentiveness, overactivity and impulsivity. These qualities arise early in childhood, are relatively chronic in nature and are not readily accounted for on the basis of gross neurological, sensory, language or motor impairment, intellectual disability or severe emotional disturbance. These difficulties are typically associated with deficits in rule-governed behaviour and in maintaining a consistent pattern of work performance over time.

Recent evidence indicates that ADHD has a predominantly biological basis, but that its manifestations are modified by family and social factors. A genetic component to ADHD is now established.

ASSESSMENT

Assessment should include some or all of the following (Table 25.1):

- Child and family interview. *Note:* Observation of the child's behaviour in the office is *not* a reliable guide to the child's behaviour in other settings and should not be used to either confirm or refute the diagnosis of ADHD
- Physical and neurologic examination
- Assessment of visual acuity
- Referral for audiological assessment, including testing in background noise and short term auditory memory
- Serum lead level in children from high-risk groups
- Standardized child behaviour checklists completed by parents and teachers enable the child's behaviour to be compared with same age children, and are important diagnostic tools
- Referral for formal cognitive achievement and testing; 25% of children with ADHD have coexistent learning disabilities

MANAGEMENT

The management of ADHD involves a combination of the following.

Medication

Stimulants

Dexamphetamine (0.15–0.5 mg/kg per day) and Methylphenidate (0.3–1.0 mg/kg per day) are usually given in two divided doses at breakfast and lunch-time, with breaks on weekends and school holidays. About 75% of ADHD children treated with stimulants display dramatic improvements in behaviour, academic performance, cognitive processing and socialization. Side-effects include decreased appetite, insomnia, tearfulness and nausea, most of which are transient.

Under some circumstances, particularly when the treatment response is equivocal, a blinded, controlled trial of medication versus placebo with

Table 25.1 Diagnostic criteria for ADHD (DSM IV)

Either inattention or hyperactivity/impulsivity

Inattention

At least six of the following symptoms have persisted for at least 6 months to a degree that is maladaptive and inconsistent with developmental level

- Often fails to give close attention to details or makes careless mistakes in schoolwork, work or other activities
- Often has difficulty sustaining attention in tasks or play activities
- Often does not seem to listen to what is being said to him or her
- Often does not follow through on instructions and fails to finish schoolwork chores or duties in the workplace (not due to oppositional behaviour or failure to understand instructions)
- Often has difficulty organizing tasks or activities
- Often avoids or strongly dislikes tasks (such as schoolwork or homework) that require sustained mental effort
- Often loses things necessary for tasks or activities (e.g. school assignments, pencils, books, tools or toys)
- Often easily distracted by extraneous stimuli
- Often forgetful in daily activities

Hyperactivity/impulsivity

At least six of the following symptoms of hyperactivity/impulsivity have persisted for at least 6 months to a degree that is maladaptive and inconsistent with developmental level

Hyperactivity

- Often fidgets with hands or feet and squirms in seat
- Often leaves seat in classroom or in other situations in which remaining seated is expected
- Often runs about or climbs excessively in situations where it is inappropriate (in adolescents or adults may be limited to feelings of restlessness)
- Often has difficulty playing or engaging in leisure activities quietly
- Often 'on the go' or acts as if 'driven by a motor'
- Often talks excessively

Impulsivity

- Often blurts out answers to questions before the questions have been completed
- Often has difficulty waiting in line or awaiting turn in games or group situations
- Often interrupts or intrudes on others

Onset no later than 7 years of age

Symptoms must be present in two or more situations (e.g. at school, at home and/or at work)

The disturbance causes clinically significant distress or impairment in social, academic, occupational functioning

Does not occur exclusively during the course of a pervasive developmental disorder, schizophrenia, or other psychotic disorder, and is not better accounted for by a mood disorder, anxiety disorder, or dissociative disorder, or a personality disorder

---

Children with ADHD should be assessed and managed by an experienced paediatrician.

standardized outcome measures (e.g. Conners Rating Scales) may be helpful.

Tricyclic antidepressants

Desipramine or imipramine (both 1–4 mg/kg per day) are useful for those ADHD children with comorbid symptoms of anxiety or depression, which generally predict a poor response to stimulants. Baseline cardiac exam and ECG is recommended before starting treatment with tricyclics in excess of 2 mg/kg per day.

Clonidine (1–4 μg/kg per day)

Useful in combination with stimulants or for those children with co-existent tic disorders, where stimulants are contraindicated.

Major tranquillizers

Thioridizine (1–2 mg/kg per day) may be beneficial in children with extreme aggressive and explosive behaviour, but has a negative impact on cognitive function because of its sedative action.

Other Therapies

- *Parent training:* involves working with parents on establishing clear routines, rules and consequences and fine tuning the way that they handle their child's difficult behaviour
- *Educational interventions:* ADHD children respond best to a highly organized and routine classroom structure with a minimum of distraction and noise. They do best if seated at the front centre of the room, as close to the teacher as possible, preferably near positive role models. Frequent adult input and stretch breaks are mandatory, as are clear rules and consequences for unacceptable behaviour. Additional input to assist with learning difficulties is often necessary.
- *Cognitive behaviour therapy:* teaches the child to delay their impulsive responding style and exert greater self-control
- *Family therapy:* opens lines of communication between family members, elicits effective responses, provides insight into the mechanisms and causes of family conflict and forges healthier interactional patterns.
- *Individual counselling:* Children and parents may each benefit from individual psychotherapy to ventilate feelings of distress and gain insight into the origins of their problems
- *Dietary therapy:* Less than 10% of ADHD children respond to a diet free of colourings, preservatives and salicylates. There is no established association between sugar intake and hyperactive behaviour, despite this being an anecdotal impression reported by many parents.

About 80% of ADHD children will have symptoms through adolescence/adulthood, with 30% having ongoing major problems with academic underachievement, early school dropout, antisocial behaviour and delinquency.

ENURESIS

The age at which children achieve urinary continence varies. For practical purposes enuresis is defined as daytime wetting (diurnal enuresis) after age 4 years or night-time wetting (nocturnal enuresis) after age 6 years, or wetting that occurs after a period of continence of at least 3 months (secondary enuresis). Sixty per cent of children with diurnal enuresis also have nocturnal enuresis, whereas only 10% of children with nocturnal enuresis also have diurnal enuresis.

Primary enuresis is usually related to a maturational delay in attaining bladder continence. A positive family history is common, as is a smaller functional bladder capacity. Rarely, medical factors may cause enuresis (see below); this is much more common in secondary enuresis than primary enuresis.

- Disorders with increased urinary output, e.g. diabetes mellitus
- Disorders causing bladder irritability, e.g. urinary tract infection
- Disorders with abnormal sphincter control, e.g. spinal dysraphism
- Structural urinary tract abnormalities, e.g. ectopic ureter

Limited medical investigation, which should always include a urine microscopy and culture, may be indicated depending on the history and examination findings.

MANAGEMENT

Diurnal Enuresis

- Urinary containment exercises. The child should go to the toilet immediately they feel the urge but sit and hold the urine stream for 1 min. They should then stop and start the flow of urine on three occasions before emptying the bladder completely, as a means of increasing sphincter strength
- Scheduled voiding. The child sits on the toilet and urinates at scheduled intervals through the day, whether or not they feel the urge, starting at 1 h intervals and increasing to 2–3 h intervals as control is obtained. This increases the functional bladder capacity progressively as well as reducing the likelihood of accidents
- Medication. Anticholinergic agents (e.g. oxybutynin or imipramine) may be useful in the short term as a means of increasing sphincter tone

Nocturnal Enuresis

- No treatment. Spontaneous resolution rate is 15% per year
- Fluid restriction before bed is of no value
- Scheduled waking. Parents may wake the child and take them to the toilet before they go to bed. Unlikely to be effective if wetting occurs at variable times through the night
- Star charts. The child receives a sticker on a chart for dry nights with a reward for a certain number of stickers.
- Conditioning alarms. When the child wets, the alarm sounds, waking the child. The parents need to ensure that the child is awake and is taken to the toilet before going back to bed. Progress is monitored on a chart. Effective in 90% of children over a 6–8 week period
- Medication. A proportion of children with enuresis may have decreased nocturnal release of antidiuretic hormone. *Desmopression acetate* nasal spray has recently been licensed for use in Australia and can be effective in resistant cases. Imipramine is effective in 50% of children, however relapse rates are high once medication is ceased. As side effects are common and it can be fatal in high doses, imipramine is no longer recommended for children with enuresis.

LEARNING DIFFICULTIES

Problems with learning affect 10–15% of the school-age population. Learning difficulties may be the result of global impairments in cognitive capacity (intellectual disability), hearing or vision problems, chronic illness, medication side-effects, severe emotional disturbance, primary attention deficits, low motivation, poor teaching, or specific deficits in the processing of spoken or written language, termed *specific learning disabilities*. Specific learning disabilities are characterized by a discrepancy between the child's overall intelligence and achievement in school that is not accounted for on the basis of conditions listed previously. Failure in school of any origin may cause secondary problems with self-esteem and behaviour.

ASSESSMENT

This should include:

- History from parents *and* teachers of the child's school difficulties. Request previous school reports, psychometric testing results and details of behaviour at home and at school

- Standardized child behaviour checklists completed by parents and teachers are an important adjunct to behavioural assessment by enabling the child's behaviour to be compared with other children the same age
- Physical and neurological examination to rule out chronic illnesses and underlying gross neurological problems. The traditional neurological examination is usually normal, although 'soft' neurological signs may be present and include subtle abnormalities of tone, reflexes, motor co-ordination and sensory function
- Referral to a paediatrician for neurodevelopmental assessment. These tests sample aspects of development that are important for learning in school, including gross and fine motor co-ordination, visual–spatial orientation, short-term auditory memory, visual sequencing and oral language. Although neurodevelopmental testing will shed further light on the child's strengths and weaknesses that might partially or fully explain their school difficulties, it is no substitute for formal psychological testing
- Referral to an educational psychologist for formal cognitive testing, including testing of intelligence and academic achievement

MANAGEMENT

- Individualized and dependent on cause(s)
- Collaborate with teachers and parents and ensure that everyone (including the child) has a common understanding of the basis of the learning difficulty, and the accommodative strategies that can be used
- Foster and promote the child's strengths
- Individualized or small group remedial educational assistance is the cornerstone of intervention for most children. There is no single best approach. The paediatrician can advocate extra resources in the classroom to assist the child or recommend outside tutoring if help at school is not available
- Behavioural counselling, social skills training, pharmacotherapy for attention deficits, etc. can be recommended depending on the associated problems identified
- Monitor progress and re-evaluate at intervals

SPEECH AND LANGUAGE DELAY

Delayed development of speech and language is common. The delay may occur alone or be associated with other conditions such as hearing impairment, general developmental delay, autism or social–emotional deprivation.

Indicators of speech and language difficulties may include parental concern, lack of babbling or vocalization, unintelligible speech, poor language comprehension, lack of speech and dysfluency (Table 25.2). Early referral to a speech pathologist is important and should be considered as part of the paediatric assessment (Table 25.3).

Table 25.2 Indicators of language delay

Age (years)	*Reason for concern*
0.5	No response to sound, not cooing, not laughing
1	Not localizing sound, no babble, no vocalization
1.5	No meaningful words except *mum/dad,* not pointing to wanted things
2	Expressive vocabulary less than 20 words
2.5	Expressive vocabulary less than 50 words or no two-word combinations, not understanding simple instructions without gesture, stuttering
3	Not understood within family, not using early syntax (e.g. verb + ing *running* noun + plural *hats*)
4	Not understood outside family, not using complex sentences (e.g. *and but because if when so before after*)
5	Speech not reasonably clear, not fluent, not complex, not understood

Table 25.3 Assessment of language delay

What to consider	*What to do*
Hearing	Audiology referral ENT referral
Developmental delay	Paediatric assessment Psychological assessment Speech pathology referral
Social–emotional context	
Family history of speech/language/ fluency problems	
Specific speech/language disorder	Speech pathology referral
Stuttering	Speech pathology referral

CHAPTER 26

DEVELOPMENTAL DELAY AND DISABILITY

Dinah Reddihough, Doug Bryan and Margaret Rowell

ASSESSMENT OF CHILD DEVELOPMENT

An integral part of paediatrics is the monitoring of children's development. *Developmental screening is not definitive but sorts out children who probably do have developmental delay from those who probably do not.* Screening may include, but is not limited to, the administration of formal developmental screening tests, such as the Denver II.

Developmental screening tests are not merely history check-lists; they need to be formally administered. Please refer to the Denver Manual for details.

Children who fail developmental screening should be referred (either to a paediatrician or to a multidisciplinary assessment team) for formal developmental assessment, using standardized assessment tools such as the *Bayley Scales of Infant Development* and the *Griffiths Developmental Scales.*

GUIDE TO DEVELOPMENTAL MILESTONES

Table 26.1 is a guide to developmental milestones. It is not a formal screening tool.

DEVELOPMENTAL DELAY AND DISABILITY

Children with a developmental delay and/or disability have the same basic needs as non-disabled children. They have a potential for further development and the principles of normal development apply.

Specific disabilities in one area may cause secondary disabilities in other areas (e.g. children with motor disabilities with reduced opportunity for exploration may have a delay in their understanding).

Table 26.1 Developmental milestones

*Age**	*Gross motor*	*Fine motor adaptive*	*Language*	*Personal–social*
1 m	Lifts head momentarily while prone (0–3 w)	Visual following to mid-line (0–5 w)		Watches face (0–4 w)
2 m	Lifts head momentarily to erect position when sitting	Hands predominantly open	Vocalizes (0–7 w)	Smiles responsively (0–7 w)
3 m	Lifts head to 90° while prone (0–10 w)	Visual following past mid-line (0–10 w)	Laughs (6–10 w)	
4 m	Head steady when held erect (6–17 w)	Plays with hands together (6–15 w)	Goos and gurgles	Excited by approach of food
5 m	No head lag when pulled to sitting (3–6 m) Rolls over	Grasps rattle (10–18 w) Reaches for object with palmar grasp (3–5½ m)	Squeals (6–18 w)	Smiles spontaneously (6 w–5 m)
6 m	Lifts head forward when pulled to sit (9–19 w)	Passes block hand to hand (4½–7½ m)	Turns to voice (3½–8½ m)	Friendly to all comers
8 m	Maintains sitting position without support		Repetition of syllables (e.g. ba ba, Dada)	Feeds self biscuit (5–8 m) Tries to get toy out of reach (5–9 m)
10 m	Stands holding on (5–10 m)	Index finger approach	'Mum', 'Dad' without meaning (6–10 m)	Shy with strangers Plays peek-a-boo

(Continued)

Table 26.1 *(Continued)*

*Age**	*Gross motor*	*Fine motor adaptive*	*Language*	*Personal–social*
12 m	Walks holding on to furniture (7½–12½ m)	Crude finger–thumb grasp (7–11 m)	Imitates speech sounds (6–11 m)	Gives up a toy
15 m	Walks alone (11½–15 m)	Neat pincer grasp of pellet (9–15 m)	'Mum', 'Dad' with meaning (9–15 m)	Indicates wants (10½–14½ m)
1½ y	Walks well (11½–18 m)	Builds tower of two blocks (12–20 m)	Three words other than 'Mum', 'Dad' (12–20 m)	Drinks from cup (10–17 m)
2 y	Walks up steps without help (14–22 m)	Scribbles (12–24 m)	Points to one named body part (14–23 m)	Feeds self with spoon (12–24 m)
2½ y	Throws ball (15–32 M)	Builds tower of four blocks (15–26 m)	Combines two words (14–27 m)	Helps in house — simple tasks (15–24 m)
3 y	Pedals tricycle (21 m–3 y)	Imitates vertical line (18 m–3 y) Copies circle (2½–3½ y)	Uses three word sentences	Puts on clothes (2–3 y)
4 y	Balances on one foot (2¾–4½ y)	Copies square	Gives first and last name (2–4 y)	Dresses with supervision (2½–3½ y)
5 y	Hops on one foot (3–5 y)	Draws person in three parts (3–5 y)	Knows some colours (3–5 y) Knows age	Dresses without supervision (2½–5 y)

w, weeks; m, months; y, years

*Age indicates when at least 90% of a normal group of children will achieve the test. Figures in parentheses represent the range from 25th to 90th centiles for achievement.

Transient developmental delay may be associated with:

- Prematurity
- Physical illness
- Prolonged hospitalization
- Family stress
- Lack of opportunities to learn

Causes of *persistent developmental delay* include:

- Language disorders
- Intellectual disability
- Cerebral palsy
- Autism
- Hearing impairment
- Visual impairment
- Degenerative neuromuscular disorders

Once suspicion regarding a child's development has been raised, a complete paediatric consultation is required. This should include full details of the family, obstetric, neonatal and developmental histories. Liason with the family doctor to obtain background information is often helpful. A history of loss of previously attained developmental skills is suggestive of *regression* rather than delay, and requires more comprehensive investigation to exclude neurodegenerative conditions. Observation of how the child looks, listens, moves, explores, plays, communicates and socializes is essential prior to formal examination. Understandably, parents will be anxious and a sensitive approach is therefore essential at all times.

Developmental assessment provides the family with an understanding of the child's development, and outlines developmental goals and strategies to facilitate development and reduce any handicapping effects of the disability. Assessment and management may include physiotherapists, speech pathologists, educationalists, occupational therapists, psychologists and social workers.

PRINCIPLES OF ASSESSMENT

- Utilization of play as a fundamental assessment tool
- Promotion of optimal performance of the child
- Gearing of the assessment towards remediation rather than merely producing a profile
- Involvement of the parents in the assessment process
- Close linking of the assessment service with those offering help and support

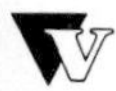

EARLY INTERVENTION

Early intervention includes prevention (through public health) and early detection of disabilities, as well as health, educational and community services which assist the child, family and community in adapting to the child's disability and developmental needs. Services are based on the principles of *normalization* and the *least restrictive alternative*.

The aims of early intervention are to minimize the handicapping effects of the child's disability on his/her development and education, and to support the family in understanding and providing their child's individual needs. Services include individual teaching and therapy (physio, speech and occupational), family support and counselling, resourcing and support to child care and preschools, and respite care. Services are regionally based and are provided by government and non-government agencies.

EDUCATION

There are a range of special educational strategies to optimize learning and development, dependent on the child's abilities and disabilities, with increasing opportunities for integration as resources are moved from special to local schools. A range of special schools are also available.

FAMILY SUPPORT

Parents need to be aware of the services that are available to them to assist in the care of their child with a disability. Supports include social security benefits, home help and respite care through foster agencies and community residential units. *Consumer organizations* can provide parent support, information and advocacy.

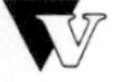

INTELLECTUAL DISABILITY

The definition of intellectual disability is comprised of three elements: (i) a significantly subaverage general intellectual functioning (i.e. two standard deviations below the mean of the intelligence quotient), existing concurrently with (ii) deficits in adaptive behaviour and (iii) manifested during the developmental period.

This definition is used by service providers, as well as academically and in legislation. The term *developmental disabilities* is being used increasingly to reflect the complexity of development.

Up to 2.5% of children have an intellectual disability: approximately 2% mild, 0.5% moderate, severe or profound.

PRESENTATION

- At birth with a known syndrome or malformation
- With associated medical complications (e.g. epilepsy)
- At follow-up of high-risk infants
- Global developmental delay
- Learning difficulties
- Language delay
- Secondary handicaps (e.g. behavioural difficulties)

Aetiological diagnosis is important to:

- Answer parents' questions such as 'Why has this happened?'
- Assist in understanding the prognosis
- Be alert for associated problems
- Provide appropriate genetic counselling

The timing and type of insult can be determined in approximately 70% of cases. The majority are caused by CNS insults during the prenatal period, with about 15% due to perinatal and 10% postnatal insults. The two most common causes are trisomy 21 and Fragile X.

INVESTIGATIONS

These should usually include:

- Screen for congenital infection: ophthalmologic examination, paired maternal–infant serology (rubella, toxoplasma), viral culture (cytomegalovirus); consider cerebral CT scan (calcification)
- Chromosomes
- Urinary metabolic screen
- Creatinine phosphokinase in boys
- Thyroid function studies

Other investigations may include:

- DNA specific probes (e.g. Fragile X, Prader–Willi and Williams syndromes)
- CT scan or MRI
- Mucopolysaccharide screen

MANAGEMENT

- Regular assessment of vision and hearing
- Investigation for associated anomalies (e.g. cardiac and thyroid status with trisomy 21)
- Treatment of associated disorders (e.g. epilepsy)
- Referral to and liaison with other practitioners, early intervention, family support and educational services
- Monitoring of development

- Support and information for parents
- Child advocacy

CEREBRAL PALSY

Cerebral palsy is a persistent but not unchanging disorder of movement and posture due to a defect or lesion of the developing brain. It occurs in about 2 per 1000 live births.

AETIOLOGY

Cerebral palsy is not a single entity but a term used for a diverse group of disorders, which may relate to events in the prenatal, perinatal or postnatal periods. The cause is unknown in many children. Perinatal asphyxia accounts for less than 10% of cases, and postnatal illnesses or injuries for a further 10%. There is a significant association with prematurity.

CLASSIFICATION

- The type of motor disorder (e.g. spasticity, athetosis)
- The distribution (e.g. hemiplegia, diplegia and quadriplegia)
- The severity of the motor disorder

ASSOCIATED DISORDERS

- Visual problems
- Hearing deficits
- Communication disorders
- Epilepsy
- Intellectual disability
- Learning disabilities
- Perceptual problems

Some children have only a motor disorder.

MANAGEMENT

Management of the child with cerebral palsy involves:

- Accurate diagnosis with genetic counselling
- Assessment of the child's capabilities and referral to appropriate services for the child and family. Liaison with kindergarten, school and general practitioner is important
- Management of the common associated disabilities and health problems

- All children require a *hearing* and *visual assessment*
- *Epilepsy*
- *Obesity* and *undernutrition* – dietary advice
- *Gastro-oesophageal reflux*
- *Constipation*
- *Drooling* with techniques employed by speech pathologists, or by the use of medication or surgery in a small group of children

Orthopaedic Management

Any operative procedure requires consultation with a physiotherapist who will be essential in the postoperative rehabilitation phase. Surgery is mainly undertaken on the lower limb, but is occasionally helpful in the upper limb. Some children require surgery for scoliosis.

The hip: Non-walkers and those only partially ambulant are prone to hip subluxation and eventual dislocation. Early detection is important. Hip X-rays should be performed at yearly intervals. Dislocation, which may cause pain and difficulty with perineal hygiene, is difficult to treat once it occurs.

The knee: Hamstring surgery may be necessary to improve gait pattern.

The ankle: Equinus deformity is commonly corrected.

Referrals

Referral to and ongoing liaison with allied health professionals is essential to enable children to achieve their optimal physical potential and independence.

- *Physiotherapists* give practical advice to parents and carers on positioning, handling and play to minimize the effects of abnormal muscle tone and encourage the development of movement skills. They also give advice regarding mobility aids, the use of orthoses or special seating. They may provide individual or group treatments or refer to appropriate community services
- *Occupational therapists* help parents to develop their child's upper limb and self-care skills, and are also involved in suggesting suitable toys as well as equipment and house adaptations for home care
- *Speech pathologists* provide guidance with severe eating and drinking difficulties, with communication and with augmentative communication systems for children with limited verbal skills
- Other professionals that may be helpful include medical social workers, psychologists, special education teachers and community nurses
- General practitioners play an important role in supporting these children and their families in the community

SPINA BIFIDA (MYELOMENINGOCELE)

Spina bifida is the commonest severe congenital malformation of the nervous system. The degree of impairment from the spinal cord pathology varies. Most children have some element of lower limb dysfunction, sensory loss and a neurogenic bladder and bowel. Eighty per cent have progressive hydrocephalus requiring surgery. Many children have specific learning problems.

PREVENTION

The 'good news' since 1992 in spina bifida care has been that periconceptional folic acid supplementation (in the month before and in the first 3 months of pregnancy) has been shown to reduce substantially the risk of recurrence in any at-risk family (by about 75%), and probably occurrence in any family. Recommended doses are:

- Low-risk women (no family history of neural tube defects): 0.5 mg daily
- Women with a previous child with a neural tube defect (or personal, partner or close family history): 4 mg daily (5 mg if 4 mg formulation not available)

Note: Multivitamin supplements are *not* recommended because of the potential risks of vitamin overdose to the developing fetus.

Fortification of staple foods with folate has been recommended in many countries.

MANAGEMENT

Management requires collaboration between health, education and welfare professionals and the child and family. Most children attend regular schools. Families require a great deal of support.

An interdisciplinary team of physicians, neuropsychologist, physiotherapist, orthotist, occupational therapist and social worker develops appropriate developmental and rehabilitation programmes, in collaboration with the family and community agencies (including local primary care service providers).

Initial Management

- Neurosurgical and paediatric assessment of the newborn infant is undertaken to determine if early surgery to close the spinal defect should be recommended. Clinical and ultrasound observation to detect and monitor the presence of hydrocephalus is important

- Orthopaedic and urological consultations and investigations are undertaken in the neonatal period to provide baseline information for subsequent management. A small number of infants require early management of talipes or a high-pressure neurogenic bladder
- The families must be fully informed about the diagnosis, natural history and prognosis, and be reassured that assistance is available

Specific Aspects of Management

Mobility

- Whatever the degree of lower limb impairment, independent mobility is the primary goal of the orthopaedic surgeon, physiotherapist and orthotist
- Almost all children learn to walk during childhood. The degree of assistance required in the form of surgery, bracing, crutches and so on varies with the level of the lesion. Those with high lesions often choose in adolescence to use a wheelchair as their primary method of mobility

Urinary tract

- The primary goals of the urologist and stomal therapist are the establishment of urinary continence (dryness) at a developmentally appropriate age, and the maintenance of satisfactory renal function
- *Clean intermittent catheterization* is now the preferred first method of treatment. Not all children become dry, and additional support may be necessary in the form of condom drainage or protective clothing. Bladder augmentation and/or the insertion of artificial urinary sphincters may be required
- Urinary tract infections (UTI) are common and should be treated in the usual way. Younger children and those with an ileal conduit present with constitutional symptoms. Recurrent UTI require investigation
- Discharge from the bladder may occur in a patient with an ileal conduit. This is usually either an infection (pyocystis) or a seminal discharge. If an infection is suspected daily neomycin bladder washouts (three to five) via a urethral catheter are required
- Children with urinary continence problems should have a urological assessment regularly: every 6–12 months in infancy and every 1–2 years in childhood

Neurological Functioning

- Depending upon the form of neonatal management undertaken after discussion between neurosurgeon, paediatrician and family, the neural tube defect is closed early or late
- If hydrocephalus becomes established a ventriculoperitoneal shunt is inserted. Problems with the ventriculoperitoneal shunt are common (see p. 173)
- In those infants for whom conservative early treatment is undertaken, a shunting procedure may precede excision of the lesion. Careful observation of the head circumference should be undertaken in all individuals surviving the perinatal period
- Careful follow-up of shunt functioning is required. Children with shunts should have neurosurgical assessment regularly (in infancy every 6–9 months; in childhood and adolescence at least every 1–2 years)
- Tethering of the spinal cord to surrounding structures occurs in most children. In a small number traction on the cord causes deterioration in neurological functioning. Regular detailed assessment of muscle strength and function is important to recognize early signs of cord tethering and traction problems. Surgical detethering may be required

Miscellaneous medical problems

- *Scoliosis*, and possibly *kyphosis*, are common management problems
- *Pressure sores* occur in all children with spina bifida at some time, most commonly on the feet or the buttocks
- *Pathological fractures* occur infrequently, and usually in those with a high lesion. Common symptoms are local swelling and erythema, with or without deformity, and usually without pain
- *Constipation* is a common long-term difficulty but may present as an acute impaction. Dietary advice, laxatives and enemas may be required
- *Epilepsy*. Some 15% of children with spina bifida have epilepsy. Treatment is along the usual lines (see p. 157).

CHAPTER 27

ADOLESCENT HEALTH

Glenn Bowes and George Patton

ADOLESCENT MEDICINE

WHAT IS ADOLESCENCE?

Adolescence is the transitional period of development between relatively dependent childhood and relatively independent adulthood.

WHAT IS AN ADOLESCENT?

Chronological age is not always a good reflection of developmental stage; however, an adolescent is generally considered to be between the age of 10 and 19 years. More recently, the term *young person* has been used in the context of health policies and *young people* are those between the age of 10 and 24 years.

MAJOR AREAS OF HEALTH PROBLEMS

Adolescent medicine has developed as a subspecialty, largely due to increased understanding of the major health problems for young people, which include:
- Injuries, including motor vehicle accidents
- Mental health problems, including attempted suicide and suicide
- Chronic illness and disability (numbers of paediatric survivors are increasing)
- Potentially health compromising behaviours, including drug use (licit and illicit) and unsafe sexual practices

A SOCIAL HEALTH PERSPECTIVE

It is clear that many of the health problems of adolescents have been exacerbated by or occur as a result of social and economic change in communities. Unemployment, poverty and increased drug use have special impact upon young people who are extremely vulnerable as a consequence of their transtional developmental stage.

ADOLESCENT DEVELOPMENTAL TASKS

Engaging adolescents in a productive therapeutic relationship requires the clinician to have a good understanding of both the social context of young people's lives and the developmental tasks they confront. The key developmental tasks include:

- Autonomy and independence
- Sexuality
- Body self-integrity and personal identity
- Peer relationships and recreational goals
- Educational and vocational goals

DEVELOPMENTAL OUTCOMES AS HEALTH OUTCOMES

Clinicians must have clear goals of therapy related to the health problems that they are trying to manage in partnership with their patients. Such clear clinical outcomes are absolutely necessary in the care of young people; however, they are insufficient. Clinicians must also have a good understanding of the developmental outcomes relevant to the young person and set treatment goals in the context of these developmental goals (see Table 27.1).

Negotiation of treatment goals in a way that takes account of the individual needs of the young person is crucial to engaging a young person in a way that engenders good compliance with treatment regimens.

A CLINICAL APPROACH TO ADOLESCENTS

Consultations with young people are likely to be relatively time consuming and allowing adequate time is essential to the conduct of a successful consultation.Young people generally perceive that they are not listened to, not given adequate time to put their view and have their opinions dismissed. *A clinician who listens respectfully and acknowledges a young person's point of view will have made an excellent start in establishing a therapeutic relationship.*

Starting the Consultation

Greet the young person by name, making eye-to-eye contact and ensuring that they are given your full name. When parents are present, be sure to greet the young person first and then introduce yourself to the parents. The young person is the patient and must be given time alone with the clinician during the consultation.

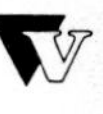

Confidentiality

Clinicians should make a clear statement that explains the issue of confidentiality at the beginning of the first contact with every adolescent. Maintenance of confidentiality enhances trust and honesty, which enables more appropriate health care. Although the adolescent may be an integral member of a family, he or she, not the family, is the patient. Young people may require added reassurance before being able to trust clinicians with important information.

- In general all information gained from an adolescent should be regarded as confidential until this issue has been discussed and clarified
- Issues of confidentiality for young people under 16 years of age require negotiation. An agreement to break confidentiality or a compromise agreement may be made by negotiation
- Exceptions to confidentiality are if there is considered to be a current and substantial risk of the adolescent committing suicide, committing homicide or being subject to physical or sexual abuse

DEVELOPMENT

Developmental Screening

Young people are most likely to present for clinical care as a consequence of a minor complaint, such as a viral illness or injury. Irrespective of the primary reason for presentation, the clinician should take the opportunity to undertake a developmental screening that is related to health promotion and disease prevention.

It may be necessary to make a second appointment to enable such a time-consuming consultation to take place. The *HEADSS* (***H***ome, ***E***ducation and employment, ***A***ctivities, ***D***rugs, ***S***exuality and ***S***uicide risk) is a psychosocial interview framework for adolescents, and is useful in the conduct of developmental screening (see Table 27.1). HEADSS involves a series of questions that move from less to more sensitive areas in a systematic manner. At the end of this interview the clinician can give a brief report to the young person, giving positive messages about their present health and highlighting areas that need some work.

Physical Examination

A thorough physical examination should be conducted gently and with consideration. Protection of the adolescent's modesty and privacy is vital. It is helpful during the examination to integrate friendly and reassuring dialogue that explains the reason for the particular examination and gives immediate feedback on the findings.

Table 27.1 Adolescent developmental screening: HEADSS*

	Area	*Questions*
H	Home	Where do you live and who lives there with you?
E	Education and employment	What are you good at in school? What grades do you get?
A	Activities	What do you do for fun? What things do you do with friends?
D	Drugs	Many young people experiment with drugs, alcohol and cigarettes. Have you ever tried them?
S	Sexuality	Most young people become interested in sex at your age. Have you had a sexual relationship with anyone?
S	Suicide risk/ depression screening	See Table 27.2, p. 315

*Goldenring and Cohen, *Contemporary Pediatrics*, July, 1988, pp. 75–80.

COMPLIANCE

Engendering compliance with treatment regimens is a challenge for clinicians irrespective of the age of the patient but may be more difficult with adolescents. This is because of the apparent contradiction that exists between the young person's (developmentally appropriate) pursuit of independence, and the clinician's desire to give clear instructions on health care. Careful and respectful negotiation is required. Practical tips include:

- Keeping language and instructions simple
- Ensuring that the treatment regimen is practical
- Considering the acceptability of treatment to peers
- Being consistent without 'nagging'
- Keeping communication open and avoiding the use of threats
- As appropriate, encouraging parents to either be more involved or to 'back off' and not be overprotective

YOUNG PEOPLE WITH CHRONIC ILLNESSES AND DISABILITIES

These young people represent a special group requiring skilled multidisciplinary teams. Young people in these categories are frequently the most experienced consumers of the health system met in the paediatric environment. Clinicians must be extremely careful to acknowledge and respect the experience and views of these young people and their families.

Conflict of Priorities

It is not uncommon for a conflict of priorities to occur between the therapeutic goals articulated by the clinician (focused on disease management), and the developmental goals that are frequently the dominant concern of young people. Clinicians need to recognize the potential for this conflict to occur, and be prepared to negotiate a successful resolution by clear and open discussion.

Multidisciplinary Teams and Mixed Messages

The value of the multidisciplinary team is well established. However, there is a considerable potential for individual health professionals who are part of the team to give conflicting and mixed messages to young people and their families, thereby confounding the achievement of satisfactory disease and developmental outcomes. Excellent communication within the team is crucial to ensure that a mutually agreed upon, common set of themes and messages is delivered to the young person and their family.

WORKING ACROSS THE SECTORS

The health of young people can be influenced by professionals working outside the health sector. Consideration needs to be given to both gaining information from and communicating information to those who work with young people in other settings:
- School and educational agencies
- Community based youth organizations
- Recreational programmes
- Peer support groups

ADOLESCENT MEDICINE REFERRALS

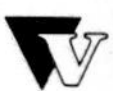

Specialist Adolescent Medicine units are a resource for general practitioners and other health professionals for early referral of adolescents with difficult problems.

Common reasons for referral include:
- Health problems that are relatively unique to the adolescent age group, including eating disorders (p. 316), deliberate self-harm and

suicide attempts (p. 315), school-based problems and behaviour disorders
- Concerns about physical growth, puberty and sexual behaviour
- Complex interactions between young people, diseases and disease treatments
- Problems occurring at the interface between adolescent general health and adolescent mental health, such as early depression and psychosomatic disorders
- Problems that involve a knowledge of and access to networks and programmes dealing with young people

ADOLESCENT MENTAL HEALTH

GENERAL INFORMATION

The notion that adolescence was a time of inevitable emotional turmoil, which had little implication for future mental health, has given way to a view that the teens and early twenties are critical years for the development of major psychiatric disorders which persist into adulthood (see also p. 324). Major disorders with peak incidence in young people include:
- Depression
- Anxiety disorders
- Obsessional neurosis
- Schizophrenia
- Bipolar affective disorders
- Substance abuse
- Personality disorders
- Anorexia and bulimia nervosa

Many of these disorders will present with less well developed features than in an adult population and thus recognition and early diagnosis present a clinical challenge. *The mounting evidence that therapeutic interventions are most effective at this early stage of illness underlines the necessity for effective early diagnosis and referral for treatment.*

Commonly adolescent psychiatric disorders arise in a context of interpersonal and social problems. In assessment and treatment consideration should be given to stresses arising from grief (e.g. death or illness in the family), interpersonal disputes (e.g. with peers, families), developmental transitions (e.g. becoming sexually active, changing or leaving school) and lack of adequate skills to deal with the tasks of adolescence (e.g. difficulties in initiating social contact or expressing emotions).

Table 27.2 Assessment of suicide risk in young people*

Area	*Questions*
Suicidal ideation: current	
Attitude to death	Is life worthless/hopeless?
Suicidal thinking	Is there a plan? (clarity, lethality) Is there access to weapons/drugs? Have any steps been taken?
Suicide attempts: previous	
Method	Potential of methods to cause death
Planning	Length of planning period. Preparing for death (e.g. bequests, wills)
Intent	What was hoped would occur? Attitude to previous attempts
Mental health disorder: current	
Substance misuse	How much? How often? Consequences of use?
Depression	Low mood. Poor concentration on studies. Tiredness. Sleep disturbance. Negative feelings. Isolated and withdrawn
Personality disorder	Disturbed past relationships and behaviours. Responses to stress

*Patton and Bowes, *General Practitioner*, 1994; **2**: 18–19.

DEPRESSION, DELIBERATE SELF-HARM AND SUICIDE

Suicide is, after motor vehicle accidents, the most common cause of death in 15–25 year olds in Australia. Factors most commonly associated with completed suicide are a history of deliberate self-harm, major depression, substance abuse and antisocial behaviour (see also p. 326).

About 1 in 200 young people present to emergency departments each year with deliberate self-harm, typically in the form of an overdose. An even greater number do not present for medical care. In most instances adolescent deliberate self-harm is associated with some psychiatric disturbance. Key features of assessment of the potentially suicidal adolescent are shown in Table 27.2. Assessment of the act of self-harm should include:

- Attention to suicidal intent
- Perceived lethality of the act

- Actual harm incurred
- Degree of planning
- Actions taken by the patient after the event

Assessment should also be made of associated psychiatric disorder and level of social and interpersonal difficulties in a teenager's life.

Depression is the commonest major psychiatric disorder of young people with symptoms similar to those developing in adults (see also p. 329). Typical symptoms include:

- Pervasive boredom
- Extended periods of low mood
- Fatigue
- Loss of self-confidence
- Social withdrawal
- Impaired concentration
- Suicidal ideas

In most instances a teenager will give a better account of these symptoms than parents or other informants. Assessment should include consideration of organic causes (e.g. recent steroid therapy, substance abuse). Both psychological (cognitive behavioural and interpersonal psychotherapies) and medication treatments have parts to play in the management of adolescent depression.

EATING DISORDERS

The commonest adolescent eating disorders presenting clinically are anorexia nervosa and bulimia nervosa.

Anorexia Nervosa

- Anorexia nervosa is characterized by a relentless pursuit of thinness through the use of extreme weight control strategies, amenorrhoea and intense fear of gaining weight
- Assessment of post-pubertal anorexia nervosa should include attention to current weight, rate of weight loss, methods employed (e.g. abstinence, self-induced vomiting, purging, exercise) and associated depression
- Consideration should be given to the exclusion of other primary psychiatric disorders (e.g. major depression, obsessional neurosis) and physical disorders (thyrotoxicosis, malabsorption).
- Admission is indicated where weight loss is extreme (to <70% standardized bodyweight for age), where physical complications

supervene (e.g. hypokalaemia, hypothermia) or where outpatient treatments have failed

Bulimia Nervosa

- Bulimia nervosa is characterized by frequent loss of control of eating (bingeing), extreme methods of weight control and fear of fatness
- Assessment should give consideration to the presence of intercurrent depression and the presence of more general difficulties with impulsive control
- Treatment is usually on an outpatient basis and focal psychotherapies such as cognitive–behavioural therapy (CBT) are effective both in individual and group treatment settings

28

CHAPTER 28

PAEDIATRIC HEALTH MAINTENANCE

Frank Oberklaid

There is increasing recognition that the burden of paediatric morbidity and mortality can be reduced significantly by focusing on the *prevention* of illness and injury, and by early detection of conditions to prevent or minimize their consequences.

SCREENING

For some conditions, community-wide screening programmes allow early diagnosis and treatment. The best known examples of successful screening tests are the ones performed shortly after birth to detect phenylketonuria and hypothyroidism.

Screening is defined as the presumptive identification of unrecognized disease or defect by the application of tests, examinations, and other procedures which can be applied rapidly. Screening tests sort out apparently well persons who may have a disease from those who probably do not. **A screening test is not expected to be diagnostic.**

A number of important criteria must be met in order that a screening programme is considered for a particular condition. These include:

- Issues to do with the condition for which the person is being screened (prevalence, importance, natural history, availability of effective treatment, ability to reliably detect its presence at an early stage)
- The screening test (sensitivity, specificity, reliability, cost, time taken for administration, acceptability to community)
- Logistic issues (feasibility of a community-wide or state-wide screening programme; availability of adequate resources for diagnosis, counselling and treatment)

Few conditions in paediatrics meet these criteria. For this reason, *surveillance* in paediatrics has come to be accepted as the most appropriate activity for the early identification of problems and the prevention or minimization of injury and disease.

SURVEILLANCE

Surveillance also involves whole populations of children, and is initiated by professionals. However, it actively involves parents and other caregivers in the process. Surveillance aims to optimize the health of all children through the ongoing overview of the physical, social and emotional health and development of all children.

Surveillance includes recording physical growth, monitoring development, ensuring complete immunization, eliciting any parental concerns, and providing health information and support to parents and caregivers. Surveillance may also include the administration of specific screening tests.

The major paradigm shift is that health professionals now focus on health maintenance and the prevention of illness and injury rather than only diagnosing and treating established conditions. In addition, the active involvement of parents in health surveillance is likely to lead to improved outcomes for children. By providing parents and caregivers with appropriate health information, they are more likely to bring their concerns to the attention of the health professional at an early stage.

Two other concepts are emerging as being central to good paediatric health maintenance: opportunistic surveillance and key times during childhood which are important for designated surveillance activities.

OPPORTUNISTIC SURVEILLANCE

Every time a health professional sees a child, in addition to addressing the presenting complaint, ideally they should use the opportunity for health surveillance. Taking into account the child's age, they could speak to parents about a range of preventive issues (such as injury prevention and immunization), and monitor the child's growth and development, as well as ensuring that the child is up to date with his/her immunization.

Many will also engage the parents in a discussion of health, developmental and behavioural issues relevant to the child's age group, as well as providing them with appropriate health information. This is called *anticipatory guidance*, and is intended to make parents more confident and competent, and to minimize the common and often distressing behavioural problems encountered in the first 5 years of life in particular.

KEY AGES FOR HEALTH SURVEILLANCE

There is an emerging international consensus regarding certain key times during childhood when it is important that children are seen by health professionals, and the specific issues to be discussed at each age group. It is suggested that if a child has no other reason to visit a doctor or nurse, they should attend at these specific ages. Table 28.1 lists the key ages for health surveillance and the suggested issues to be discussed at each visit.

NOTES ON HEALTH SURVEILLANCE ACTIVITIES

At each visit, any parental concerns are actively elicited and addressed. A general question such as 'Is there anything else about Johnny that you are concerned about at this time?' is followed by the discussion of specific issues relevant to the particular age group (Table 28.1).

Immunization and *injury prevention* are raised at every visit. Injury prevention topics will depend on the age of the child, and will vary from choosing a safe cot or pram in infancy through to water safety and tricycles/bicycles in the toddler age group. Travelling safely in the car is raised at each age group.

At each age group, parents are asked a set of specific questions designed to elicit concerns about the child's *development, vision* and *hearing.* **Parental concern or suspicion of deafness, visual problems or developmental delay must be taken very seriously and is usually an indication for referral for formal screening and/or assessment.**

Finally, there is a range of *childhood behaviours* that are invariably of concern to parents at different ages. Many of these behaviours are transient and seemingly of little importance when compared to other causes of morbidity. However, it is surprising the extent to which they cause parental distress and can adversely affect the parent/child relationship, often diminishing parental confidence and sometimes setting the stage for ongoing behavioural and emotional problems.

SUMMARY

- In addition to the traditional challenge of accurate diagnosis and effective treatment of illness and injury in children, health professionals are now faced with another challenge – could this condition have been prevented in the first place?

Table 28.1 Health surveillance issues in the first 5 years

Specific questions for parent(s) appropriate to developmental age	Birth/1–2 weeks	6–8 weeks	6–9 months	18–21 months	3–3½ years	School entry
Issues in infancy						
Vitamin K	★					
SIDS	★	★	★			
Feeding	★	★	★			
Crying/temperament	★	★	★			
Injury and disease prevention						
Immunization		★	★	★	★	★
Injury prevention	★	★	★	★	★	★
Sun protection	★	★	★	★	★	★
Care of teeth			★	★	★	★
Special senses, development						
Hearing	★	★	★	★	★	★
Vision	★	★	★	★	★	★
Development	★	★	★	★	★	★

(Continued)

Table 28.1 *(Continued)*

Specific questions for parent(s) appropriate to developmental age	Birth/1–2 weeks	6–8 weeks	6–9 months	18–21 months	3–3½ years	School entry
Behaviour, parenting issues						
Sleep problems			★	★	★	
Sibling rivalry	★	★	★	★	★	
Temper tantrums				★	★	
Parenting practices (discipline, setting limits)				★	★	★
Toilet training				★	★	
Transitions						
Day care			★	★		
Kindergarten					★	

At each of these visits, and at other visits where possible, doctors and nurses should actively elicit parental concerns about any aspect of their child's health and development, and address them as appropriate.

- There is increasing emphasis on maintaining optimal health of children in the community
- Doctors and nurses must become familiar with concepts of health surveillance and function in an opportunistic way to ensure full immunization, prevent injury, detect health and developmental problems at the earliest opportunity, and provide parents with accurate and timely information about their child's health, development and behaviour
- *Anticipatory guidance* is a concept that is now seen as increasingly important in paediatric health maintenance. Health professionals anticipate that most, if not all, parents will be faced with these common childhood behaviours, and they provide appropriate information and guidance to parents at each of the specified visits. If parents are given good information and the support of the health professional, these behaviours will be less likely to develop into major problems

29

CHAPTER 29

CHILD PSYCHIATRY

Robert Adler and Ernest S. L. Luk

About 10–15% of the child and adolescent population have adjustment/ behaviour disorders. The majority of them are helped by their families, relatives, friends, school, primary health-care workers, general practitioners and paediatricians. Only a small proportion are seen by mental health services.

Successful use of mental health services requires preparation for the referral process.

PREPARATION FOR REFERRAL

The social stigma of attending a mental health service still exists. It is important that parents understand that they are not blamed for their child's problem; that it is not a sign of failure and it is positive that they seek help; that it is not unusual for children to have such problems; and that it may take some time to find the best way to help their child.

It should be explained directly to the child that referral is not a punishment but a means to overcome difficulties. A number of discussions may be needed.

It is best to know the setting and the clinical approach of the person to whom you are referring the child. Phoning the professional is often useful.

INTERVIEWING FOR PSYCHIATRIC PROBLEMS IN CHILDHOOD

- As well as interviewing the parent(s) and child together, see each separately, if possible, to get a more complete picture. Determine why the family have presented at this particular time. *Note that children, the less intelligent or educated, and those with language and cultural disadvantages, are more likely to be misunderstood and to misunderstand questions, to be afraid or hostile and to use somatic complaints to communicate distress*

- Use simple language, and try to understand the predicament of the child and the family. One's own response to the child and the family is a vital aspect of the assessment
- Assess the details of the problem behaviour: history, frequency, context and the responses of family members. Assess the meaning of the problem behaviour to the family and the ways in which they have attempted to solve the problem, including professional advice previously sought
- Inquire about: pregnancy, delivery, nursing relationship, early development, preschool and school life (educational progress, peer relations), interests, family structure, recent stresses, marital relationship, family supports and extended social network, intergenerational difficulties, illnesses and separations

Observe the following:

- *Affect:* range, variability and form (e.g. flat, anxious)
- *Play:* confidence, competence, co-ordination, activity, creativity
- *Thinking:* content (including suicidal thoughts), concentration, organization, orientation, form of thoughts, dreams, wishes, etc.
- *Personality:* behaviour style, adaptability/rigidity, openness/defensiveness, ability to engage in a relationship

Often it is very helpful to obtain information from the school. Seek parents' consent before doing so.

FAMILY CRISIS

Children's self-perception, emotional life, understanding of people and relationships and behaviours are intimately connected with the views and the behaviour of their families. Parental responsibilities and obligations include: nurturance, care and protection of children; the establishment of limits and rules; the provision of security and emotional space to play and develop; appropriate education, stimulation and involvement.

Where parental competence is undermined by illness, poverty, ignorance, stress, lack of supports and other factors, children may show evidence of behaviour disturbance. Overactivity, aggression, self-stimulation, destructive behaviour, stealing, running away and suicidal behaviour may all be evidence of family difficulty. While these behaviours bring the predicament of the child to the attention of others, they are also often perceived by parents as 'bad' and in turn punished or rejected. A cycle of unsatisfactory interactions develops where the parents feel bad and angry and the child feels bad and angry.

It is very useful to differentiate families who have been functioning well, but present in crisis because of some recent stresses, from those who have had difficulties for a long period of time, e.g. more than 6 months. The latter often require longer-term treatment.

At various points in the crisis-filled lives of some families, children may be presented at emergency departments with adjustment problems. They may carry such labels as 'hyperactive', 'suicidal', 'possessed', 'bad' or 'out of control'. At such times, it is helpful to focus on the difficulties of the caretakers, as well as on those of the child, and clarify the interactional cycles or habits that characterize their lives.

One should balance the disadvantages of offering crisis admission with the benefits of being able to establish appropriate responsibilities and community supports once the problem becomes clearer

Action

- Crisis social work/psychiatry referrals for assessment
- Liaison and referral to appropriate community agencies
- Liaison with general practitioner

ATTEMPTED SUICIDE

- This most often presents as a drug overdose in children over 9 years old, but may take more violent forms such as wrist laceration or attempted hanging
- Most are an expression of long-standing difficulties between parent(s) and child where care, co-operation and communication are unsatisfactory
- Up to 50% are more serious expressions of suicidal intent, often in association with depressed mood and other depressive symptoms
- *It is always dangerous simply to dismiss a self-injurious act as attention seeking.* The most worrying profile is a male adolescent who has a history of attempted suicide, has access to firearms and shows depressive symptoms

Action

- Do not delay necessary medical attention
- Interview the child alone, parent(s) alone and family together and evaluate underlying difficulties, strengths and likely responses of the family to this crisis
- Consult the local Mental Health Service to determine whether urgent psychiatric assessment, admission or referral for outpatient assessment is required
- Involve the general practitioner in the management plan

ANXIETY DISORDERS

These present with high levels of autonomic arousal and subjective fear or panic. It may occur in attacks or as a persistent state, and may lead to avoidance behaviour.

Childhood anxiety may be related to over-worrying, separation from carer, excessive shyness in social situations and following stress or trauma. *Anxiety problems in children often present as somatic complaints such as headache, abdominal pain and nausea.* Diagnosis is based on the absence of an organic cause, a history of other anxiety symptoms and examination. (see also Recurrent Abdominal Pain, p. 94 and Headache, p. 166).

Action

- After defining the origin of the fear, explanation and planned follow-up with the family doctor is usually sufficient
- More difficult cases should be discussed with the child psychiatric service for emergency psychiatric assessment or urgent outpatient appointment

CONVERSION REACTIONS

These may be associated with paralysis, blindness, deafness, pains or other sensory changes which have no organic basis.

They usually occur in association with recent stresses, family difficulties with emotional communication and difficulties in providing emotional support.

Action

- Admission may be required for full medical and psychiatric assessment
- Otherwise, consider elective consultation with the local Mental Health Service, referral to medical outpatients or follow-up with general practitioner

SCHOOL REFUSAL

The child is brought with the complaint of panic and distress on being sent to school. The presenting symptom is often some somatic problem or complaint of abdominal pain. This should be distinguished from *truancy* where the child avoids school without the accompanying anxiety symptoms and often without parents' knowledge.

Action

- Full physical examination should precede psychiatric referral
- *Urgent return to school is a high priority*

AGGRESSIVE BEHAVIOUR

Anxious children may present with problems of aggressive behaviour, which is often confined to the home situation in children with a history of dependency. The parent/child relationship may become very confrontational and the child is seen as 'out of control'.

Action

- Helping the carers to understand the underlying basis of the aggression goes a long way towards reducing their anxiety
- Further work to change the parent/child relationship is needed
- Severe cases should be referred for emergency psychiatric assessment or urgent outpatient appointment

OBSESSIVE–COMPULSIVE BEHAVIOUR

This presents with checking, rituals, compulsive behaviour or intrusive thoughts. Obsessive–compulsive *disorder* is relatively uncommon. Obsessive–compulsive *behaviour* is more common, and is often associated with anxiety or depression, and pervasive developmental disorder.

Action

- Explanation and support to the child and family
- Referral for assessment and management by a psychiatrist is indicated
- These children respond well to cognitive behavioural therapy alone or in combination with medication

GRIEVING

Grieving may occur in response to loss of support (if parents are unavailable or are themselves grieving) as well as following more obvious losses. Protest at the loss with overactivity and rage may be followed by sadness, depression and withdrawal.

Action

- Parents need explanations and the children need support by adults who can understand their response to the loss
- Assist family to access appropriate support and counselling

DEPRESSION

Depression occurs in childhood, but it is often missed. Depressive phenomena are often modified because of age and developmental stage. They may present with low mood, difficulty in sleep onset, not enjoying meals, low self-esteem, negative thoughts including suicidal ideas, poor concentration and irritability.

Depressed adolescents are at increased risk for suicide. Co-morbidities are common including oppositional defiant/conduct disorder, anxiety disorders and attention deficit hyperactivity disorder.

Action

- It is very important to recognize depression in children and adolescents, because if untreated they run a much higher risk of depression in adulthood
- Psychiatric referral for an early outpatient appointment is often needed
- The general practitioner plays an important role in management

DISRUPTIVE BEHAVIOUR DISORDERS

Separation of attention-deficit hyperactivity disorder (ADHD) and conduct problems is essential. Many families with a child suffering from ADHD may appear to be coping poorly. This is often secondary to the ADHD and, once the diagnosis is made and appropriate treatment provided, the family functioning improves (see p. 290).

Chronic conduct problems (more than 6 months) in childhood have serious consequences for the social adjustment in adult life. They require long-term and multiple forms of treatment.

Action

- The management of ADHD should be left in the hands of experienced paediatricians or psychiatrists

- Chronic conduct problems should be referred to the local Mental Health Service

PSYCHOSIS

Psychosis is a general term for states in which mental function is grossly impaired, so that reality testing and insight are lacking and delusions, hallucinations, incoherence, thought disorder and/or disorganized behaviour may be apparent.

In the case of 'organic' psychosis there may also be clouding of consciousness, confusion and disorientation as well as perceptual disturbances. Short-term memory impairment is common in organic brain syndromes.

Anticholinergic, anticonvulsants, antidepressants, antimalarial and benzodiazepines have been associated with psychotic reactions in young people, as have substances of abuse (amphetamines, cocaine, opiates, hallucinogens). Organic brain syndromes may follow even minor head injury.

Adolescents may occasionally present in an acutely psychotic state with no prior history of drug ingestion or head injury. In this case the possibility of a 'functional' psychosis, schizophrenia or manic-depressive disorder should be considered. The latter often presents with elated mood, grandiose ideas, increased energy and reduced sleep requirements.

Action

- The doctor should make a clinical evaluation and psychiatric referral. Most of these children will require admission for full psychiatric and medical examination
- Do not sedate the child before complete assessment unless essential

SEXUAL AND EMOTIONAL ABUSE OF CHILDREN

This is an increasingly recognized phenomenon (see also p. 333). Signs of neglect and emotional abuse are often non-specific, but suspicion should be raised when infants, pre-schoolers or school-age children behave in the following ways:

- Persistently angry, socially avoidant, defiant, disobedient and overactive
- Anxiously attached, watchful of their patients, limited ability to enjoy things, intensely ambivalent to parents

- Low self-esteem, depressed or unresponsive, developmental and emotional retardation, poor social skills and over-inhibition

Signs of sexual abuse are also usually non-specific, but may include the above and various behaviour problems (phobias, bad dreams, eating and sleeping disorders, depression, school problems, delinquency). There may be overt manifestations of sexual preoccupation, including precocious and inappropriate sexual activity, promiscuity and aggressive sexual behaviour

Action

Psychiatric consultation is often useful in conjunction with involvement of local child protection services (see p. 333).

BASIC TREATMENT PRINCIPLES IN PSYCHIATRIC PROBLEMS

EXPLANATION

- Treatment should involve collaboration of parents, the child and the professional
- The *parents* should be informed of the diagnosis, the formulation of the problem, the treatment plan and the steps it takes to achieve the treatment goals
- The *child* should also be informed, using age-appropriate language
- With parents' consent, the *school* and *family doctor* should be contacted to share relevant information and to help the child whenever appropriate

SUPPORTIVE PSYCHOLOGICAL WORK/BASIC BEHAVIOUR MODIFICATION

- Some families will improve by explanation, advice and referral to appropriate reading materials
- Behaviour modification based on observation, recording and learning principles can also be used
- Consultation or advice from psychologists or psychiatrists should be sought, as described above

USE OF PSYCHOTROPIC DRUGS

- Psychotropic drugs should be used with care. They are only part of the whole package of treatment. However, in some cases they can be extremely important

- Before prescribing, it is advisable to consult with an experienced paediatrician or child psychiatrist. The common indications are psychosis, some cases of ADHD, tic disorder and severe behaviour problems in children with brain damage or mental retardation
- Anxiety problems are rarely treated with drugs except when related to severe pain, in some cases of severe separation anxiety, in severe acute stress and before surgical operation
- Psychological treatment is the first line of treatment for depression. Medication should be considered for melancholia, psychotic depression and refractory depression

MONITORING AND REFERRAL

- Monitoring of progress is essential. Initially families should be seen weekly or bi-weekly
- The more severe, chronic or refractory cases should be referred

CHILD ABUSE AND NEGLECT

Anne Smith and Karen Hogan

DEFINITIONS

Physical Abuse

Physical abuse includes inflicted physical violence directed against children, such as bruises, burns and scalds, head injuries, fractures, abdominal injuries, suffocation and drowning. It also includes intentional poisoning with drugs or other substances and Munchausen's syndrome by proxy.

Neglect

The failure of parents to adequately provide for and safeguard the health, safety and well-being of the child.

Sexual Abuse

The involvement of dependent, developmentally immature children and adolescents in sexual activities that they do not fully comprehend and to which they are unable to give consent.

Emotional Abuse

The distortion of the parent–child relationship that deprives children of the consistent nurturing of body and mind that would enable them to develop fully.

INTERVIEWING PARENTS

- A non-judgemental, sensitive approach is essential
- Ask open, not leading questions
- Use verbatim quotes whenever possible

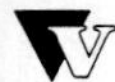

MANDATORY REPORTING

In most states of Australia notification to the relevant statutory authorities is mandatory for suspicion of child abuse or neglect.

PHYSICAL ABUSE AND NEGLECT

PRESENTATIONS

- *Bruises and welts*, especially:
  - Sides of face, behind the ears, the upper lip and fraenulum
  - Buttocks and lower back
  - Upper arms and legs
  - Scalp
  - Genitalia
  - Bruises in different stages of healing
  - Multiple bruises of same age on different parts of the body
  - Linear bruises
  - Bruises made by belt buckles, ropes, hand prints or fingerprints
- *Burns*, especially if:
  - Circumferential
  - Absence of splash pattern
  - Spare skin folds (e.g. held in hot water with hips flexed)
  - Shape of instrument (e.g. cigarette burn)
- *Fractures*, especially if:
  - Old, untreated fractures
  - Different stages of healing in multiple fractures
  - Metaphyseal fractures
  - Epiphyseal separations
  - Unusual fracture sites (ribs, vertebrae, scapulae, sternum, metacarpals)
  - Fractures in long bones in children <1 year old
- *Brain injury/whiplash injury (commonest cause of death due to child abuse)*. The whiplash shaken infant syndrome should be considered in any young infant with an unexplained impairment of consciousness. Shaking leads to shearing forces on cerebral vessels causing scattered subdural haemorrhages
  - Examine for retinal haemorrhages and dislocated lenses. Bloody CSF from an atraumatic tap suggests intracranial haemorrhage. Tin ear syndrome = ipsilateral subdural haemorrhages. Consider in a child with a bruised pinna and decreased conscious state
- *Abdominal injury*. Second commonest cause of death due to child abuse

  - Ruptured liver
  - Ruptured spleen
  - Traumatic pancreatitis
  - Renal injury
- *Thermal injury*
- *Poisoning*
- *Inadequate nutrition, failure to thrive:* from insufficient food or fad diets
- *Inadequate growth (psychosocial dwarfism)*
- *Poor hygiene*
- *Developmental delay* due to lack of stimulation
- *Munchausen syndrome by proxy*

EXAMINATION

A thorough physical examination must be performed.

- Record measurements
- Estimate ages of lesions (colour of bruise is only a rough guide to age)
- Use diagrams whenever possible

Note the following:

- Skin markings – lacerations, burns, ecchymoses, linear contusions, contusions with shapes resembling an instrument, circular contusions on trunk or limbs (finger pressure points), bites
- Torn fraenulum, contused gums, loose teeth, dental trauma, petechiae on soft palate
- Nasal trauma, septal haematoma in an infant
- Ear trauma, including barotrauma
- Eye trauma, including hyphaema, periorbital haematoma, haemorrhage
- Chest injuries
- Blunt abdominal trauma
- Limb trauma – fractures, dislocations, limp, localized tenderness
- Head trauma – haematomas, lacerations, conscious state
- Growth – percentiles
- Development
- Emotional state
- Parent–child interaction

INVESTIGATIONS

Full Blood Examination (Include Platelets), Clotting Studies (PT, APTT)

Indicated if bruising or blunt abdominal trauma.

Imaging for Fractures

- X-ray clinically suspected site of fracture or hot spots on bone scan
- Bone scan: children less than 3 years with suspected physical abuse; more sensitive than X-ray for recent undisplaced fracture with minimal soft tissue swelling, as well as for older radiologically remodelled fractures; may miss metaphyseal fracture (difficult to distinguish from 'hot' growth plate)
- Skull X-ray is better than bone scan at detecting skull fracture
- Skeletal survey of skull, thorax and abdomen (not pelvis), limbs; may be alternative if bone scan is not available (note large dose of irradiation to the child); may miss posterior rib fractures

Photographs

Photographs should be taken at the time of presentation. A picture speaks a thousand words.

MANAGEMENT

Psychosocial Assessment of Child and Family

Always involve social worker; multidisciplinary assessment may be indicated; liaise with family doctor.

Admission to Hospital

Children with moderate or severe injuries should be admitted. When a child is not admitted, a decision should be made as to where and with whom the child should be discharged.

Case Conference

- Should be held for each child admitted to hospital
- Should be arranged by the regional protective services team after notification
- Should be attended by hospital staff as requested

Medical Reports

- Should be prepared on request by the senior medical person responsible for the child's care
- Should be in language appropriate for non-medical professionals
- Should be clear, concise and informative, and include an opinion

about the injury and its cause(s), as well as recommendations for continuing care of the child

Mandatory Reporting

The legislation of many states mandates professionals to notify the child protection authorities if they suspect child abuse. Practitioners should become familiar with the relevant local legislation.

Court Appearances

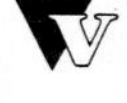

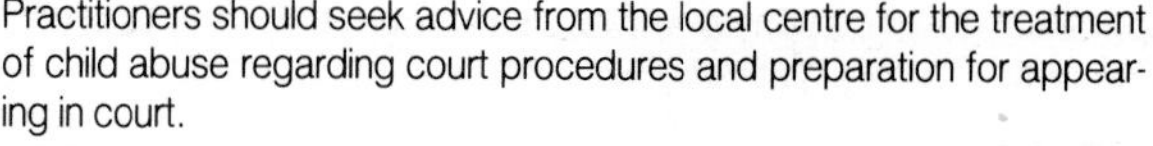

Practitioners should seek advice from the local centre for the treatment of child abuse regarding court procedures and preparation for appearing in court.

SEXUAL ABUSE

HISTORY

A full paediatric assessment is required. Evaluation should include:

- The nature of sexual contact (oral, rectal, penile, vaginal)
- The time and circumstances of the abuse
- Identification of the perpetrator(s)
- Vaginal discharge or perineal complaints; including treatment for constipation
- Non-specific complaints and behavioural patterns, which may be indicators of sexual abuse

EXAMINATION

Note: **The physical examination of suspected sexually abused children should be conducted by trained, experienced personnel with adequate light and magnification, after careful explanation to the child and family. These guidelines are for the uncommon situation where the examination cannot be deferred and a clinician with experience in this examination is not available.**

Take note of the child's emotional state and signs of trauma (e.g. bruising, abrasions, lacerations, fractures).

- Girls <2 years can be examined in 'frog leg' position on a parent's lap. Grasp the labia and apply traction forward and downward to inspect the hymen
- The external genitalia should be carefully examined for bruises, oedema, lacerations and erythema
- Ask the child to point with a finger to the area or areas of the alleged assault

- The lateral buttocks separation test needs to be performed with the child in the left lateral position
- Adequate visualization of the posterior hymenal rim can often be achieved with the child in the prone knee–chest position
- An otoscope is superior to the naked eye in examining the hymen when a colposcope is not available
- Record any abnormalities, including details of size and colour, and estimate of age. Photography (stills or video) provides excellent documentation

Notes:

Speculum examination is not usually required in prepubertal girls or adolescent girls who have not had intercourse.

In the majority of sexually abused children the genitalia are normal.

SPECIMEN COLLECTION

- The collection of forensic specimens should be considered for children sexually abused within the preceding 72 h
- Semen fluoresces under a Wood's lamp
- Forensic swabs should be air-dried, labelled and handed to police. Document the chain of transmission of forensic evidence
- Swabs and serum should be collected for *STD screening* whenever forensic swabs are collected, when a vaginal discharge is noted, or when factors in the history lead to suspicion of STD. Urethral, anal and pharyngeal swabs should be sent for Gram stain and culture for *Neisseria gonorrhoeae*, and for *Chlamydia* culture (low vaginal swab in prepubertal children). Send blood for hepatitis B, hepatitis C and HIV serology. If vesicles are present, send fluid for IF and viral culture

MANAGEMENT

- Consider pregnancy prophylaxis if within 72 h of assault (two contraceptive pills containing 50 µg ethinyl oestradiol plus two metoclopramide 10 mg stat.; repeat 12 h later)
- Treatment and follow-up should be arranged as needed. All abused children and their parents should have access to appropriate counselling

Note: Remember:

SUSPECT CHILD ABUSE
RECOGNIZE CHILD ABUSE
CONSULT THE CHILD PROTECTION AUTHORITIES

THE DEATH OF A CHILD

Peter McDougall, Margaret Loughnan, John Rogers, Gerry Silk

The death of a child precipitates an intense grieving process in surviving family members which may last for years. It is very important for the family's future well-being that the health-care team ensure that the processes surrounding death are carried out in a sensitive and caring manner. The purpose of this chapter is to provide some guidelines.

ANTICIPATED DEATH

The death of a child can often be anticipated by hospital staff. This occurs in preterm infants with multiple problems or term infants with major congenital abnormalities, overwhelming sepsis or metabolic disease. Death occurs in the older child following a chronic illness or trauma. The majority of these children spend time in hospital and become involved with many members of staff.

THE INTERVIEW

Personnel: The consistency of the health-care team in a child's final illness is essential. Medical interviews with families are best led by a senior doctor together with a junior doctor, nurse, social worker or member of the clergy. The presence of more than two of these people at an interview may be threatening to the family. Other health-care team members, especially the family doctor and others outside the hospital, need to be closely involved.

Be comfortable: Choose a physically comfortable location where interruptions can be avoided. The open ward or corridor are not the places for interviews.

Information Must be Clear and Simple

- Begin by asking the family to give *their understanding* of the situation
- *The prognosis* is usually best given early
- *Give an explanation* of the disease process
- *Avoid* the use of *unexplained medical jargon*

- *Avoid information overload unless requested.* There is time to deal with complex medical issues at later interviews
- *Avoid ambiguous phrases* such as 'we might lose the battle' or 'he's passed away'. The words *death*, *die* and *dying* should be used

Respect silences: When bad news is delivered it is best to remain silent until the parent responds. This sometimes takes minutes and can be very uncomfortable. These are important moments and should not be interrupted.

Responsibilities of the accompanying members of the health-care team: *The accompanying members of the health-care team* at a medical interview need to be sensitive to the parents' needs and be watchful for misunderstandings. If they do not understand the medical message, it is unlikely that the parents will. At an appropriate time, the accompanying team member may ask the doctor to clarify some of the explanations given, but it is important not to interrupt a train of conversation or the silences that occur.

The senior doctor should inform the family that *all possible reasonable measures* were taken to preserve their child's life. It is not necessary to repeat this message.

Adequate relief of pain and distress of the child: This needs to be attended to and the parents assured of its importance.

Interpreters: The availability of trained interpreters for those with a language other than English is essential. Do not use other family members or friends as interpreters.

PREPARATIONS FOR DEATH

Time and space: The health-care team must not overwhelm families. Parents need to spend time alone together and with their child, either in the hospital ward, a quiet room or at home.

Arrangements: Arrangements need to be made for: baptism; religious advice; photographs; videos; and other memories of the child.

Permission: Many families have specific needs and sometimes they are unsure whether these are permissible. If these issues can be anticipated and discussed, the family's wishes may be facilitated with the least amount of interference to the continuing care of other children and families in the hospital.

The child: The preparation for death is largely dependent on the age and particular illness of the child. The older child with a chronic illness is often aware of impending death, and the health-care team needs to be sensitive to the family's and child's wishes in the delivery of information.

The place of death: Decisions need to be made about where the child will die. This largely depends on the family, but may be at home, in a hospice or the hospital. When appropriate the child may be included in this planning.

SUDDEN UNEXPECTED DEATH

The sudden death of a child from a wide variety of causes may occur in the community, the emergency department or the ward of a hospital. Sudden infant death syndrome (SIDS; see p. 344) is particularly traumatic because it is the unexpected and unexplained death of a previously well infant. Although most of the preceding guidelines are applicable, there are some additional considerations regarding sudden death.

Resuscitation

This is frequently attempted either at home or in hospital. Some parents may wish to be present and they should not be excluded, but an experienced staff member needs to be available to provide them with support.

When it becomes clear that further resuscitative attempts are futile, it is the responsibility of the senior hospital doctor or general practitioner to inform the family. **A member of staff should be available to:**

- Establish a relationship of trust
- Listen to the family's account of the events
- Allow the family freedom to express their emotions
- Provide non-judgemental understanding of any pre-existing difficult family relationships
- Provide access to telephones for notification of relatives
- Facilitate the attendance of siblings and other important family members at the hospital

In the case of a death in the community, the general practitioner should assume the above responsibilities.

The Family Response

The immediate responses to sudden death vary from emotional withdrawal to outbursts of profound grief. Unexpected reactions commonly occur. *Any response is appropriate*, provided it does not threaten other people.

BRAIN DEATH

Occasionally, it becomes clear that a child who is dependent on mechanical ventilation is brain dead.

- The senior doctor needs to explain the *meaning of brain death.* Avoid the use of confusing words. The unambiguous message that death has occurred, together with the *distinction between brain death and coma* need to be clearly explained
- It frequently helps parents to understand that their child has died by encouraging them to witness some or all of the brain death tests
- *Request for organ donation* generally requires a separate interview, made in a positive manner, without coercion, and with clear acknowledgement of the family's vulnerability. Issues related to donation need to be discussed in order to provide informed consent

AFTER DEATH

The moment of death: Although usually anticipated, the moment of death is an important event and needs medical confirmation.

Mementoes: Offer the family mementoes such as photographs, locks of hair, hand and footprints together with personal belongings.

- Black and white photographs of the dead child produce better results than colour
- If parents do not initially want mementoes, these need to be stored as some families request them at a later date

Viewing the Body: This can be valuable for family members. It is particularly important for the family of a child whose organs have been donated as it provides a visible reality of death, and may eliminate the fantasy or haunting fear of possible body mutilation.

- Provide a private area where the family can spend uninterrupted time with their child
- Families should be offered the opportunity to wash and dress their dead child as a last act of care

Autopsy: Discussion is often best done before anticipated death. Explanations should include the following:

- The autopsy procedure
- The potential future benefit to the parents

- A doctor will perform the autopsy like an operation, with care and respect
- The process does not interfere with funeral arrangements
- The results may not be available for some weeks after death

Coroner's cases: Following a sudden death, referral to the coroner is a statutory requirement. The coroner then decides whether or not an autopsy is to be performed. Parents can request (on a special form) that the coroner does not direct that an autopsy be performed. In many cases where the cause of the death is not in doubt (e.g. severe head injury), the coroner will respect the wishes of the family.

Funeral options: These need to be discussed and the family assisted to make their own arrangements with a funeral director. Encouragement is given to the family to involve siblings in this important ritual.

Sedation: Unless a parent has a well-defined psychiatric illness, sedation is best avoided for the acute stages of grief.

Breast feeding: Advice needs to be given to the breast feeding mother regarding suppression of lactation.

The surviving siblings: Children react in their own way to their sibling's death. They may blame themselves and/or fear their own death. Parents often need help and support to understand the responses of their surviving children.

Availability of the health-care team: Availability of the health-care team to the family after death needs to be assured, and follow-up arranged. In particular, notify health professionals who have been and will continue to be involved with the family following the child's death, including the referring doctor or institution, the family's general practitioner, and the maternal and child health nurse.

On leaving the hospital: It is usually important to both families and staff that farewells be made. For families new to the hospital, appropriate assistance and guidance from the premises is important.

Other families in the ward: The death of a child often affects the parents of other children in the hospital ward. The acknowledgement of a child's death with these families is very important.

Care of staff: The death of a child, whether anticipated or sudden, often deeply affects closely involved staff members. Some members of staff may not have been present at the time and it is important to ensure that they are notified. *Debriefing sessions* can be therapeutic in these circumstances.

FOLLOW-UP

Medical interview: Whether an autopsy is performed or not, it is essential that an appointment be made for the parents to see the child's treating doctor. Some parents are reluctant to attend, but most see the interview as a 'final farewell'. The discussion should include the autopsy results, the child's period of illness, future child bearing and issues related to bereavement.

Although the child's doctor should see the family for one or more follow-up visits, he or she may not be the best person to conduct ongoing *bereavement counselling*. It is necessary for the doctor to ensure that appropriate subsequent follow-up is arranged, often via the family doctor.

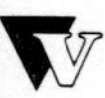

Support groups: Information needs to be provided to families regarding the support groups that are available both at the hospital and in the community.

SUDDEN INFANT DEATH SYNDROME

Sudden infant death syndrome (SIDS) is the sudden death of any infant or young child, which is unexplained by history, and in which a thorough post-mortem evaluation fails to demonstrate an adequate cause of death.

EPIDEMIOLOGY

Until 1990, around 550 babies a year died of SIDS in Australia (approximately 140 of these in Victoria) which correlated with the national and international average of two SIDS cases per 1000 live births. Following the 'Reducing the Risks' campaign, the rate has steadily fallen to 0.76 per 1000 live births in 1993. A drop in incidence has also been observed in Europe and New Zealand where similar campaigns have been conducted.

SIDS accounts for 43% of deaths that occur between the ages of 1 month and 1 year. SIDS most commonly occurs under 6 months of age. It rarely occurs after the age of 12 months. Although the risk of SIDS is slightly higher in subsequent siblings of a SIDS infant, when matched for birth order with controls there is no difference in incidence.

'REDUCING THE RISKS' CAMPAIGN

The campaign advises that babies should:

- Be slept on their back or side
- Not be allowed to get too hot
- Kept in a smoke-free environment, pre- and postnatally
- Be fed breast milk if possible
- Further information on the campaign can be obtained from the local SIDS organization.

APPARENT LIFE-THREATENING EPISODE

An apparent life-threatening episode (ALTE) is defined as an episode that is frightening to the observer and that is characterized by some combination of apnoea, colour change, marked change of muscle tone, choking or gagging. The terms 'near miss SIDS' and 'aborted cot death' should not be used, as they imply a close association between ALTE and SIDS, which does not exist.

- Less than 7% of infants who die from SIDS have a preceding history of ALTE
- No cause is found in over 50% of cases presenting under the age of 6 months

Associations that have been found with ALTE are:

- *Gastro-oesophageal reflux:* a small number of infants with this common condition experience coughing and choking episodes, and occasionally apnoea. These episodes occur most frequently when the infant is awake, and are often recurrent. Most resolve within a month but some persist for up to a year
- *Respiratory syncytial virus:* can cause apnoea particularly in preterm infants. Other viruses and *pertussis* can also be associated
- *Upper airways obstruction:* due to mid-nasal narrowing or adenoidal hypertrophy, and usually suspected by a history of snoring and sleep disturbance
- *Epilepsy:* usually suggested by a good history. Investigation of ALTE by EEG is usually fruitless
- *Cardiac arrythmias:* an uncommon cause

Most infants with ALTE need minimal resuscitation. However, some need cardiopulmonary resuscitation, and these infants have at least a 10% chance of further episodes.

A cause will usually be found in infants presenting with ALTE over the age of 6 months. If no cause is found in this age group and the episodes are recurrent, consider Munchausen syndrome by proxy.

All infants presenting with ALTE who needed resuscitation at home should be admitted to hospital for monitoring, investigation and counselling of the parents.

HOME APNOEA MONITORING

No study has been able to demonstrate that widespread home apnoea monitoring programmes reduce the incidence of SIDS.

Although we do not recommend widespread home apnoea monitoring, there is a community awareness of its existence and, despite some medical advice to the contrary, a small demand for its use. The following are our recommendations for consideration of home apnoea monitoring:

- *Twin of a SIDS victim*
- *Subsequent siblings of SIDS victims:* many of these parents conduct a 24 h watch on their infants and, for these families, home monitoring might be appropriate
- *ALTE:* particularly if mouth-to-mouth resuscitation was used
- *Extremely premature infants:* most of these families have a high exposure to monitors and the reality of death in the intensive care nursery

For a home monitoring programme to be useful the following are essential:

- Counselling
- Instruction of cardiopulmonary resuscitation
- Complete medical and service backup

CHAPTER 32

FLUID AND ELECTROLYTE THERAPY

Frank Shann
In collaboration with Neil Campbell

There are marked differences between children and adults in fluid and electrolyte composition and maintenance requirements.

Table 32.1 Fluid distribution

	Total body water (mL/kg)	*Intracellular fluid (mL/kg)*	*Extracellular fluid (mL/kg)*	*Blood volume (mL/kg)*
Neonate	750	350	450	85
Infant	700	400	300	80
Child	650	400	250	70
Adult	600	400	200	60

Table 32.2 Daily maintenance intravenous fluid requirements

Bodyweight	*Requirements*
3–10 kg	100 mL/kg per day
10–20 kg	1000 mL + (50 mL/kg per day for each kg over 10 kg)
20 kg and over	1500 mL + (20 mL/kg per day for each kg over 20 kg)

Table 32.3 Hourly maintenance intravenous fluid requirements

Weight (kg)	4	6	8	10	12	14	16	20	30	40	50	60	70
mL/h	16	24	32	40	45	50	55	65	70	80	90	95	100

Table 32.4 Adjustments to maintenance intravenous fluid requirements

Condition	*Adjustment to fluid intake*
Renal failure	× 0.2 + urine output
Basal state	× 0.7
High ADH (e.g. brain injury, meningitis)	× 0.7
High room humidity	× 0.7
Breathing humidified gas	× 0.75
Fever/hypothermia	± 12% per °C from 37 °C
Burns	
Day 1	+ 4% per 1% burn
Subsequent days	+ 2% per 1% burn

For example, a 6 kg comatose child with meningitis and a temperature of 38 °C needs 24 × 0.7 (basal) × 0.7 (high ADH) + 12% (fever) = 13 mL/h for full intake; fluid restriction requires a lower intake (monitor the serum sodium; low levels suggest overhydration).

DEHYDRATION

Dehydration without shock can usually be managed with oral rehydration fluid plus food (see p. 84). Children with shock (hypotension and acidosis) caused by hypovolaemia should be given parenteral fluid immediately: give 20 mL/kg repeatedly until plasma volume is restored (this may need 20–100 mL/kg). The fluid can be given intravenously or into bone marrow (see p. 26); nasogastric or intraperitoneal fluid is not effective in shock.

In general, an isotonic saline solution or Haemaccel is suitable for rehydration in hypovolaemic shock. If other factors such as septicaemia or blood loss are involved, 5% albumin solution or blood may be required. Five per cent dextrose with low sodium concentrations (e.g. 5% dextrose in 0.225% NaCl) must not be used for rapid infusion as severe hyponatraemia with fitting may occur.

In states of hyponatraemia or hypernatraemia, correction of serum sodium towards normal should not occur at more than 1–2 mmol/L per h.

REPLACEMENT THERAPY

Three basic aspects are considered:
- Existing deficit
- Continuing losses during therapy
- Maintenance requirements

Existing Fluid Deficit

This is calculated from the bodyweight according to the degree of dehydration, estimated by the clinical features:
- Decreased peripheral perfusion (pallor or reduced capillary return)
- Deep (acidotic) breathing – not useful in diabetic ketoacidosis
- Decreased skin turgor
- Increased thirst

A history of oliguria, restlessness, lethargy, sunken eyes, dry mouth, sunken fontanelle and the absence of tears are poor signs of mild to moderate dehydration in children. In general:
- <4% bodyweight loss: no clinical signs
- 4–10% bodyweight loss: clinical signs present, and the severity of the signs is a guide to the degree of dehydration
- >10% bodyweight loss: hypotension and severe acidosis

In general, fluids to replace the existing deficit are given over the first 24 h. In hypernatraemic or hyponatraemic dehydration, at least 48–72 h should be taken for replacement.

Electrolyte Deficit

The type and amount of electrolyte deficit depends on the diagnosis: for example in gastroenteritis, loss of base leads to acidosis; in pyloric stenosis, loss of acid and chloride leads to hypochloraemic alkalosis.

The rate of infusion of potassium must not exceed 0.4 mmol/kg per h. Concentrations of potassium greater than 40 mmol/L should be used with extreme caution.

Electrocardiographic monitoring should be considered in massive potassium replacement, and infusions of concentrated solutions should be controlled with the use of a pump.

Continuing Losses

It is essential to have an accurate recording on a fluid balance chart of the volumes of vomitus or gastric aspirates, drainage from fistulae, diarrhoea, urine output and other fluid losses. These will determine both the volume and type of fluid and electrolyte replacement required.

Maintenance Requirements

These are given in addition to replacement of the existing deficit and continuing losses.

ACID–BASE PROBLEMS

The maintenance of pH within narrow limits is by two mechanisms.

- Buffer systems: the bicarbonate system is quantitatively the most important in plasma (70% of the total)
- Excretory mechanisms: via the kidneys and lungs

Acidosis (low pH) and alkalosis (high pH) may be respiratory or non-respiratory (metabolic) in origin. Respiratory disorders result from changes in the excretion of volatile carbon dioxide, and consequently in the levels of carbonic acid. Metabolic disorders occur with changes in concentrations of non-volatile acids, and consequently in the concentration of buffer base – mainly bicarbonate.

The four primary disorders are:

- *Metabolic acidosis.* This arises from increased production of non-volatile acid (e.g. ketoacids and lactic acid), failure of the kidney to excrete non-volatile acid or conserve base, or excess loss of buffer base (e.g. gastroenteritis or intestinal fistula)
- *Metabolic alkalosis.* This arises from excess loss of non-volatile acid (e.g. pyloric stenosis), excess intake of buffer (e.g. bicarbonate infusion), or potassium depletion where an extracellular alkalosis occurs as hydrogen ions are lost in the urine (e.g. renal tubular syndromes, pyloric stenosis or diuretic therapy)
- *Respiratory acidosis.* Hypercapnoea is the result of alveolar hypoventilation from any cause (e.g. central, neuromuscular or pulmonary)
- *Respiratory alkalosis.* This is caused by hyperventilation

INDICATORS OF ACID–BASE STATUS

pH

This reflects the actual hydrogen ion concentration and alters in response to both respiratory and metabolic changes.

P_{CO_2} (Partial Pressure of Carbon Dioxide)

In arterial and capillary blood samples, this represents the P_{CO_2} in blood leaving the lungs. Alterations reflect disturbance in the *respiratory component* of the acid–base state (and not the metabolic component).

Base Excess

This is an estimate of the change in total buffer base that would be present if the P_{CO_2} were normal (40 mmHg). Changes in base excess reflect disturbance in the *metabolic component* of acid–base status (and not the respiratory component). In metabolic alkalosis, total buffer base is increased, and thus base excess is positive. Other calculated measures of the metabolic component are the standard bicarbonate and the total buffer base.

Actual Bicarbonate

This is the plasma concentration of bicarbonate; it is influenced by both metabolic and respiratory components.

In practice, isolated metabolic and respiratory disorders are uncommon. Most disorders have a metabolic and a respiratory component. Usually one is the primary disorder, and the other occurs secondarily and tends to correct the change in pH. However, sometimes primary metabolic and respiratory disturbances occur together, e.g. in respiratory distress syndrome, when hypoxia leading to lactic acid accumulation produces metabolic acidosis, and carbon dioxide retention produces a respiratory acidosis.

The interpretation of changes in base excess and P_{CO_2} as primary or secondary changes must be made clinically.

Table 32.5 Changes in arterial or capillary blood (before compensation)

	pH (mmol/L)	*P_{CO_2} (mmol/L)*	*Base excess (mmol/L)*	*Actual bicarbonate*
	7.36–7.44	36–44	− 5 to + 3	18–25
Metabolic acidosis	Decrease	Normal	Decrease	Decrease
Metabolic alkalosis	Increase	Normal	Increase	Increase
Respiratory acidosis	Decrease	Increase	Normal	Increase
Respiratory alkalosis	Increase	Decrease	Normal	Decrease

Table 32.6 Changes in indicators of acid–base status seen in combined disorders

	pH	P_{CO_2}	*Base excess*	*Actual bicarbonate*
Primary metabolic acidosis + compensatory respiratory alkalosis (e.g. gastroenteritis, diabetic ketosis)	Decrease or normal	Decrease	Decrease	Decrease
Primary metabolic alkalosis + compensatory respiratory acidosis (e.g. pyloric stenosis)	Increase or normal	Increase	Increase	Increase
Combined primary respiratory and metabolic acidosis (e.g. respiratory distress syndrome)	Decrease	Increase	Decrease	Normal

CORRECTION OF METABOLIC ACIDOSIS

Metabolic acidosis will often resolve rapidly once the cause has been corrected, and administration of bicarbonate is often not required.

A guide to the amount of bicarbonate required is given by: mmol of HCO_3 required = basic deficit (mmol/L) × weight (kg) × 0.3. The factor (weight × 0.3) represents the volume of extracellular fluid through which the base deficit (negative base excess) is distributed. In babies less than 5 kg, the factor is weight × 0.5 due to the greater percentage of extracellular fluid. It is usual to give only half the amount of bicarbonate suggested by these formulae, and then repeat the blood gas measurement before giving any more.

The rate of administration of bicarbonate will be determined by the cause of the metabolic acidosis and the clinical state of the patient; for example in cardiac arrest infuse bicarbonate rapidly, in gastroenteritis correction should usually be undertaken over at least 6 h (and mild to moderate acidosis will resolve with rehydration alone). Rapid correction of metabolic acidosis will cause a fall in extracellular potassium.

The principles of correction of metabolic alkalosis are discussed in the section on pyloric stenosis (p. 355).

COMMONLY USED INTRAVENOUS SOLUTIONS

SALINE BICARBONATE

This solution is made up by adding 60 mL of sodium bicarbonate 8.4% to each litre of 1/2 isotonic saline and 2.5% dextrose. The solution is stable for only 24 h.

5% NORMAL SERUM ALBUMIN (5% NSA)

This solution contains human albumin 50 g/L, sodium 140 mmol/L, chloride 125 mmol/L and octanoate 8 mmol/L; it has an osmolality of 260 mmol/kg and a pH of 6.7–7.3.

ALBUMIN (20%)

This solution contains albumin 200 g/L, sodium 46–58 mmol/L and octanoate 32 mmol/L; it has an osmolality of 80 mmol/kg and a pH of 7.0.

Table 32.7 Commonly used intravenous solutions

	Na^+ (mmol/L)	*Cl^- (mmol/L)*	*K^+ (mmol/L)*	*Lactate (mmol/l)*	Ca^{2+} (mmol/L)	*Glucose (g/L)*
Isotonic or normal saline (0.9% NaCl)	150	150	–	–	–	–
1/2 isotonic saline with 5% glucose	75	75	–	–	–	50
1/5 isotonic saline with 4% glucose	30	30	–	–	–	40
1/5 isotonic saline with 4% glucose and KCl 20 mmol/L	30	30	20	–	–	40
Hartmann's solution	130	110	5	30	2	–
Hartmann's solution with 5% glucose	130	110	5	30	2	50

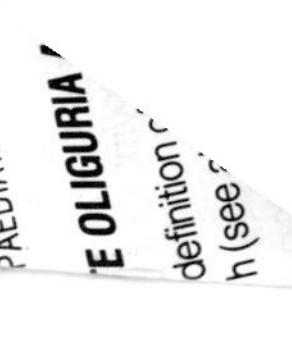

ADDITIVES

- Molar potassium chloride (0.75 g ir
  Cl^-
- 20% sodium chloride = 3.4 mmol/mL
- Molar sodium bicarbonate (8.4%) = 1
- Calcium gluconate 10% = 0.22 mmo
  mg/mL of Ca^{2+}
- Magnesium chloride for injection (0.48 g
  1 mmol/mL of Mg^{2+}

MANAGEMENT OF SOME SPECIAL CONDITIONS

PYLORIC STENOSIS

Hydrogen ion and chloride loss predominate, with consequent hypochloraemic alkalosis. Losses of potassium in vomitus and urine can lead to significant hypokalaemia. In severe cases, hypokalaemia will lead to a renal compensatory mechanism, in which additional hydrogen ion is lost in an attempt to conserve potassium. This leads to paradoxical acidaemia.

The duration and severity of vomiting will, to a large extent, determine the degree of fluid and electrolyte imbalance.

Assessment

All patients require biochemical assessment, but not all will require intravenous therapy. Any child who is clinically dehydrated or has significant biochemical derangement requires intravenous therapy.

Intravenous Therapy

In *severe dehydration* (>10%), commence with *isotonic saline* until adequate circulation has been established and then continue with 1/2 isotonic saline and 5% dextrose.

In *moderate dehydration* (4–10%), commence with *1/2 isotonic saline with 5% dextrose.* Await electrolyte results before commencing therapy if only mildly dehydrated.

Adequate potassium and chloride replacement is necessary for correction of the acid–base abnormality. As soon as urine flow is established, potassium chloride is given up to a maximum of 0.4 mmol/kg per h. Usually 20–40 mmol/L is adequate.

ANURIA

...vere oliguria is a urine output of less than 0.5 mL/kg ... p. 137).

...al Management

...hree clinical situations occur:

- Sudden and complete anuria should arouse suspicion of urinary obstruction provided the catheter is correctly placed and not blocked
- Renal hypoperfusion causing oliguria should be suspected in the presence of clinical dehydration or septicaemia leading to hypotension; the urinary sodium is usually less than 20 mmol/L. Blood volume expansion is necessary
- Renal tissue injury (e.g. acute post-streptococcal glomerulonephritis or secondary to hypoperfusion or nephrotoxin). The urinary sodium is usually more than 40 mmol/L. Frusemide (1–2 mg/kg) should be given intravenously and, if there is no response, treatment for continuing anuria should be instituted

Continuing Anuria

Fluid intake is restricted to the previous 24 h urine output and any abnormal losses; approximately 20% of normal maintenance requirements must also be given to replace insensible water loss.

At least 20% of full calorie requirements are given as carbohydrate to spare tissue protein from catabolism for energy, which accentuates the rise in blood urea. Intravenous 10–20% glucose, or oral Caloreen or Polyjoule are suitable.

Peritoneal dialysis or haemofiltration will be required for hyperkalaemia, severe uraemia (blood urea >50 mmol/L), acidosis, or water overload leading to hyponatraemia, oedema or hypertension, and should always be considered if anuria persists for more than 24 h.

HYPERKALAEMIA

The management of hyperkalaemia depends on its cause. Serum potassium is increased by acidosis, and reduced by alkalosis. In acute oliguric renal failure, if urine is not formed after intravenous frusemide (see above), the presence of hyperkalaemia (>7.0 mmol/L) is an indication for dialysis. High values (up to 7.0 mmol/L) not requiring treatment may be found in the neonatal period.

If cardiac arrhythmias are present, rapid but temporary benefit may be achieved by giving:

- *Sodium bicarbonate* 2 mmol/kg, i.v.
- *Short-acting (regular) insulin* 0.1 unit/kg given with 2 mL/kg of 50% dextrose, i.v.
- *Calcium gluconate* 10% 0.5 mL/kg, i.v. given slowly
- *Sodium polystyrene sulfonate* (Resonium) 1 g/kg, p.r. or n.g.

OTHER CONDITIONS

See acute infectious diarrhoea (p. 83), haemorrhagic shock (p. 5), burns (p. 269), diabetes mellitus (p. 197) and *Meningococcal septicaemia* (p. 8).

THE NEWBORN

Babies are different from older age groups because they have:

- More body water in all compartments
- Greater insensible water losses
- Reduced renal capacity to compensate for abnormalities
- Less integrated and responsive endocrine controls

These differences are of practical importance only in very sick babies — those requiring inpatient care in Level 2 or Level 3 nurseries.

This section highlights major practical differences between the sick newborn and older age groups. However, any baby needing intravenous therapy should be in a Level 2 or Level 3 nursery.

Insensible water losses can vary from around 30 mL/kg per 24 h at term to >200 mL/kg per 24 h below 27 weeks gestation.

The newborn kidney is less able to concentrate or dilute urine, less able

Table 32.8 Body water

	<28 weeks	*Term*
Total body water	85% (of bodyweight)	75%
Extracellular water	55%	45%
Circulating blood volume	90–100 mL/kg	85 mL/kg

Intermediate gestations lie between these figures.

to retain Na^+ and K^+ or shed excess loads, and less able to excrete H^+ to shed acid loads.

WATER REQUIREMENTS

There is often confusion between babies' *water* requirements and *milk* requirements. For normal nutrition, babies need 150–200 mL/kg per 24 h of milk. For most babies this is two to three times their water requirements. This difference is only of practical importance in babies suffering illnesses which are made worse by excess water administration, for example acute and chronic lung disease, heart failure or renal impairment.

Water requirements depend on:

- Gestational age: skin losses are greater and renal concentration poorer the earlier the gestation
- Postnatal age: skin losses decrease and renal function improves steadily from day 1
- Conditions of nursing: dressed babies lose least; naked babies under radiant heaters lose most. Humidified respiratory circuits (e.g. ventilators) reduce respiratory losses

Water requirements are summarized in Table 32.9.

Below 27 weeks gestation requirements are too variable to tabulate: start at 120 mL/kg and modify 6–12 hourly according to clinical state, serum Na^+ and urine osmolality.

SODIUM

Babies are less able to conserve sodium or excrete excess loads.

Daily requirements are 2–4 mmol/kg per 24 h; the earlier the gestation, the higher the need.

Table 32.9 Infant water requirements

	Days 1–2	*Days 6–7*
Mature 35 weeks +	40–50 mL/kg per day	60
Immature 27 weeks	80–120	60–80

Intermediate gestations lie between these figures. Lower figures are for babies on ventilators.

Hyponatraemia (Serum Na^+ <132 mmol/L)

This may be due to excess water administration, inadequate sodium administration, excess sodium loss or inappropriate ADH secretion. The cause should always be defined; do not just treat blindly.

It is easy to overload sick babies with water in the first days after birth. This is a common cause of hyponatraemia. In general, intravenous rates >60 mL/kg per 24 h in sick mature babies will provide excessive water in the first 48 h.

When the cause is water overload serum Na^+ correction by water restriction alone is very slow in the newborn. As serum Na^+ <125 mmol/L can result in fits and may be injurious to the CNS, it should be treated with Na^+ administration, even when the primary cause is water overload. The dose required can be calculated as follows:

Dose of Na^+ (mmol) = bodyweight × 0.8 × (140 – current serum Na^+)

The aim is to correct slowly over 36 h, once the level of 125 mmol is reached. Using this regimen Serum Na^+ should be checked every 6 h: if correction is occurring rapidly, Na^+ administration can be ceased once serum levels are safe.

Hypernatraemia (Serum Na^+ >154 mmol/L)

This may be due to excess Na^+ administration, inadequate water administration or excess loss of water in relation to sodium. The cause should always be defined.

It is easy to overload sick babies with sodium-containing intravenous fluids; for example 1 mL/h of normal saline = 4 mmol Na^+/24 h — the entire Na^+ requirements of a 1000 g baby, and more than half the daily requirements of a 2000 g baby. The use of sodium bicarbonate for correction of acidosis also often leads to sodium overload.

Hypernatraemia may be injurious to the CNS and should be avoided if possible.

Na^+ should be added to intravenous maintenance fluids from the beginning of day 2, taking into account separate sodium administration as sodium bicarbonate or heparinized saline.

POTASSIUM

Potassium requirements are 2–4 mmol/kg per 24 h. Serum K^+ does not reflect body K^+. With high or low levels the cause should be defined.

Except with anuria, K^+ should be added to maintenance intravenous fluids from the beginning of day 2.

With *diuretic therapy* Na^+ and K^+ losses are much greater in babies than older age groups.

GLUCOSE

Blood glucose levels are unstable in sick babies. Fasting babies require intravenous solutions containing at least 10% Dextrose. Average glucose requirements are 4–7 mg glucose/kg per min (6–10 g/kg per day), but some sick babies require more, and others less.

ACID–BASE PROBLEMS

Metabolic acidosis is the commonest acid–base disturbance in sick babies. The cause should always be defined. Correction with sodium bicarbonate is controversial, but it is reasonable to begin correcting pH <7.10 fairly quickly, that is over 30–60 min, and pH 7.10–7.20 slowly, that is over 2–4 h.

Dose of sodium bicarbonate (mmol) = bodyweight × 0.5 × base deficit.

Acid–base status should be re-evaluated once half the dose of bicarbonate has been given, and the dose adjusted if necessary. When given at the rates recommended there is no need to dilute 8.4% sodium bicarbonate before administration. Other measures to control the acidosis (e.g. volume expansion) should be instituted at the same time.

FORMULAS AND DEFINITIONS

CONVERSION FACTORS

- Sodium chloride 1 g contains 17 mmol Na and 17 mmol Cl
- Potassium chloride 1 g contains 13 mmol K and 13 mmol Cl
- Sodium bicarbonate 1 g contains 12 mmol Na and 12 mmol HCO_3

MOLARITY

Osmolality is the number of osmotically active molecules in solution per kilogram of solute (usually mmol/kg of water).

Osmolarity is the number of osmotically active molecules in solution per litre of solute (usually mmol/L of water).

USEFUL FORMULAS

Anion gap = Na – (bicarbonate + Cl); normal <12

Number mL/h, i.v. = microdrops/min = 4 × drops/min

Number mmol = mEq/valence = mass (mg)/mol. wt

Sodium deficit: mL 20% NaCl = wt × 0.2 × (140 – serum Na)

Water deficit (mL) = 600 × wt (kg) × [1 – (140/Na)]
(if body Na normal)

Non-catabolic anuria: urea rises 3–5 mmol/L per day

Bicarbonate dose (mmol) = base excess × wt/3 (give 1/2 this)

Osmolality serum = 2 Na + glucose + urea (normal 270–295 mmol/L)

CHAPTER 33

INFANT AND CHILD NUTRITION

Julie Bines, Kay Gibbons, Michelle Meehan, Neil Campbell and Helen Anthony

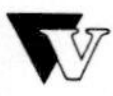

BREAST FEEDING

Breast milk alone is adequate nutrition for infants for the first 6 months of life. Breast feeding is the best feeding for babies and all efforts should be made to promote, encourage and maintain breast feeding for as long as possible.

NORMAL VARIATIONS OF BREAST FEEDING

Frequency of Feeds

Breast fed infants usually feed from 2 to 5 hourly. Young babies feed frequently but demand feeding (i.e. feeding when hungry) will usually have the baby settle into a fairly predictable pattern of feeds. The frequency of the feeds is determined by the baby's appetite and gastric capacity, as well as the amount of mother's milk available. If the baby is feeding very frequently, seems hungry or is not gaining weight as expected, ensure baby is being offered both breasts at each feed.

Length of Feeds

The duration of the feed is determined by the rate of transfer of milk from the breast to the baby, which in turn depends on the baby's suck and the mother's 'let down'. This may vary from 5–6 min to 20–30 min. It is the cessation of strong drawing sucks, and the appearance of shorter duration bursts of sucking that indicate the 'end' of the feed – *not the time.*

If mother feels the baby is on the breast 'all the time' it is better to look at the point where the pauses between bursts of sucking are longer than the sucking, and take the baby off or swap sides at this time (rather than timing it).

Appetite Spurts

Babies seem to experience appetite spurts at 2 weeks, 6 weeks and 3 months. It is crucial that parents are aware of this or the baby's natural increase in frequency of feeds may be mistaken for diminution of milk supply. This is specially true at 6 weeks when breasts are no longer carrying extra fluid and the supply is settling to the demands of the baby. Unfortunately, many women wean at this time through poor advice. Let the baby feed on demand, even 2 hourly, and this should settle in 48 h.

Appearance of Breast Milk

Breast milk is naturally thinner in consistency than artificial formula and may have a bluish tinge – this is **normal, healthy and nutritious.**

The presence of *blood in the milk* may cause a red or pinkish brown discoloration. If this is present when the mother first starts expressing colostrum, it may be due to *duct hyperplasia*. This gradually disappears and is of no significance. The most common cause of blood-stained milk (usually first noticed when the baby possets) is *trauma* to the nipple.

Bowel Actions

The motions of breast-fed infants are normally bright yellow and soft to loose. The baby may have a bowel action with every feed (strong gastro-colic reflex) or once every 5–8 days.

TEMPORARY CESSATION OF BREAST FEEDING

If the feeding pattern is interrupted due to illness, a planned fast for a procedure or the mother's absence, the mother will need to express to maintain the milk supply.

- Milk can be expressed by hand or by pump
- Express as often as the baby would normally feed (i.e. six to eight times a day). Several volumes of expressed milk can be added to the same bottle or storage bag (bags are available from commercial pharmacies), but a new container should be used every 24 h
- Milk may be kept in the freezer section of the refrigerator for 2 weeks or in the deep freeze for 3 months
- *To thaw frozen milk*, place bag/bottle in container of cool water and run hot water in until it is standing in hot water. When the milk is thawed it will be cold; continue to heat in hot water or place in the fridge until required for a feed
- Thawed milk should be used within 24 h

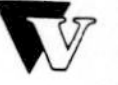

How Much Milk to Express?

If the mother wants to express to give a feed by bottle or to substitute a feed as she is weaning, how much will the baby need?

Daily requirements of milk are:
- *0–6 months:* 150 mL/kg per day
- *Over 6 months:* 120 mL/kg per day

Divide this amount by the usual number of feeds to calculate the amount required per feed.

Growth patterns differ between breast-fed and artificially fed infants. Average weights of breast-fed babies are similar to formula-fed until 4–6 months, after which breast-fed babies slow significantly in their weight gains. Length and head circumference remain similar.

There are as yet no standard weight charts for breast-fed infants. It is not appropriate to interpret their naturally slower weight gain, taken in isolation, as abnormal.

MATERNAL ILLNESS

When the mother is unwell, breast feeding should continue. In the case of maternal infection antibodies will be passed on in the breast milk to protect the baby.

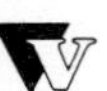

MATERNAL DRUGS

If the mother has to take medication, the cost–benefit ratio should be carefully weighed by the prescriber. The mother should continue to breast feed unless the use of the drug is absolutely contraindicated during lactation and there is no safe alternative. **There are very few drugs that are absolutely contraindicated and almost all have a safe alternative.** If the mother is concerned about continuing breast feeding even if the drug is safe, suggest taking the drug after a feed to minimize the concentration or dividing the dose if possible.

FORMULA FEEDING

If breast milk is not available, either from the breast or as expressed milk, a commercially prepared iron fortified formula should be chosen. These are based on cow milk, modified to lower the protein, calcium and electrolytes to levels better suited to the human infant, and have added amino acids, vitamins and trace minerals.

Table 33.1 How to assess good breast feeding

	Good	*Bad*
Baby's body position	On side-chest to chest	On back angled away from mother
Mouth	Open wide	Lips close together
Chin	Touching or pressing into the breast	Space between chin and breast
Lips	Flanged out	Tucked in, inverted
Cheeks	Well rounded	Dimpled or sucked in
Nose	Free of or just touching the breast	Buried in breast, baby pulls back
Breast in mouth	Good mouthful, more of bottom part of breast in mouth	Central, little breast tissue in mouth or only nipple in mouth
Jaw movement	Rhythmic deep jaw movement	Jerky or irregular shallow movement
Sounds	Muffled sound of swallowing milk	No swallowing, clicking sounds
Body language of the baby	Peaceful, concentrated	Restless, anxious
Body language of the mother	Comfortable, relaxed	Tense, hunched, awkward
Awareness of feelings during feed	Pain-free, may feel a drawing feeling deep in breast or 'let down'	Nipple or breast pain
Nipple, post-feed	Nipple elongated, well shaped	Not elongated, compressed 'stripe' or blanched

Source: Murray S, *Breast Feeding Information and Guidelines for Paediatric Units*, Royal Children's Hospital, Melbourne, 1992.

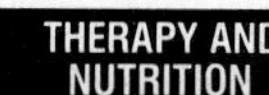

Table 33.2 Formula composition (per 100 mL)

Feed (20 kcal/30 mL, or 280 kJ/100 mL, unless specified)	*Manufacturer*	*Scoops per water volume*	*Protein (g)*	*Fat (g)*	*CHO (g)*	*Fe (mg)*	*Protein source*	*CHO source*
Human milk			1.1	4.2	7.4	0.08		Lactose
Infant formulas								
Nan 1	Nestle	1 : 30 mL	1.5	3.4	7.6	0.8	Whey/casien 60 : 40	Lactose
S26	Wyeth	1 : 60 mL	1.5	3.6	7.2	1.2	Whey/casien 60 : 40	Lactose
Enfalac Infant	Mead Johnson	1 : 30 mL	1.5	3.7	7.0	0.7	Whey/casien 60 : 40	Lactose
Enfalac Reduced Iron	Mead Johnson	1 : 30 mL	1.5	3.7	7.0	0.3	Whey/casien 60 : 40	Lactose
Karicare Infant	Douglas	1 : 50 mL	1.5	3.8	7.0	0.7	Whey/casein 60 : 40	Lactose
Formula								
Lactogen	Nestle	1 : 30 mL	1.7	3.4	7.4	0.8	Casein/whey 70 : 30	Lactose
SMA	Wyeth	1 : 60 mL	1.5	3.6	7.0	1.2	Casein/whey 82 : 18	Lactose
Enfamil	Mead Johnson	1 : 30 mL	1.5	3.7	6.9	1.2	Casein/whey 80 : 20	Lactose
Similac	Abbott	1 : 60 mL	1.5	3.6	7.4	1.2	Casein/whey 80 : 20	Lactose
Karicare Goats Milk — Infant Formula	Douglas	1 : 50 mL	1.4	3.8	7.3	0.8	Goat milk	Lactose

Table 33.2 *(Continued)*

Follow-on formulae								
Nan 2	Nestle	1 : 30 mL	2.3	3.2	7.3	1.2	Casein/whey 70 : 30	Lactose
S26 Progress	Wyeth	1 : 60 mL	2.2	3.2	7.2	1.2	Casein/whey 82 : 18	Lactose
Enfa–Pro 6	Mead Johnson	1 : 30 mL	2.5	2.7	8.3	1.2	Casein/whey 82 : 18	Lactose
Karicare Follow – on Milk Food	Douglas	1 : 50 mL	2.1	3.6	6.6	0.7	Casein/whey 40 : 60	Lactose
Karicare Goat Milk Follow-on	Douglas	1 : 50 mL	2.2	3.7	6.6	0.8	Goat milk	Lactose
Karicare Soya Follow - on	Douglas	1 : 30 mL	2.2	3.6	7.7	0.8	Soy	Maltodextrin
Prem formula								
Prem Enfalac (20 cal/30 mL)	Mead Johnson	1 : 30 mL	2.0	3.4	7.5	0.15	Whey/casein 60 : 40	Lactose, maltodextrin
(24 cal/30 mL)		1 : 25 mL	2.4	4.1	9.0	1.3	Whey/casein 60 : 40	Lactose, maltodextrin
S26 LBW	Wyeth	1 : 60 mL	2.0	4.3	8.6	0.3	Whey/casein 60 : 40	Lactose, maltodextrin
Prenan	Nestle	1 : 30 mL	2.0	3.4	8.0	1.1	Whey/casein 70 : 30	Lactose, maltodextrin

(Continued)

Table 33.2 *(Continued)*

Feed (20 kcal/30 mL, or 280 kJ/100 mL, unless specified)	*Manufacturer*	*Scoops per water volume*	*Protein (g)*	*Fat (g)*	*CHO (g)*	*Fe (mg)*	*Protein source*	*CHO source*
Soy formula								
Prosobee	Mead Johnson	1 : 30 mL	2.0	3.6	6.6	1.2	Soy	Maltodextrin
Infasoy	Wyeth	1 : 60 mL	1.8	3.6	6.9	1.2	Soy	Sucrose, maltodextrin
Isomil	Abbott	Conc. liquid	1.8	3.7	6.9	1.2	Soy	Sucrose, maltodextrin
Karicare – soya formula	Douglas	1 : 30 mL	1.8	3.6	6.7	0.8	Soy	Maltodextrin

Protein hydrolysate formulas: Pregestimil, Alfare and Nutramigen.
Breast milk fortifiers: FM 85 or Human Milk Fortifier.
Glucose polymer products: Polyjoule, Polycose or Energy Plus.
Fat emulsions: Liquigen (MCT oil) or Calogen (LCT).

COW MILK-BASED FORMULAS

- Formulas may be classified as whey-dominant or casein-dominant, describing the main protein type in the formula
- Changes to formula are made for a variety of reasons. In the normal thriving infant there is little indication to change formula

STRENGTHENING FORMULA FEEDS

Standard formulas provide 65–70 kcal/100 mL or 20 kcal/30 mL (270–280 kJ/100mL). To increase energy to 25 kcal/30 mL (350 kJ/100 mL):

- Use **additional formula powder** (i.e. for formulas where standard dilution is 1 scoop to 30 mL water use 1 scoop to 15 mL water, or for formulas where standard dilution is 1 scoop to 60 mL water use 1 scoop to 50 mL water). This will also increase protein and other nutrient intakes. Care should be taken with infants with renal or liver impairment

or

- Add **glucose polymer** (Polyjoule, Polycose) using 2 level teaspoons to 100 mL formula **or** 5 mL **fat emulsion** (Calogen, Liquigen) to 100 mL formula. *These additions will increase energy value only.*

To increase energy to 30 kcal/30 mL (420 kJ/100 mL):

- Use **additional formula powder** as above with the addition of either **glucose polymer** or **fat emulsion** (as above).

CHILDREN OVER 6 MONTHS

For infants over 6 months, follow-on formulas can be used. They have a higher protein and renal solute load and are not suitable for infants under 6 months of age.

SOY FORMULAS

If a soy-based feed is chosen, a soy *infant formula* should be chosen. These are nutritionally adequate for infants.

NUMBER OF FEEDS

Babies under 6 weeks of age usually feed every 3 h; however, they may take more each time and feed 4 hourly. Babies rarely sleep through the night before 6–8 weeks. When they miss a night feed (usually sleeping 5–6 h straight) they will have five feeds. They will consequently have more milk each feed. Babies that sleep longer in the day (e.g. 5 h between feeds) often need to feed overnight to maintain adequate intake. Parents may need to wake the baby after 4 h in the daytime. There is no need to wake a baby overnight if intake and weight gain are adequate.

INTRODUCTION OF WHOLE COW MILK

The introduction of cow milk products as part of an expanding diet is appropriate but the main milk intake should be breast milk or formula until 12 months, because of the risks of iron deficiency and allergy. Small amounts can be used on cereal, in custard and yoghurt from about 7 to 8 months.

Full cream dairy products should be used for children up to 2 years; skim milk should not used for children under 5 years.

INTRODUCTION OF SOLIDS

Breast milk or formulas will meet all nutrient needs for the first 4–6 months. From this time solids can be introduced, to increase intake of nutrients such as iron and as part of the educational process of learning to eat.

First solids can be iron-fortified baby cereal, smooth vegetables or fruits. Foods should be introduced one at a time to allow observation of tolerance. Meat can be introduced at about 7 months. Texture should be increased so that by about 8–9 months the infant is managing lumps and varying textures, and is starting to manage finger foods. By about 12 months most family foods can be offered. By 12 months the intake of milk should have reduced to about 600 mL. Much higher intakes limit the intake of other foods; in infants continued high intakes of cow milk with its low iron content are associated with the development of iron deficiency.

Iron deficiency and associated anaemia is the commonest nutrient deficiency in children in Australia. It is associated with the early introduction of cow milk, high intake of cow milk in the second year and low intake of iron-rich foods, such as meat and pulses.

WEANING

There is no set rule for weaning time. Solids should be introduced by 6 months and cup drinking started as a skill by 7–9 months. There is no need for the baby to be weaned to a bottle – if he/she is old enough they can go straight on to a cup.

Sudden cessation of breast feeding leaves the breasts at risk of developing mastitis. Ideally, weaning is achieved by reducing the feeds by one a week. Start by offering a drink in a cup or bottle instead of a breast feed at midday, then gradually increasing these other drinks. Many mothers retain the early morning feed or the last feed at night for a little longer.

Persistent difficulty weaning usually requires someone to support the mother, giving the baby a feed and allowing the baby some time away from the mother to help them with mutual separation. Both need to be ready to let go. Mother and baby units, especially those with a day-stay programme, are helpful here.

TODDLERS WHO WILL NOT EAT

Assessment of the toddler who refuses food includes:
- Plotting weight and height to assure the parents of normal growth
- **Demonstrating by the chart that the growth rate normally slows in the second year**
- Linking this to lessened need for food and subsequent drop in appetite
- Emphasizing the developmental progress

Advise parents:
- A healthy child will eat when hungry – *quit the fight!*
- Showing independence is an important part of toddler development – choosing and refusing food is an expression of independence
- Serve small portions – lower your expectations
- Serve food that you know they like. Cereal is OK for lunch! Lack of variety is not a major worry at this age
- Try to avoid arguments over food. Remember 'It's my job to offer food, it's the child's job to eat it'
- Avoid filling up on milk and juice – large volumes of milk (over 600 mL a day) can make the child feel full
- Give the child time to enjoy the meal without comment. Remove the food after 1/2 hour or if they dawdle or lose interest
- Learning to eat is fun. Switch to finger food if they refuse to be fed
- Try not to use food as a punishment or reward. It only increases its potential power

FOOD NEEDS OF PRESCHOOLERS

The following is a guide to the quantities suitable for the 2–5 year old. Many parents are surprised at how little children of this age need. However, because total needs are small there is relatively little place for high-fat, high-sugar extras such as savoury snack foods and soft drinks.

DAILY

Milk Group

Three serves (one serve = 250 mL milk, 200 g yoghurt, 35 g cheese). *Full cream products are recommended.*

Bread and Cereal Group

Four to five serves (one serve = one slice bread, 1/2 cup pasta, two wheat biscuit cereals).

Vegetable and Fruit Group

Four or more serves (one serve = one piece fruit, two tablespoons vegetables).

Meat or Protein Group

Two serves (one serve = 30 g lean meat, fish or chicken, 1/2 cup beans, one egg).

ENTERAL FEEDING

Enteral nutrition is the provision of nutrients to the alimentary tract via a feeding tube. It can be used to provide the total nutritional needs of a patient (either short or long term), or to provide additional nutrients when voluntary oral intake is inadequate.

Enteral feeding has certain advantages over Total Parenteral Nutrition:
- Less risk of infection
- Less risk of metabolic abnormalities
- Nutrients provided to the alimentary tract enhance intestinal growth and function
- Cheaper method

INDICATIONS

Enteral feeding is used for patients who:
- Cannot feed orally (eg. neurological damage, prematurity)
- Have increased metabolic requirements for nutrients (e.g. burns, CHD)
- Fail to achieve their nutritional requirements (e.g. FTT, cystic fibrosis)
- Require unpalatable specialised feeds to treat their medical condition (e.g. metabolic disorders, liver disease)

CONTRAINDICATION

Non-functioning GI tract

ROUTES OF ADMINISTRATION

The most commonly used route is *nasogastric*, its main benefit being ease of intubation. When long term feeding is required, a *gastrostomy tube* may be indicated.

When gastric motility is poor or when gastric residues are persistently high, a *nasojejunal tube* may be of benefit. However feeding directly into the jejeunum limits the choice of formula and may increase the risk of bacterial overgrowth.

IMPLEMENTATION OF FEEDS

In choosing a method consider the feeding route, the length of time the feed is expected to be required and the type of feed to be used. Introduction of hyperosmolar feeds should be done gradually.

Table 33.3 Types of feeding regimes

	Advantages	*Disadvantages*
Bolus feedings	Most closely mimics physiological feeding Increases patient mobility Little equipment is needed Volume given can be precisely measured	Can be time consuming for care giver May decrease voluntary oral intake
Gravity drip	Little equipment needed	Rate of delivery cannot be closely monitored
Pump assisted continuous	Feeding most likely to be tolerated Feeding can be delivered while patient sleeps Larger volumes can be tolerated than if given by bolus method	Requires feeding pump

SELECTION OF FEED

A full *nutritional assessment* (current nutritional status, current intake, requirements and consideration of medical condition/fluid restrictions) should be carried out by a dietitian to establish which feed would be optimal.

In general, infants can be managed using breast milk (if available) and/or infant formula. The formula will usually require additional fortification with both energy and other nutrients at around 6 months of age; this is suitable for up to about 2 years of age.

Children over 2 years can be managed adequately using a proprietary product (see Table 33.4).

It is generally inappropriate to put pureed foods down feeding tubes as the amount of fluid required to achieve a suitable consistency dilutes the energy and nutrient content, while increasing the risk of microbial contamination and tube blockage.

MONITORING ENTERAL NUTRITION

When monitoring patients on enteral feeds, mechanical, metabolic, gastrointestinal, nutritional and growth parameters must be assessed routinely. In the early stages of feeding, the patient's tolerance of the feeding regime is critical to the success of feeding.

Once the feeding plan has been fully implemented, assessment of the patient's nutrient requirements is needed regularly to ensure that adequacy of the nutritional support is maintained and also to indicate when enteral feeding can be ceased.

TRANSITION FROM TOTAL PARENTERAL NUTRITION (TPN) TO ENTERAL FEEDING

Initiation of enteral feeds in critically ill patients (even in small amounts), helps to preserve gut function and structure, and to minimize the hypermetabolic response to stress. When initiating enteral feeds in patients maintained on TPN, an isotonic, lactose free formula perfused at a low constant rate is usually best tolerated. The transition from parenteral to enteral nutrition should be gradual with tapering of TPN and advancing enteral feeds. This helps to prevent hypoglycaemia and fluid overload. TPN should be ceased when enteral feeds provide approximately 75% of nutritional requirements.

TRANSITION FROM ENTERAL TO ORAL FEEDING

The goals for enteral feeding should be set at the onset. Once the patient is able and willing to eat by mouth the enteral feed can be reduced in proportion to the amount consumed orally. Transition from continuous feeds to overnight feeds may help establish oral intake while ensuring the patient is not nutritionally compromised.

HOME ENTERAL FEEDING

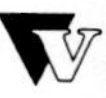

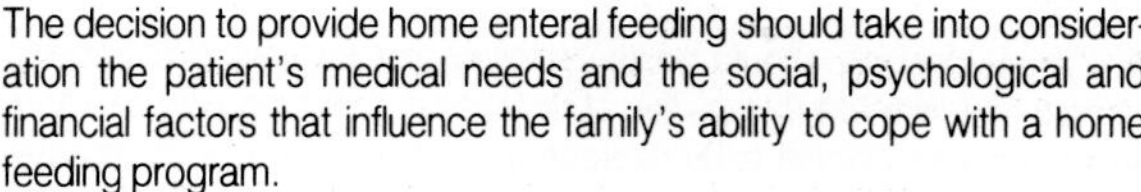

The decision to provide home enteral feeding should take into consideration the patient's medical needs and the social, psychological and financial factors that influence the family's ability to cope with a home feeding program.

Children on home enteral feeding, especially those who have minimal or no voluntary oral intake, require close monitoring of their growth and need their feeding regimes altered appropriately.

COMMON PROBLEMS

- *Gastrointestinal* disturbance is the most common problem (diarrhoea, cramping, nausea, vomiting). These problems can be minimized with the correct formula selection and administration in conjunction with a review of medications and their content. High gastric residues should be treated by reducing the rate of feed given or feeding small volumes continuously, reassessing concentration of feed and assessing GI function. Directing feed into the jejunum alleviates the problems caused by slow gastric emptying
- Other problems include *overhydration*, *dehydration*, *electrolyte imbalance*, *hyperglycaemia*, *hypoglycaemia* and *constipation*. These need to be assessed and managed appropriately
- *Malnutrition* is associated with major changes in electrolyte balance. Patients with significant and long standing undernutrition should be enterally fed with caution and serum phosphate, potassium, magnesium and glucose levels assessed regularly (see Refeeding Syndrome, p. 391).
- *Psychomotor development*. Young children who have been fed enterally during infancy or for long periods of time may miss important developmental steps in self feeding. Non-nutritive sucking or taking small amounts of appropriate food/fluid orally help establish and/or maintain eating and feeding skills. A speech pathologist may be of assistance in this area

FEEDING THE SICK NEWBORN

FEED TYPE

Feed types available are:
- Breast milk, including expressed breast milk (EBM)
- Artificial formulas, including specialized 'low birthweight' formulas
- Specialized feeds for pathological states

Breast Milk

Breast milk feeding should be the primary aim for very sick babies. When babies are too ill to suckle at the breast, most mothers can and wish to establish lactation by expression. EBM can be fed by gavage (nasogastric or orogastric) tube or other artificial means until the baby is well enough to be put to the breast.

In this way breast milk feeding can be achieved in extremely premature babies, and those with most major malformations, birth defects and other serious illnesses. The only situations in which breast milk feeding is not possible are:
- When an informed mother chooses not to express
- Inborn errors of metabolism, which require exclusion formulas
- Some complex malabsorption syndromes (e.g. short bowel syndrome). However, even some of these can succeed with EBM

Evidence is accumulating that EBM feeding of sick babies reduces morbidity and mortality and improves developmental outcome compared with artificial feeding.

Lactation by expression

Every mother embarking on this course needs ready access to nurses trained in lactation or lactation consultants.

Expression by hand or pump should be started within 24 (preferably 4–8) h of delivery. Episodes should be every 3–4 h, lasting about 30 min with a break for sleep. Hand expression is best until lactation is established. Using clean straightforward techniques, EBM does not have to be sterilized or pasteurized.

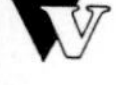

General

- EBM for sick babies should be from the baby's mother rather than a bank

- EBM for sick babies should not be frozen; the freshest EBM available at the time should be used first

Supplements and fortifiers

'Fortifiers', derived from cow milk, are available to add to EBM to increase its content of protein, energy and other nutrients. The effects of adding such substances on the biological properties of breast milk are unknown and may be deleterious; however, it is common practice.

Babies who may benefit from fortifiers are those with greatly increased nutritional requirements (e.g. very low birthweight babies, VLBW), and those requiring fluid restriction (i.e. babies with heart failure or chronic lung disease). For babies with greater nutritional requirements it is not appropriate only to add calories (i.e. glucose polymer or MCT oil); such babies need a range of additional nutrients.

VLBW babies may need folate and iron, in addition to fortifier, extra sodium, Vitamins C, D and E. Addition of fortifier should be delayed until feeds are fully established (i.e. 150–200 mL/kg per 24 h).

Iron should not be started until 12 weeks of age. VLBW babies who receive multiple blood transfusions may not need supplemental iron.

Phototherapy

Phototherapy for jaundice can impede breast feeding by placing physical and psychological barriers between mother and baby, and by causing diarrhoea. Breast feeding should be protected by interrupting the phototherapy frequently. Diarrhoea or sugar in bowel fluid are not reasons to suspend breast feeding. Although insensible water loss is increased by some phototherapy devices, the increase is only 10–20 mL/kg per 24 h. Thus, as long as usual amounts of breast milk are available by suckling or expression, supplements of water or formula are not necessary.

Artificial Formulas

These must be used when breast milk is not available. For those sick babies with greater nutritional requirements or in need of fluid restriction formulas can be strengthened (by adding extra formula powder) from the standard 66 kcal/100 mL strength to 82–100 kcal/100 mL.

Low birthweight (LBW) artificial formulas are designed for very premature (<32 weeks) babies. In general these contain extra protein,

Table 33.4 Commonly used enteral feeds

Type	*Example*	*Notes*
Polymeric foods	Paediasure	
1 kcal/mL (4.2 kJ/mL)	Osmolite	
	Ensure	
	Isocal	
	Jevity	Contains fibre
	Pulmocare	High fat, low CHO
High energy polymeric		
1.5 kcal/mL (6.3kJ/mL)	Ensure Plus	Hypertonic
2.0 kcal/mL (8.4 kJ/mL)	Twocal HN	Hypertonic
Specialised formula (elemental)	Vital HN Elemental 028	Contain short chain peptides; not suitable for infants under 1 year
	Neocate*	Suitable for infants
	Generaid Plus	Used in hepatic disorders
Modular feeds		
Protein source	Promod, Maxipro HBV	Nutritionally incomplete; require vitamin and mineral supplement
CHO source	Polyjoule, Polycal Douglas Energy Plus	
Fat source		
LCT	Calogen	
MCT	Liquigen, MCT Oil*	
Fat and CHO source	Duocal	

All feeds are lactose free
*Australian Pharmaceutical Benefits Schedule listed

more easily assimilated additional calories and increased calcium, phosphorus, trace elements, and some (but not all) vitamins.

LBW formulas may also be used in sick *mature* babies who need more nutrients or fluid restriction, instead of the concentrated standard formulas described above.

Specialized Feeds

Specialized feeds for pathological states are available for the treatment of complex malabsorption, allergy, inborn errors of metabolism, and liver and renal disease.

FEED VOLUMES, FREQUENCY AND DELIVERY

For sick babies who cannot be fed to appetite or 'demand' fed, schedules specifying volume, frequency and delivery method are required.

Factors determining schedules include:

- Intestinal motility and gut enzyme and hormonal activity are low at birth and take time to switch on. This process is depressed by hypoxia, acidosis and sepsis and drugs, especially narcotics. This limits the feed volumes that sick babies can tolerate
- Full stomach and bowel can press on the diaphragm, impairing breathing
- Sick babies reflux or vomit more often and are less able to protect their airways so that milk aspiration is an ever present risk
- Aggressive schedules appear to increase the risk of necrotizing enterocolitis

Mature babies need 150 mL milk/kg per 24 h. This is usually reached over 5–7 days, starting at 30–40 mL/kg per 24 h and increasing by 30 mL/kg per 24 h as tolerated. Formula is used at three-quarters strength in the first 24–48 h, but EBM should not be diluted this way. Feed frequency should be 3–4 hourly, although with reflux or abdominal distension, smaller volume and more frequent feeds may help.

By using LBW formulas or concentrated standard formulas, adequate nutrition may be achieved with 120–150 mL/kg per 24 h. LBW formulas should be given diluted (15–20 kcal/30 mL or 210–280 kJ/100 mL) until full daily volumes are achieved. Standard strength (24 kcal/30 mL) should then be introduced.

VLBW babies require 180–200 mL/kg per 24 h of EBM or standard formula, or 150–180 mL/kg per 24 h of fortified EBM or LBW formula, starting at 20–30 mL/kg per 24 h and increasing by 30 mL/kg per day as tolerated. LBW formula should be used diluted (15–20 kcal/30 mL or 210–280 kJ/mL) until close to maximum daily volumes are reached (usually after 2 weeks); LBW formulas are not designed to be given in full strength to sick or unstable VLBW infants. Initial feed frequency should be 1–2 hourly. Hourly feeds may be necessary in babies <1000 g.

Intragastric feeding tubes are necessary for sick babies who cannot suck: use No. 5–6 French for babies <2000 g and No. 6–8 French for bigger babies. Nasogastric tubes should not be used in babies <1250 g as they cause significant airways obstruction (use orogastric).

Continuous intragastric infusion of milk rather than intermittent boluses may help if reflux, gastric distension or apnoea are persistent. Transpyloric duodenal or jejunal feeding provide no advantages and additional risks.

THE NUTRITIONAL MANAGEMENT OF THE UNWELL CHILD

Deciding the most appropriate nutritional therapy for infants and children to prevent or treat a nutritional deficiency requires an evaluation of the medical history and nutritional status in order to define specific nutritional requirements and to determine the optimal method of providing these requirements. Dietary manipulation with or without supplementary enteral feeding should always be considered as the preferred route in any patient with a functioning gastrointestinal tract.

BASIC INFORMATION HELPFUL IN DETERMINING NUTRITIONAL RECOMMENDATION

Medical History

- Type of illness
- Duration
- Degree of metabolic stress
- Treatment (medications, surgery)

Nutritional Status

Clinical examination

- *Anthropometry:* weight, height, head circumference; growth velocity; skinfold thickness and arm circumference (in selected patients)
- *Sexual maturation* (in selected patients)
- *Specific nutrient deficiency:* hair, skin, mucous membranes; bruising, bleeding, pallor; eye and neurological assessment

Biochemical assessment

- Sodium, potassium, chloride
- Urea, creatinine
- Calcium, phosphate, magnesium
- Albumin, total protein
- Full blood examination
- Vitamins A, D and E (in selected patients)
- Prothrombin time (in selected patients)
- Delayed hypersensitivity testing (in selected patients)

Dietary/feeding assessment

- 24 h dietary recall or 3 day prospective diet diary
- Evaluation of feeding skills and mealtime routine

CALCULATING NUTRITIONAL REQUIREMENTS

Energy (Calories)

The energy requirement can be calculated based on the requirements for a *normal* child of the same sex and age *or* by calculating specific requirements, based on an estimation of basal metabolic rate and adding a factor to account for increased metabolic demands due to activity, disease and stress.

Recommended dietary intake (RDI)

See Tables 33.5a,b. *Note:* Energy and protein requirements for the unwell child have been based on FAO/WHO/UNU recommendations. For Australian recommendations for the normal child, refer to *Recommended Nutrient Intakes* Australian Papers, Professional Publications, Mosman, 1990.

Calculation of specific needs

Estimating basal energy requirement (MJ/day)

- $<$ 3 years:
  - Male: BMR = 0.249 wt − 0.127
  - Female: BMR = 0.244 wt − 0.130
- 3–10 years:
  - Male: BMR = 0.095 wt + 2.110
  - Female: BMR = 0.085 wt + 2.033
- 10–18 years:
  - Male: BMR = 0.074 wt + 2.754
  - Female: BMR = 0.056 wt + 2.898

Source: Schofield W.N., Schofield C, James WPT. *Hum. Nutr. Clin. Nutr.* 1985; **396** (Suppl. 1): 1–96.

Factors that increase energy requirements

- *Activity:* bed rest, + 10%; light, + 30% (sitting, playing with hands); moderate, + 50% (standing and playing); heavy, + 75%
- *Fever:* 12% for each degree >37 °C
- *Cardiac failure:* 12–25%
- *Major surgery:* 20–30%

THERAPY AND NUTRITION

Table 33.5a Daily average energy requirements and safe level of protein intake for infants and children

Age	*Daily energy requirement*		*Daily protein intake*
	(kJ/kg)	*Total (kJ)*	*(g/kg)*
Months			
3–6	414	2760	1.86
6–9	397	3280	1.65
9–12	418	3920	1.50
Years			
1–2	444	4890	1.21
2–3	418	5690	1.13
3–5	398	6510	1.07
5–7	367	7360	1.00
7–10	303	8150	1.01

Source: Energy and protein requirements: Report of a joint FAO/WHO/UNU expert consultation. *Technical Report Series 724*. WHO, Geneva 1985.

Table 33.5b Daily average energy requirements and safe level of protein intake for young people (10–18 years)

Age (years)	*Daily energy requirement* BMR (kJ/kg)	*BMR factor*	*Total (kJ)*	*Daily protein intake (g/kg)*
Boys				
10–12	153	1.75	9 160	1.00
12–14	136	1.68	9 930	1.00
14–16	123	1.64	11 060	0.95
16–18	115	1.60	11 860	0.90
Girls				
10–12	138	1.64	8 140	1.00
12–14	119	1.59	8 720	0.95
14–16	111	1.55	8 990	0.90
16–18	107	1.53	8 930	0.80

Source: Energy and protein requirements: Report of a joint FAO/WHO/UNU expert consultation. *Technical Report Series 724*. WHO, Geneva 1985.

- *Severe burns:* up to 100%
- *Long-term growth failure:* 50–100%

Catch-up growth

kcal/kg = RDI for chronological age × ideal wt for actual height/actual wt

Protein

Recommended dietary intake

See Tables 33.5a,b. Refer to *Recommended Nutrient Intakes*, Australian Papers, Australian Professional Publications, Mosman, 1990.

Specific needs

- *Failure to thrive:* 1.5–2 times the RDI for age
- *Human immunodeficiency virus infection:* 1.5 times RDI for age
- *Burns:* increase in protein requirement depends on surface area, severity and complications of burn; aim calorie to nitrogen ratio of 150 : 1 for <10% burn surface area and 100 : 1 for >10% burn surface area. *Initial aim:* 0–6 years 3 g/kg per day; 6–18 years 2.5 g/kg per day
- *Hepatic encephalopathy:* 0.4–0.5 g/kg per day

Fat

- Preterm and nutritionally depleted infants will develop essential fatty acid deficiency within days if they receive fat-free parenteral nutrition
- Essential fatty acid deficiency is prevented by an intake of linoleic acid of 1–2% of total dietary calories. This can be provided as either intravenous fat (0.2–1 g/kg per day) or an enteral supplement with corn oil, sunflower oil or safflower oil

Micronutrients

Recommended dietary intake

Refer to *Recommended Nutrient Intakes*, Australian Papers, Australian Professional Publications, Mosman, 1990.

Specific needs

Increased requirements:

- Zinc: inflammatory bowel disease, burns
- Vitamin C: burns
- Vitamins A, D, E and K: chronic cholestasis, pancreatic insufficiency
- Vitamin K: antibiotics
- Vitamin B_{12}: malabsorption, Crohn's disease, intestinal worm infestation, bacterial overgrowth, intrinsic factor deficiency
- Folate: prematurity, malabsorption, Crohn's disease, drugs (methotrexate, phenytoin)
- Calcium: chronic diarrhoea, renal disease, Vitamin D, magnesium or PTH deficiency
- Phosphate: refeeding in malnutrition
- Magnesium: chronic diarrhoea, chemotherapy, amphotericin B, aminoglycosides
- Iron: chronic blood loss, chronic disease

PARENTERAL NUTRITION

Indications

- Unable to tolerate enteral feeding due to gastrointestinal dysfunction
- Increased metabolic requirements, which are unable to be adequately treated with enteral therapy

Composition

THERAPY AND NUTRITION

Parenteral nutrition is usually provided as a combination of a nutrient solution and a fat emulsion.

Nutrient solution

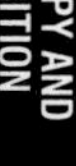

Carbohydrate D-glucose provides 14.3 kJ/g (3.4 kcal/g). Slowly advance concentration (≤5% dextrose concentration per day) to allow an appropriate endogenous insulin response and decrease the risk of glycosuria (see p. 389). When ceasing parenteral nutrition the solution should be reduced in volume or concentration gradually over hours to days, depending on glucose concentration and patient response. A dislodged intravenous catheter should be immediately replaced. If a replacement nutrient solution is unavailable an infusion of a similar concentration of dextrose (i.e. 20% dextrose in 1/4 normal saline with potassium) should be commenced. Table 33.6 gives the maximum

Table 33.6 Maximum dextrose intake

Fluid intake (mL/kg per 24 h)	*Intake of amino acid (g/kg per 24 h)*			
	1.0	*1.5*	*2.0*	*2.5*
Vamin (7% solution)				
20	2	–	–	–
30	9	4	–	–
40	15	10	6	–
50	22.5	17.5	12.5	7.5
60	29	24	19	14
70	36	31	26	21.5
Synthamin (10% solution)				
20	5	15	–	–
30	11	7.5	5	–
40	18	15	11	7.5
50	25	20	17.5	14
60	32	27.5	25	20
70	39	35	30	27.5

dextrose intake compatible with different intakes of parenteral amino acid (g/kg per day) provided in the nutrient solution.

Dextrose concentration (%) = amount of dextrose (g/kg per day)/fluid volume of nutrient solution (mL/kg per day)

Complications:
- Phlebitis: risk increased if concentration of dextrose is >10% in a peripheral vein or >30% in a central vein
- Glucose intolerance
- Hepatic steatosis: increased risk if >20% dextrose solution at 150 mL/kg per day. Neonate: avoid initially exceeding the hepatic rate of glucose production (6–8 mg/kg per min)
- Water retention: increased risk if sole source of calories
- Increased CO_2 production: relevant in patients with compromised respiratory status or who are ventilator dependent

Protein Amino acid requirements of parenterally fed patients:
- Premature neonates: 2.0 g/kg per day
- Infants, 0–1 year: 2.5 g/kg per day
- Children, 2–13 years: 1.5–2.0 g/kg per day

- Adolescents: 1.0–1.5 g/kg per day

Some stable LBW babies may tolerate higher amino acid loads.

Initiate amino acids at 1–1.5 g/kg per day are gradually increased (see Table 33.6). Tolerance and adequacy of protein can be assessed by blood urea, creatinine, pH/CO_2, ammonia and 24 h urinary urea/nitrogen/creatinine.

Calorie–nitrogen ratio: To promote the optimal use of protein and prevent its use simply as another source of energy, approximately 150–200 non-protein calories are required per gram of nitrogen.

N (g) = protein (g)/6.25

1 g protein = 0.16 g nitrogen

Therefore,

1 g/kg per day protein requires 24–32 non-protein calories

2 g/kg per day protein requires 48–64 non-protein calories

Electrolytes and minerals

- Sodium: 2–4 mmol/kg per day (average 3 mmol/kg per day) or as ordered
- Potassium: 2–3 mmol/kg per day (average 2 mmol/kg per day) or as ordered
- Calcium: <5 kg order as maximum to 12 mmol/L; >5 kg 7.5 mmol/L or as ordered
- Phosphate: <5 kg order as maximum to 12 mmol/L; >5 kg 7.5 mmol/L or as ordered
- Magnesium: 4 mmol/L or as ordered

Trace elements

- Chromium: 0.005 µmol/kg
- Copper: 0.5 µmol/kg
- Iodide: 0.04 µmol/kg
- Manganese: 0.2 µmol/kg
- Zinc: 3.0 µmol/kg
- Selenium: 0.025 µmol/kg per day if TPN for >3 months

Vitamins

- B and C group: thiamine 20 mg/L, riboflavin 10 mg/L, sodium pantholene 10 mg/L, nicotinamide 100 mg/L, pyridoxine 5 mg/L, ascorbic acid 100 mg/L

- Cyanocobalamin: 20 μg/L
- Folic acid: 100 μg/day
- Vitamin K: 2 mg/L if not receiving MV1 Paediatric
- Multivitamin preparation. Added 5 days/week (Mon.–Fri.) for patients receiving >7 days TPN:
    - Patients <1 kg: MVI Paediatric 1.5 mL/24 h
    - Patients 1–3 kg: MVI Paediatric 2.5 mL/24 h
    - Patients >3 kg and <12 years: MVI Paediatric 5 mL/24 h
    - Patients >12 years: MVI 12 10 mL/bag

MVI Paediatric 5 mL contains: Vitamin A 2300 IU, Vitamin D 400 IU, Vitamin E 7 IU, thiamine 1.2 mg, riboflavin 1.4 mg, pyridoxine 1 mg, nicotinamide 17 mg, cyanocobalamin 1 μg, ascorbic acid 80 mg, pantothenic acid 5 mg, folic acid 140 μg, biotin 20 μg, Vitamin K 200 μg.

MVI 12 10 mL contains: Vitamin A 3300 IU, Vitamin D 200 IU, Vitamin E 10 IU, thiamine 3 mg, riboflavin 3.6 mg, pyridoxine 4 mg, nicotinamide 40 mg, cyanocobalamin 5 μg, ascorbic acid 100 mg, pantothenic acid 15 mg, folic acid 400 μg, biotin 60 μg

Other additives

Heparin: 1 unit/mL

Fat emulsion

- Intravenous fat is a concentrated isotonic source of calories and prevents or reverses essential fatty acid deficiency. Twenty per cent Intralipid contains 8.4 kJ/mL (2 kcal/mL) or 42 kJ/g (1g in 5 mL)
- Aim to provide 30–40% (not >60%) of non-protein calories as fat
- Infusion should be increased gradually (Table 33.7). Fat should be infused continuously whenever possible. The dose should not exceed 0.15 g/kg per h particularly in preterm infants
- In patients with high bilirubin levels and low serum albumin, intravenous fats should be infused to meet essential fatty acid requirements only (0.5–1.0 g/kg per day)
- Tolerance depends on hepatic clearance and can be estimated by the measurement of serum triglycerides which should be routinely assessed with advancement of fat infusion rates. Other measures of fat tolerance include serum free fatty acids, prothrombin time and platelet count

Prescribing Parenteral Nutrition

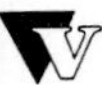

Determine:

- *Intravenous route:* central versus peripheral. Maximum dextrose concentration: peripheral 10%; central 30%
- *Fluid requirement.* Fluid volume is determined by calculating:
  - Daily maintenance

3–10 kg	100 mL/kg per day
10–20 kg	1000 mL + (50 mL/kg per day for each kg over 10 kg)
20 kg and over	1500 mL + (20 mL/kg per day for each kg over 20 kg)

  - Specific considerations: replacement of deficit and/or ongoing losses; fluid restriction (cardiac disease, renal failure, head injury); and other sources of fluid intake (blood products, intravenous medications)
- *Establish nutritional aims* (see previous section)
  - energy
  - protein
  - fat
  - specific requirements
- *Advancement protocol.* A typical advancement schedule is shown in Table 33.7
- *Monitoring.* See Table 33.8
- *Cycling parenteral nutrition*

For patients who require long-term parenteral nutrition and are clinically stable, it may be desirable to limit the time that the patient is connected to the intravenous line while still maintaining complete nutrition support.

The amount of time for which it is feasible to disconnect a patient depends on age, nutritional and medical status and the relative contribution of enteral feeds to their nutritional and fluid requirements. In general, infants and young children tolerate cycling less predictably than adolescents and particular care must be taken to avoid hypoglycaemia, acid–base and fluid imbalance. Usually the establishment of a cycling protocol takes 3–7 days.

To avoid hypoglycaemia it is recommended that the rate of infusion is decreased during the last hour of the infusion with the first 30 min running at 50% of the original rate and the final 30 min running at 25% of the original rate. A Dextrostix or serum glucose should be taken 1 h after cessation of the infusion or if symptoms are suggestive of hypoglycaemia. The infusion should then be recommenced at 50% of the original

Table 33.7 Suggested advancement schedule

	Premature/ SGA infant	*Term AGA infant*	*<10 kg*	*10–20 kg*	*>20kg*
Dextrose (g/kg per day)					
Start	5–10	10	10	5	5
Increase daily by	2–5	2–5	5	5	5
Final maximum dose	15–20 (≤6–8 mg/kg/min)	15–20	15–20	10–15	10
Amino acids (g/kg per day)					
Start	1.5	1.5	1.5	1	1
Increase daily by	0.5	0.5	0.5	0.5–1	1
Final maximum dose	1.5–3	2.5	2	2	1–2
Fat (g/kg per day)					
Start	0.5	0.5–1	0.5–1	0.5–1	0.5–1
Increase daily by	0.25–0.5	0.5	0.5	0.5	0.5
Final maximum dose	2–3	3	3	3	2–2.5

Table 33.8 Parenteral nutrition monitoring

	Baseline/ pre-TPN	*Daily*	*Twice weekly*	*Weekly*	*1–3 monthly*
Weight	X	X			
Height/length	X				X
Head circumference (<2 years)	X				X
Triceps skin fold thickness	X				X
Mid arm circumference	X				X
Fluid balance	X	X			
Inspect intravenous site	X	X			
Urinanalysis	X	X			
Electrolytes	X	X (until stable)		X	
Urea	X	X (until stable)		X	
Creatinine	X	X (until stable)		X	
Acid–base	X	X (until stable)		X	
Glucose	X	X (until stable)	X		
Calcium	X	X (until stable)		X	
Phosphate	X	X (until stable)		X	
Magnesium	X		X (until stable)	X	
Triglycerides	X	X (with advancement of fat)		X	
LFT	X		X (until stable)	X	
FBE	X			X	
Zinc/ALP					X
Iron, ferritin					X

B_{12}, folate, selenium, manganese, molybdenum, copper, aluminium — 6 monthly or as indicated

rate for the first 30 min of the infusion. Long-term glucose stability may be assessed by haemoglobin A1c levels.

- *Discontinuing parenteral nutrition.* Once a patient is receiving ≥60% of their estimated energy requirements via the enteral route, parenteral nutrition can generally be weaned. This is performed over hours to days depending on the clinical setting and the composition of the parenteral nutrition formula

Drug Compatibilities

As parenteral nutrition solutions are individually made to specific patient requirements drug compatibilities can never be guaranteed. Where possible any drug should be administered through a separate intravenous line or catheter lumen. If a separate intravenous site is not available, certain drugs may be administered through a separate line entering the parenteral nutrition line at a Y connection as close to the patient as possible. The drug should not be administered while the parenteral nutrition is running and the common tubing should be flushed before and after drug administration. In patients who require uninterrupted parenteral nutrition certain drugs may administered concurrently. Drugs that may be suitable for concurrent administration include:

Ampicillin	Hydrocortisone	Metoclopramide
Cefazolin	Heparin	Morphine
Cimetidine	Insulin	Noradrenaline
Clindamycin	Iron dextran	Penicillin G
Cloxacillin	Isoproterenol	Piperacillin
Dopamine	Lidocaine	Ranitidine
Frusemide	Meperidine	Ticarcillin
Gentamicin	Methyl prednisolone	Tobramycin

Drugs which are **not compatible with parenteral nutrition solutions** may *not* be run concurrently under any circumstances include:

Acetazolamide	Cisplatinum	Mannitol
Acyclovir	Cyclosporin	Metronidazole
Amphotericin	Desferroxamine	Phenytoin
Antithymocyte globulin	Doxorubin	Sodium bicarbonate

REFEEDING SYNDROME

After a period of prolonged starvation, aggressive nutritional therapy may precipitate a cascade of potentially fatal metabolic complications. These include:

- Hypokalaemia

THERAPY AND NUTRITION

- Hypophosphataemia
- Hypomagnesaemia
- Glucose intolerance
- Cardiac failure
- Seizures
- Myocardial infarction/arrhythmias

At particular risk are patients with:

- Anorexia nervosa
- Classical marasmus
- Kwashiorkor
- No nutrition for 7–10 days in adolescents (much less in infants and children) with significant metabolic stress
- Acute weight loss of ⩾10–20% of usual bodyweight, and possibly metabolic stress, or >20% of usual bodyweight
- Morbid obesity with massive weight loss (i.e. post-operative)

Treatment

- Identify risk and chronicity
- Identify and treat metabolic stress if present (i.e. infection)
- Establish baseline status: weight, height/length, head circumference, fluid status, electrolytes, urea, creatinine, calcium, phosphate, magnesium, albumin, glucose, acid–base, full blood examination
- Correct any electrolyte or mineral disturbance, particularly with potassium, phosphate, magnesium, prior to commencing nutritional rehabilitation
- Establish modest nutritional goals initially (i.e. basal requirements until stability is assured), then aim to provide for catch-up growth
- Monitor closely over the first week until a nutritional plan is established with: pulse rate; fluid balance; weight; caloric intake; glucose; electrolytes; urea; creatinine; phosphate; magnesium
- Administer vitamin and mineral supplement

CHAPTER 34

ACUTE PAIN MANAGEMENT

Philip Ragg

GENERAL PRINCIPLES OF PAEDIATRIC ANALGESIA

- Unrelieved pain has negative physiological and emotional consequences, including adverse effects on respiratory, cardiovascular and endocrine systems
- To manage pain adequately, its intensity and relief must be assessed regularly
- Children's and parents' desires must be considered when choosing an appropriate treatment
- Children's pain is often masked and may present differently from pain in adults. They often will not report pain
- Prevention is better than treatment. Analgesic requirements are lower if treatment is pre-emptive
- Paediatric analgesia must be calculated as a dose per kg bodyweight, and routes of administration must be appropriate for age
- Children do not like intramuscular injections
- Severe pain is best treated with continuous intravenous or subcutaneous infusions or regional blocks using local anaesthesia. Long-acting drugs are also useful for severe pain
- Parents and children must have realistic expectations of analgesia. It may not be possible to eliminate all pain, but it should be possible to allow normal daily activities
- Two misconceptions which contribute to undertreatment of paediatric pain are:
    - A belief that all children are 'sensitive' to analgesics
    - A belief that p.r.n. dosing regimens mean 'as little as possible as infrequently as possible'

PAEDIATRIC PAIN ASSESSMENT

- Routine assessment enables better titration of an individual child's analgesic needs
- Unexpected or severe pain, especially if associated with other physi-

cal signs such as tachycardia or shortness of breath, should be evaluated immediately
- Any assessment of a child's pain must take into account the child's age, cognitive ability and personality. Family traditions and preferences and words used by the child should be considered. Smaller children or those with developmental delay warrant particular attention as they have less mature communication skills

After eliciting a careful history of the pain (onset, duration, site, character, etc.) and having examined the child, the following are useful assessment tools:
- *Behavioural observation:* vocalization, facial expressions, posture, movement, personality, depression, fatigue. Remember that a child lying still and withdrawn may be in severe pain
- *Pain rating scales:* older children can assess their own pain with linear analogue scales using a 10 cm line, with '0' meaning no pain and '10' the worst pain ever experienced. Under 7 years of age similar scales of faces (Wong Baker Faces Pain Rating Scale) are useful
- *Physiological signs:* vital signs may add information, especially in smaller children where assessment can be difficult

GENERAL USE OF ANALGESICS

The three most commonly used analgesics in children are paracetamol, non-steroidal anti-inflammatory agents and opioids.

PARACETAMOL

Paracetamol is a very useful analgesic and antipyretic with little anti-inflammatory action.

Note: Paracetamol may reduce the antibody response to infection, prolonging minor illness and possibly increasing mortality in severe infection. It should be used to reduce pain or discomfort, but not simply to treat fever.
- *Routes of administration:* oral, rectal
- *Dosage:* 20 mg/kg 4 hourly, p.r.n. (maximum 5 doses/day), or 30 mg/kg 8 hourly, p.r.n. Do not exceed 100 mg/kg per day. (Previously recommended doses of 10–15 mg/kg are probably less effective than 20 mg/kg in relieving pain)

If a child requires continuous pain relief over a 24 h period (i.e. pain is interfering with sleep), a stronger analgesic is indicated.

Paracetamol should be used with caution in patients with severe liver disease or jaundice.

NON-STEROIDAL ANTI-INFLAMMATORY DRUGS (NSAID)

NSAID have analgesic and anti-inflammatory properties, both of which may be useful in the management of acute pain in children. Several studies have confirmed their efficacy postoperatively after tonsillectomy, orthopaedic surgery, and dental extraction.

- *Routes of administration:* oral, rectal
- *Dosage: Naproxen:* 5–7.5 mg/kg (max. 500 mg) 12 hourly; *Indomethacin:* 0.25–1.0 mg/kg (max. 50 mg) 8 hourly; *Diclofenac:* 1 mg/kg (max. 50 mg) 8 hourly; *Ketoprofen:* 0.5–2.0 mg/kg (max. 100 mg) 8–12 hourly

Parenteral NSAID, such as ketorolac, are not recommended in children. All NSAID must be used with caution in patients with bleeding disorders as they all have antiplatelet effects. Renal dysfunction has been reported in children with NSAID, in particular diclofenac and piroxicam. *Aspirin* has been implicated in Reye syndrome and it should not be used as an analgesic in children.

OPIOID ANALGESICS

Oral preparations

Most opioids undergo significant metabolism either in the gastrointestinal tract or on first pass through the liver, making their bioavailability low when taken orally.

Codeine: is a partial agonist opioid, which is very useful as an oral analgesic.

Dosage: 0.5–1.0 mg/kg 4 hourly, p.r.n.

Buprenorphine: Buprenorphine is a useful partial agonist opioid that can be a very effective analgesic in older children when administered sublingually, thereby avoiding first-pass metabolism.

Dosage: (sublingual) 5 μg/kg 6 hourly, p.r.n.

Parenteral Opioids

Opioids remain the most powerful parenteral analgesics for children in severe pain (see Table 34.1). These drugs bind to opioid receptors producing analgesia, as well as respiratory and psychomimetic effects. Infants under 6 months may be more sensitive to opioids. To ensure safe administration in this age group, morphine should be titrated to effect up to a maximim of 50 μg/kg, and the infant should be continually monitored for respiratory depression (e.g. pulse oximetry).

Table 34.1 Equipotent doses of opioids for children over 12 months (mg)

	Intravenous (mg)	*Recommended maximum dose (mg/kg)*
Morphine	1	0.2
Pethidine	10	2
Fentanyl	0.01	0.002
Methadone	1	0.2
Codeine		1 (usually oral 0.5–1.0)

Administration

Administration of parenteral opioids may be as:

- Intermittent boluses (intramuscular, intravenous or subcutaneous)
- Continuous infusion (intravenous or subcutaneous)

In general, infusions optimize analgesia by enabling the child to remain in the 'analgesic corridor' without fluctuations in plasma level.

The *subcutaneous* route is very effective and often convenient in the child with difficult intravenous access. Although absorption is not as predictable as the intravenous route, the deltopectoral groove has been successfully employed for continuous infusions. An intravenous cannula can be safely placed under the skin without risk of trauma. **Parenteral opioids should not be administered without the availability of oxygen, resuscitation equipment and naloxone to reverse the opioid effect.**

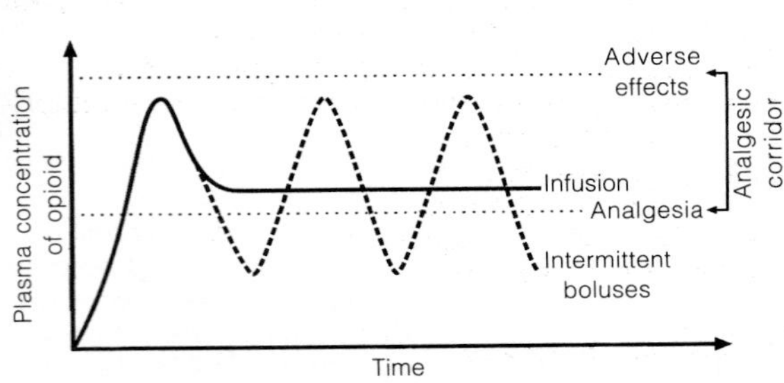

Figure 34.1 The analgesic corridor

Common effects of parenteral opioids

- *Central nervous system:* euphoria, sedation, nausea, miosis
- *Respiratory:* hypoventilation, bronchospasm
- *Cardiovascular:* bradycardia, hypotension
- *Alimentary:* constipation, vomiting, biliary colic
- *Skin:* histamine release, itch

Maximum dosage

Maximum doses of *intramuscular* opioids are:

- *Morphine:* 0.2 mg/kg 4 hourly, p.r.n.
- *Pethidine:* 2 mg/kg 3 hourly, p.r.n.

Intermittent Intravenous Opioids

Children dislike intramuscular injections, and intravenous administration is preferred. The following is a suggested protocol to minimize drug calculation error:

- Before boluses are given, ensure:
    - The patient is awake and stable
    - The intravenous line is patent
    - The child is older than 12 months
- Morphine 10 mg or Pethidine 100 mg is diluted in a 100 mL bottle of normal saline connected to a burette. Final concentration is thus:
    - 100 μg/mL morphine
    - 1 mg/mL pethidine
- The bolus dose and maximum dose to be given are checked. Only the bolus dose volume should be placed in the burette
- The bolus dose must be administered over at least 5 min, and administration ceased if the respiratory rate or oxygen saturation decreases
- Monitoring during administration should be by continuous pulse oximetry, and 5 minutely BP, HR and RR for 20 min
- After a bolus, allow 15 min before considering another bolus
- If oxygen saturation falls below 93% or airways obstruction or respiratory depression is suspected:
    - Cease infusion immediately
    - Administer 100% O_2 by mask
    - Give *naloxone* 0.01 mg/kg stat, i.v.
    - Resuscitate as necessary

Continuous Opioid Infusions

Should a child require ongoing opioid analgesia or more than two intermittent boluses, an infusion should be commenced if practical.

Figure 34.2 Opiate infusions instructions and record

OPIATE INFUSION INSTRUCTIO

ROYAL CHILDREN'S HOSPITAL, MELBOURNE OPIATE INFUSION INSTRUCTION Five hundred (500) mL dilution Weight	AFFIX PATIENT IDENTIFICATION LABEL

TICK ☐ IF INSTRUCTIONS DIFFER FROM GUIDELINES

GUIDELINES

MORPHINE Add **0.5 mg/kg** to **500 mL** diluent of choice (any i.v. maintenance solution of electrolytes and/or glucose) to make infusion
Infuse at 0–40 mL/h equivalent to 0–40 µ/kg/h. Commonly used 20 mL/h (20 µg/kg/h)
Recommended initial bolus: 50–100 mL (0.05–0.10 mg/kg) of infusion
Recommended bolus for pain or painful procedure 10–20 mL (0.01–0.02 mg/kg) of infusion at intervals of at least 5–10 min

PETHIDINE Add **5.0 mg/kg** to **500 mL** diluent of choice (any i.v. maintenance solution of electrolytes and/or glucose) to make infusion
Infuse at 0–40 mL/h equivalent to 0–400 µ/kg/h. Commonly used 20 mL/h (200 µg/kg/h)
Recommended initial bolus: 50–100 mL (0.5–1.0 mg/kg) of infusion
Recommended bolus for pain or painful procedure 10–20 mL (0.1–0.2 mg/kg) of infusion at intervals of at least 5–10 min

MEDICAL INSTRUCTIONS

1. Add .... **mg** of .... to **500 mL** of ....
2. Infuse at .... **mL/h** to .... **mL/h** as required for analgesia
3. Administer initial bolus .... **mL** of infusion
4. Administer .... **mL** bolus of infusion *prn* for pain or painful procedures, at intervals of no less than .... min
5. Notify doctor if respirations less than .... per min or systolic blood pressure less than .... mmHg

N RECORD MR 68 (A) (500 ml)

IF OPIATE TOXICITY SUSPECTED (slow or shallow respirations or hypotension or coma)

- Stop the Infusion
- Administer **NALOXONE** .... i.v. or i.m. (0.01–0.1 mg/kg)
- Call ICU Registrar (extensions 5211, 6555) and ward HMO

Doctor's signature .... Date .... Printed Name .... ID Number ....

INFUSION RECORD

INFUSION PREPARATION	Time and Date	Registered Nurses' Signatures	
Bag 1	....	....	....
Bag 2	....	....	....
Bag 3	....	....	....
Bag 4	....	....	....
Bag 5	....	....	....
Bag 6	....	....	....
INFUSION DISCARDED			
Bag No ___	....	....	....
Bag No ___	....	....	....
INITIAL BOLUS GIVEN	....	....	....

A copy of the Royal Children's Hospital Protocol is shown in Fig. 34.2 and may be used for intravenous or subcutaneous infusion. Please note that the volume used may be either 500 mL or 50 mL.

Patient-controlled Analgesia (PCA)

PCA usually requires a microprocessor-controlled injector pump. PCA is suitable for children older than 8 years with the ability to understand the concept of pressing a button to relieve pain and the willingness to use it. It has the advantage of involving patients in their own care, and is safe, as children will fall asleep and stop bolusing when plasma levels rise. It also saves nursing time. Indications include postoperative pain, oncology, burns and frequent painful procedures.

Protocol

Dilute 0.5 mg/kg morphine in 50 mL saline (i.e. 10 μg/kg per mL). Set PCA to: (i) 5 min lockout interval; (ii) 2 mL boluses (20 μg/kg). May run background infusion (0.5 mL/h or 5 μg/kg per h) concurrently.

Observations and resuscitation protocols are as per opioid infusions.

LOCAL ANAESTHESIA

Local anaesthesia in children provides very effective analgesia for acute trauma (e.g. fractures), lacerations and postoperative wounds. Although central blocks such as epidurals, spinals and caudals are the domain of anaesthetists in operating theatres, several other applications of local anaesthesia exist.

LOCAL INFILTRATION

The skin and subcutaneous tissues can be effectively infiltrated with local anaesthetic solutions as shown in Table 34.2.

The addition of *adrenaline* 1 in 200 000 may increase the duration of action and slow absorption by up to 50%. **Adrenaline should not be used in end organs such as fingers or toes due to the risk of ischaemia.**

Table 34.2 Local anaesthetic solutions

	Maximum dose (mg/kg)	*Duration (h)*
Bupivacaine (0.25% or 0.5%)	2	2–3
Lignocaine (1% or 2%)	5	1–2

COMMON PERIPHERAL NERVE BLOCKS

Femoral nerve: Immediately lateral to the femoral artery, this nerve can be blocked under the fascia lata and fascia iliacus at the mid-inguinal point (see p. 30). This block will give analgesia of the anteromedial thigh and is very useful for a fractured femur.

Lateral cutaneous nerve of thigh: Can be blocked by fanning local anaesthetic subcutaneously below the anterior superior iliac spine through 180° and is useful for painful conditions of the outer thigh (e.g. lacerations, abrasions, burns and grafting).

Intercostal nerve blocks: Pain from rib fractures or chest wall or abdominal wounds may be relieved by intercostal nerve blocks. The nerves run under each rib in a neurovascular bundle, and both anterior and posterior divisions can be blocked if the needle is placed posteriorly within a few centimetres of the vertebral column. As pneumothorax is a potential complication of this block, it should be performed cautiously by experienced staff.

TOPICAL LOCAL ANAESTHETIC CREAM

The insertion of intravenous drips, lumbar punctures and blood sampling are all potentially distressing for children. Application of local anaesthetic cream 1 h before these procedures ensures an area of analgesia of the skin.

EMLA is a mixture of prilocaine 5% and lignocaine 5% and often vasoconstricts the area under application.

NITROUS OXIDE

Increasing use is being made in burns and oncology units of nitrous oxide, which is a very useful inhalational analgesic.

Methods of delivery include:

- Entonox (a mixture of 50% nitrous oxide and 50% oxygen)
- Quantiflex (variable demand delivery system of nitrous oxide and oxygen)

Nitrous oxide provides potent short-term analgesia for painful procedures such as wound dressings, removal of catheters, etc. It has a rapid onset and offset. Side-effects may include sedation, nausea and bone marrow depression with prolonged exposure.

It should *not be used* in head injuries, pneumothorax, obtunded patients or cardiac patients.

ALTERNATIVE TECHNIQUES

Non-pharmacological strategies can be used alone for less painful procedures, or as adjuncts to drugs for better analgesia.

Intervention needs to be tailored to the child and family, as encouragement is often critical to their success. Some suggested techniques are listed.

INFANTS

Sensorimotor aids such as pacifiers, feeding, warm blankets, holding and rocking.

OLDER CHILDREN

Guided imagery and cognitive techniques such as hypnosis, relaxation, distraction, music, art, play, positive encouragement and rehearsal all may be useful. The use of calico dolls to simulate the procedure has been shown to be effective.

PHYSICAL TECHNIQUES

Application of heat or cold, massage, exercise, rest or immobilization.

CHAPTER 35

PHARMACOPOEIA

Frank Shann

Considerable care has been taken to see that the information in this pharmacopoeia is accurate, but the user is advised to check the doses carefully. The authors shall not be responsible for any errors in this publication.

Acarbose 1–4mg/kg per dose (max. 200mg) 8 hourly oral with food.
Acebutolol 4–8mg/kg per dose (max. 400mg) 8–24 hourly oral.
Acemetacin 1.2mg/kg per dose (max. 60mg) 8–12 hourly oral.
Acetaminophen See paracetamol.
Acetazolamide 2–7.5mg/kg per dose (max. 350mg) 8 hourly oral.
Acetyl sulfisoxazole 1.16g = 1.0g sulphafurazole (qv).
Acetylcysteine *Paracetamol poisoning* (irrespective of time elapsed): 150mg/kg in 5%D i.v. over 15 min, then 10 mg/kg per h for 72h (longer if still encephalopathic); monitor serum potassium. Give if paracetamol >1000μmol/L (150μg/mL) at 4h, >500 μmol/mL 8h, >250μmol/mL 12h. *Meconium ileus equivalent:* 5mL per dose (NOT/kg) of 20% solution 8 hourly oral. *CF:* 4–8mg/kg per dose 8 hourly oral.
Acetylcysteine 5% + hypromellose 0.35% eye drops 1–2 drops/eye 6–8 hourly.
Acetylsalicylic acid See aspirin.
Acipimox 5mg/kg per dose (max. 250mg) 8–12 hourly oral.
Acitretin 0.5–1.5mg/kg (max. 75mg) daily oral.
Aclarubicin 60mg/m^2 per day for 3–5 days by i.v. infusion, then 25–100mg/m^2 infusion every 3–4 weeks (usual total dose 300–600mg/m^2). Lower doses in combination regimens.
Acrivastine 0.15mg/kg per dose (max. 8mg) 8 hourly oral.
Acrosoxacin 3mg/kg per dose (max. 150mg) 8 hourly oral.
ACTH (Corticotrophin) 1unit/kg (max. 40u) i.m. daily.
Activated charcoal See charcoal.
Acyclovir *Cutaneous herpes:* 250mg/m^2 per dose 8 hourly i.v. over 1h. *Herpes encephalitis, varicella or EB virus:* 500 mg/m^2 per dose 8 hourly i.v. over 1h; neonate 10mg/kg per dose i.v. over 1h daily (<30 weeks gestation), 18 hourly (30–32 weeks), 12 hourly (1st week of life), 8 hourly (2–12 weeks). *Genital herpes* (NOT/kg): 200mg per dose oral ×5/day for 10 days, then 200mg per dose ×2–3/day for 6 months if required. *Zoster* (NOT/kg): 400mg per dose (<2 years) or 800mg per dose (≥ 2 years) oral ×5/day for 7 days.

Reprinted with permission of Dr Frank Shann from *Drug Doses, 9th Edition*, Royal Children's Hospital, 1995.

Adenosine 0.05mg/kg (max. 3mg) stat rapid i.v. push, increase by 0.05mg/kg (max. 3mg) every 2min to max. 0.25mg/kg (max. 12mg).
Adrenaline *Croup:* 1% (L isomer) or 2.25% (racemic) 0.05 mL/kg per dose diluted to 4mL by inhalation; or 1 in 1000 0.5mL/kg per dose (max. 5mL) by inhalation. *Cardiac arrest:* 0.1 mL/kg of 1 in 10 000 i.v. or intracardiac or via ETT (up to 1 mL/kg per dose if no response). *Anaphylaxis:* 0.05–0.1 mL/kg per dose of 1 in 10 000 i.v. *s.c.:* 0.01mg/kg (0.01 mL/kg of 1 in 1000), × 3 doses 20min apart if required. *Infusion:* see [X-REF].
Agar See paraffin (and phenolphthalein) and agar.
Albendazole 400mg per dose (NOT/kg) 12 hourly for 3 days. *Enterobiasis:* 400mg (NOT/kg) once, repeat in 2–4 weeks.
Albumin *20%:* 2–5mL/kg i.v. *5:* 10–20mL/kg.
Albuterol See salbutamol.
Alclometasone, cream or ointment 0.05% Apply 8–12 hourly.
Alcuronium *ICU:* 0.3mg/kg i.v. p.r.n. *Theatre:* 0.3mg/kg i.v. stat, then 0.05mg/kg per dose.
Aldesleukin (synthetic interleukin–2) See interleukin–2.
Alfacalcidol 0.05μg/kg (max. 1μg) daily oral or i.v., adjusted according to response.
Alfentanil 10μg/kg i.v. or i.m. stat, then 5μg/kg p.r.n. *Theatre* (ventilated): 30–50μg/kg i.v. over 5min, then 15μg/kg prn or 0.5–1μg/kg per min. *ICU:* 50–100 μg/kg i.v. over 10min, then 0.5–4μg/kg per min.
Alfuzosin 0.05mg/kg per dose (max. 2.5mg) 6–12 hourly oral.
Alginic acid (Gaviscon) *Infants:* 1–2g powder with feed 4 hourly. *1–12 years:* liquid 5–10mL, or granules ½ sachet after meals. *>12 years:* liquid 10–20mL, or granules 1 sachet after meals.
Alglucerase Initially 60u/kg i.v. over 2h every 1–4 weeks according to response, reducing every 3–6 months.
Allopurinol *Gout:* 2–12mg/kg per dose (max. 600mg) daily oral. *Cancer therapy:* 2.5–5mg/kg per dose (max. 200mg) 6 hourly.
Allyloestrenol *Adult:* 5mg per dose (NOT/kg) 8 hourly (threat abtn), 12–24 hourly (habit abtn), 3–6 hourly (prem labour) oral.
Alprazolam 0.005–0.02mg/kg per dose (adult 0.25–1mg) 8 hourly oral.
Alprenolol 1–4mg/kg per dose (max. 200mg) 6–12 hourly oral.
Alprostadil (prostaglandin E1, PGE1) 0.01–0.1μg/kg per min (10–100ng/kg per min). To maintain PDA with 0.01 μg/kg per min (10ng/kg per min): <16kg put 30μg/kg in 50mL saline, run at 1mL/h; >16kg put 500μg in 830/wt mL saline, run at 1mL/h (e.g. 20kg child, 500μg in 41.5mL saline at 1mL/h). Pulmonary vasodilation with 0.1μg/kg per min (100 ng/kg per min) put 500μg in 83/wt mL saline and run at 1mL/h (5.0 μg/kg per min nitroglyc = 2.0 μg/kg per min nitropr = 0.1 μg/kg per min PGE1 approx).
Alteplase (tissue plasminogen activator) 0.2mg/kg (max. 10mg) over 2min, then 1mg/kg (max. 50mg) for 1h, then 0.5mg/kg (max. 25mg per h) for 2h i.v. (keep fibrinogen >100mg/dL). *Local IA infusion:* 0.05mg/kg per h for 4–8h.
Altretamine 150–300mg/m^2 daily oral.
Aluminium acetate, solution 13% (Burrow's lotion) For wet compresses, or daily to molluscum contagiosum.

Aluminium chloride hexahydrate, lotion 20% Daily at night for 1 week, then × 1–2/week.

Aluminium hydroxide 5–50mg/kg per dose (adult 0.5–1g) 6–8 hourly oral. Gel (64mg/mL) 0.1mL/kg per dose 6 hourly oral.

Aluminium hydroxide 40mg/mL, magnesium hydroxide 40mg/mL, simethicone 4mg/mL (Mylanta) 0.2–0.4 mL/kg per dose (adult 10–20mL) 4–6 hourly oral. *ICU:* 0.5mL/kg per dose 3 hourly oral if gastric pH <5.

Alverine 1–2mg/kg per dose (max. 120mg) 8 hourly oral.

Amantadine 2mg/kg per dose (max. 100mg) 12–24 hourly oral. *Flu A prophylaxis:* 100mg daily (5–9 years), 100mg 12 hourly (>9 years).

Amcinonide, 0.1% lotion, cream, ointment Apply 8–12 hourly.

Amethocaine, eye drops 0.5%, 1% 1–2 drops.

Amikacin *Single daily dose i.v. or i.m.:* 7.5mg/kg (<30 weeks gestation), 10mg/kg (30–35 weeks gestation), 15mg/kg (1st week of life), 22.5mg/kg (2 + weeks), 18mg/kg (>10 years). Trough <5mg/L.

Amiloride 0.2mg/kg per dose (max. 5mg) 12 hourly oral.

Aminobenzoate 60mg/kg per dose (max. 3g) 6 hourly oral.

Aminocaproic acid 100mg/kg (max. 5g) stat, then 30 mg/kg per h (max. 1.25g per h) until bleeding stops (max. 18 g/m^2 per day) oral or i.v. *Prophylaxis:* 70mg/kg per dose 6 hourly.

Aminoglutethimide *Adult:* 250mg (NOT/kg) daily oral, increase over 4 weeks to 250mg 6 hourly.

Aminophylline (100mg aminophylline = 80mg theophylline) *Load:* 10mg/kg (max. 500mg) i.v. over 1h. *Maintenance:* 1st week of life 2.5mg/kg per dose 12 hourly; 2nd week of life 4 mg/kg per dose 12 hourly; 3 weeks–12 months ((0.12 × age in weeks) + 3) mg/kg per dose 8 hourly; 1–9 years 1.1mg/kg per h (55mg/kg in 50mL at 1mL/h), or 6mg/kg per dose i.v. over 1h 6 hourly; 10–16 years or adult smoker 0.7mg/kg per h (<35kg 35mg/kg in 50mL at 1mL/h; >35kg 25mg/mL at 0.028mL/kg per h), or 4mg/kg per dose i.v. over 1h 6 hourly; adult non-smoker 0.5mg/kg per h (25mg/mL at 0.02 mL/kg per h), or 3mg/kg per dose i.v. over 1h 6 hourly; elderly 0.3 mg/kg per h (15mg/kg in 50mL at 1mL/h), or 2mg/kg per dose i.v. over 1h 6 hourly. *Monitor theophylline level:* 60–80µmol/L (neonate), 60–110 (asthma) (× 0.18 = µg/mL).

5-Aminosalicylic acid See mesalazine.

Amiodarone *i.v.:* 25µg/kg per min for 4h, then 5–15µg/kg per min (max. 1.2g/24h). *Oral:* 4mg/kg per dose (max. 200mg) 8 hourly 1 week, 12 hourly 1 week, then 12–24 hourly. After starting tablets, taper i.v. infusion over 5 days. Reduce dose of digoxin and warfarin.

Amitriptyline Usually 0.5–1.0mg/kg per dose (max. 100mg) 8 hourly oral. *Enuresis:* 1.0–1.5mg/kg nocte.

AmLodipine 0.05–0.2mg/kg (adult 2.5–10mg) daily oral.

Amodiaquine *Treatment:* 10mg/kg daily for 3 days oral. *Prophylaxis:* 5mg/kg once a week.

Amoxapine 0.5–2mg/kg per dose (max. 100mg) 8 hourly oral.

Amoxicillin See amoxycillin.

Amoxycillin 10–20mg/kg per dose 8 hourly i.v., i.m. or oral. *Severe infection:* 50mg/kg per dose (max. 2g) i.v. 12 hourly (1st week of life), 6 hourly (2–4 weeks), 4–6 hourly or constant infusion (4 + weeks).

Amoxycillin and clavulanic acid Dose as for amoxycillin.

Amphetamine See dexamphetamine.

Amphotericin B Test dose 0.1mg/kg i.v. over 1h, then 0.5–1.0mg/kg i.v. over 6h daily; total dose 30–35mg/kg over 4–8 weeks. *Oral* (NOT/kg): 100mg 6 hourly treatment, 50mg 6 hourly prophylaxis. *Bladder washout:* 25μg/mL. *Cream or ointment 3%:* apply 6–12 hourly.

Amphotericin, liposomal 1mg/kg daily i.v. over 1h, increase over 2–4 days to 2–3mg/kg daily. Total dose typically 20–60mg/kg over 2–4 weeks.

Ampicillin 15–25mg/kg per dose 6 hourly i.v., i.m. or oral. *Severe infection:* 50mg/kg per dose (max. 2g) i.v. 12 hourly (1st week of life), 6 hourly (2–4 weeks), 3–6 hourly or constant infusion (4 + weeks).

Ampicillin 1g + sulbactam 0.5g 20–40mg/kg per dose (max. 2g) of ampicillin 6 hourly i.m. or i.v. over 30min.

Amrinone *<4 weeks old:* 4mg/kg i.v. over 15 min, then 3–5 μg/kg per min. *>4 weeks old:* 1–3mg/kg i.v. over 30min, then 5–15μg/kg per min.

Amsacrine. 450–600mg/m^2 i.v. over 2h daily for 3–5days.

Amylobarbitone 0.3–1mg/kg per dose 8–12 hourly, or 2–4mg/kg at night, oral.

Anistreplase *Adult:* 30u (NOT/kg) i.v. over 5min.

Anthraquinone See Sennoside.

Antithrombin III. No. IU = (desired – actual level) × wt / 1.4.

Antithymocyte (lymphocyte) globulin See immunoglobulin, lymphocyte.

Antivenom to jellyfish (box), snakes (black, brown, death adder, sea, taipan, tiger) spiders (funnel-web) and ticks Dose depends on amount of venom injected, not size of patient. Higher doses needed for multiple bites, severe symptoms or delayed administration. Give adrenaline 0.005mg/kg (0.005mL/kg of 1 in 1000) s.c. Initial dose antivenom usually 1–2 amp diluted 1/10 in Hartmann's solution i.v. over 30min. Monitor PT, PTT, fibrinogen, platelets. Give antivenom repeatedly if symptoms or coagulopathy persist.

Antivenom, red back spider 1amp i.m., may repeat in 2h. *Severe envenomation:* 2amp diluted 1/10 in Hartmann's solution i.v. over 30min.

Antivenom, stonefish 1000u (2mL) per puncture i.m. *Severe envenomation:* 1000u/puncture diluted 1/10 in Hartmann's solution i.v. over 30min.

Apraclonidine, 1% eye drops 1–2drops/eye 12 hourly.

Aprobarbital 1–3mg/kg oral at night.

Aprostadil See prostaglandin E1.

Aprotinin (1kiu = 140ng = 0.00056epu) *Shock:* 10 000 kiu/kg (max. 1 000 000kiu) i.v. over 1h, then 1 000 kiu/kg per h (max. 50 000kiu per h). *Hge proph:* 4 000kiu/kg slow i.v., then 2 000kiu/kg per dose 6 hourly. *O&G hge* (NOT/kg): 1 000 000kiu over 30min, then 200 000kiu per h.

Aqueous cream; pure, buffered or with 5% or 10% olive oil or peanut oil A base for other ingredients, or before cold compresses.

Arginine HCl mg/kg = BE × 70 (give ½ this) i.v. over 2h.

Ascorbic acid *Scurvy:* 100mg per dose (NOT/kg) 8 hourly oral 10 days. *Urine acidification:* 10–30mg/kg per dose 6 hourly.

Asparaginase-L Test 2–50u intradermal. Typical dose 6000u/m^2 every 3rd day × 9 doses i.v. over 4h, i.m. or s.c.

Aspirin 10–15mg/kg per dose (adult 300–600mg) 4–6 hourly oral. *Antiplatelet:* 2–5mg/kg daily. *Kawasaki:* 25mg/kg per dose 6 hourly 14 days (monitor levels), then 4mg/kg daily. *Arthritis:* 25mg/kg per dose (max. 2g) 6 hourly for 3 days, then 15–20 mg/kg per dose 6 hourly. Salicylate level (arthritis) 0.7–2.0 mmol/L (× 13.81 = mg/100mL).

Astemizole 0.2mg/kg (max. 10mg) daily oral.

Atenolol *Oral:* 1–2mg/kg per dose (max. 100mg) 12–24 hourly. *i.v.:* 0.05mg/kg every 5min till response (max. 4 doses), then 0.1–0.2 mg/kg per dose (max. 10mg) over 10min 12–24 hourly.

Atracurium 0.3–0.6mg/kg stat, then 5–10µg/kg per min i.v.

Atropine 0.02mg/kg (max. 0.6mg) i.v. or i.m., then 0.01 mg/kg per dose 4–6 hourly. *Organophosphate poisoning:* 0.05 mg/kg i.v., then 0.02–0.05mg/kg per dose every 15–60min until atropinized (continue 12–24h). *Colic:* see phenobarbitone.

Auranofin *Adult:* 6–9mg (NOT/kg) daily oral.

Aurothioglucose 0.25mg/kg weekly i.m., increase to 1mg/kg (max. 40mg) weekly for 20 weeks, then every 1–4 weeks.

Azapropazone 10mg/kg per dose (max. 600mg) 12 hourly oral. *Acute gout:* day 1 6 hourly, day 2 8 hourly, then 12 hourly.

Azatadine 0.02–0.04mg/kg per dose (max. 2mg) 12 hourly oral.

Azathioprine 25–75mg/m^2 (approx 1–3mg/kg) daily.

Azelaic acid (micronised) 20% cream applied 12 hourly.

Azidothymidine (AZT) See zidovudine.

Azithromycin 10mg/kg per dose (max. 500mg) day 1, then 5 mg/kg per dose (max. 250mg) days 2–5 oral.

Azlocillin 40mg/kg per dose 8 hourly i.v. *Severe infection:* 100mg/kg per dose (max. 5g) i.v. 12 hourly (1st week of life), 8 hourly or constant infusion (2 + weeks).

Aztreonam 30mg/kg per dose 8 hourly. *Severe infection:* 50mg/kg per dose 12 hourly (1st week of life), 8 hourly (2–4 weeks), 6 hourly or constant infusion (4 + weeks) i.v.

Bacampicillin 15–25mg/kg per dose 8–12 hourly oral.

Bacillus Calmette–Guerin (BCG) vaccine (CSL) Live. *Intradermal* (1mg/mL): 0.075mL (<3mo) or 0.1mL (>3mo) once. *Percutaneous* (60mg/mL suspension): 1 drop on skin, inoculated with Heaf apparatus, once.

Bacillus Calmette–Guerin (BCG) suspension, about 5×10^8 cfu/vial *Adult:* 1 vial (OncoTICE) or 3 vials (ImmuCyst) left in bladder for 2h each week for 6 weeks, then at 3, 6, 12, 18 and 24 months.

Bacitracin 400u/g + neomycin 5mg/g + polymyxin B 5000u/g (Neosporin) *Ointment or eye ointment:* apply × 2–5/day. *Powder:* apply 6–12 hourly (skin infections), every few days (burns). *Eye drops:* see gramicidin.

Baclofen 0.1mg/kg per dose 8 hourly oral, increase by 0.1 mg/kg per dose every 3 days. Effective dose about 0.5 mg/kg per dose 8 hourly (max. 1mg/kg per dose 8 hourly). *Intrathecal infusion:* 2–20µg/kg (max. 1000µg) per day.

Bambuterol 0.2–0.4mg/kg (max. 20mg) daily at night oral.

BCG vaccine See Bacillus Calmette–Guerin vaccine.

Beclomethasone *Rotacap or aerosol* (NOT/kg): 100–200µg (<8 years), 150–500µg (>8 years) × 2–4/day.

Beclomethasone dipropionate, nasal *Aerosol or pump* (50μg/spray): 1spray 12 hourly (<12 years), 2spray 12 hourly (>12 years).
Benazepril Usually 0.2mg/kg per dose (max. 10mg) oral daily.
Bendroflumethiazide See bendrofluazide.
Bendrofluazide 0.1–0.2mg/kg (max. 10mg) daily oral.
Benorylate 30mg/kg per dose (max. 1.5g) 8 hourly oral.
Benperidol 5–15μg/kg per dose (max. 1.5mg) 12–24 hourly oral.
Benserazide See levodopa and benserazide.
Benzhexol 0.02–0.3mg/kg (max. 15mg) daily oral.
Benzocaine, topical 1–20% Usually applied 4–6 hourly.
Benzoic acid 6% + salicylic acid 3%, ointment (Whitfield's) Apply 12 hourly.
Benzonatate *Adult:* 100mg per dose (NOT/kg) 4–8 hourly oral.
Benzoyl peroxide, liquid or gel 2.5–10% Apply × 1–3/day.
Benzphetamine 0.5–1mg/kg per dose (max. 50mg) 8–24 hourly oral.
Benzquinamide *i.m.:* 1mg/kg (max. 50mg) stat and repeat in 1h if needed, then 3–4 hourly p.r.n. *i.v. over 1min:* 0.5mg/kg (max. 25mg) once.
Benzthiazide 0.5–2mg/kg per dose (max. 100mg) 12–24 hourly oral.
Benztropine 0.02mg/kg stat i.m. or i.v., may repeat in 15min. 0.02–0.1mg/kg per dose (max. 6mg) 12–24 hourly oral.
Benzylpenicilloyl polylysine See penicilloyl polylysine.
Benzyl benzoate, lotion 25% *Scabies:* apply from neck down after a hot bath, remove in bath after 24h; repeat after 5 days. *Lice:* apply to infected region, wash off after 24h; repeat after 7 days.
Benzylpenicillin See penicillin G.
Bepridil 4–8mg/kg (max. 400mg) daily oral.
Beractant (bovine surfactant, Survanta) 4mL/kg intratracheal 4 times in 48h (each dose in 4 parts: head and body inclined down with head to right, body down head left, body up head right, body up head left).
Betacarotene *Porphyria:* 1–5mg/kg daily oral.
Betahistine 0.15–0.3mg/kg per dose (max. 16mg) 8 hourly oral.
Betamethasone 0.01–0.2mg/kg daily oral. Betamethasone has no mineralocorticoid action, 1mg = 25mg hydrocortisone in glucocorticoid action.
Betamethasone; gel 0.05%; cream, lotion or ointment, 0.02%, 0.05%, 0.1% Apply sparingly 12–24 hourly.
Betamethasone acetate 3mg/mL with betamethasone sodium phosphate 3.9mg/mL (Celestone Chronodose) *Adult:* 0.25–2mL (NOT/kg) intramuscular, intra-articular, or intralesional injection.
Betaxolol 0.2–0.8mg/kg (max. 40mg) daily oral. *Eye drops* 0.25–0.5%: 1–2 drops per eye 12 hourly.
Bethanecol *Oral:* 0.2–1mg/kg per dose (max. 50mg) 6–8 hourly. *s.c.:* 0.05–0.1 mg/kg per dose (max. 5mg) 6–8 hourly.
Bezafibrate 4mg/kg per dose (max. 200mg) 8 hourly oral with food.
Bicarbonate *Under 5kg:* dose (mmol) = BE × wt/4 slow i.v. *Over 5kg:* dose (mmol) = BE × wt/6 slow i.v. These doses correct half the base deficit.
Bifonazole 1% cream Apply daily for 2–4 weeks.
Biperiden 0.02–0.1mg/kg per dose (max. 4mg) 6–12 hourly oral.

Bisacodyl NOT/kg: <12 months 2.5mg p.r., 1–5 years 5mg p.r. or 5–10mg oral, >5 years 10mg p.r. or 10–20mg oral.

Bismuth subcitrate See tripotassium dicitratobismuthate.

Bisoprolol 0.1–0.4mg/kg (max. 20mg) daily oral.

Bitolterol *Respiratory solution* (0.2%): 1mL per dose diluted to 4mL 3–6 hourly (mild), 2mL per dose diluted to 4mL 1–2 hourly (moderate), undiluted constant (severe, in ICU). *Aerosol 370µg/puff:* 1–2 puff 4–6 hourly.

Bleomycin 10–20u/m^2 i.m., s.c. or i.v. over 15min × 1–2/week. Max. total dose 250u/m^2.

Blood products See albumin, cryoprecipitate, factor 8, fresh frozen plasma, packed cells, platelets, prothrombinex and whole blood.

Bretylium 5–10mg/kg i.v. over 1h, then 5–30µg/kg per min.

Bromazepam 0.05–0.25mg/kg per dose 8 hourly oral.

Bromocriptine 0.025mg/kg per dose (max. 1.25mg) 8–12 hourly, increase weekly to 0.05–0.2mg/kg per dose (max. 2.5–10mg) 6–12 hourly oral. *Inhibit lactation:* 2.5mg per dose (NOT/kg) 12 hourly for 2 weeks.

Brompheniramine 0.1–0.2mg/kg per dose (max. 10mg) 6–8 hourly oral, s.c., i.m. or slow i.v.

Buclizine 0.25–1.0mg/kg per dose (max. 50mg) 8–24 hourly oral.

Budesonide *Metered dose inhaler* (NOT/kg): <12 years 50–200µg 6–12 hourly, reducing to 100–200µg 12 hourly; >12 years 100–600µg 6–12 hourly, reducing to 100–400µg 12 hourly. *Nebuliser* (NOT/kg): <12 years 0.5–1mg 12 hourly, reducing to 0.25–0.5mg 12 hourly; >12 years 1–2mg 12 hourly, reducing to 0.5–1mg 12 hourly. *Nasal spray or aerosol* (NOT/kg): 100–200µg/nostril daily.

Bumetanide 25µg/kg (max. 1mg) daily oral, may increase to 8–12 hourly.

Bupivacaine *Max. dose:* 2–3mg/kg (0.4–0.6mL/kg of 0.5%). *With adrenaline:* max. dose: 3–4mg/kg (0.6–0.8mL/kg of 0.5%). *Epidural infusion:* 0.2–0.4mg/kg per h.

Buprenorphine 3–9µg/kg per dose (max. 600µg) 6–8 hourly sublingual, i.m. or slow i.v.

Bupropion 2–3mg/kg per dose (max. 150mg) 8–12 hourly oral.

Buserelin (gonadorelin analogue) Adult. *Intranasal:* 100 µg per dose (NOT/kg) 4 hourly, or 150µg (NOT/kg) each nostril 8 hourly. *s.c.:* 0.5mg per dose (NOT/kg) 8 hourly.

Buspirone 0.1mg/kg per dose 8 hourly oral, increase to max. 0.4 mg/kg per dose (max. 15mg) 8–12 hourly.

Busulfan *Induction:* 0.06mg/kg (max. 4mg) daily oral if leucocytes >20 000/mm3 and platelets >100 000/mm3. *Maintenance:* 0.01–0.03mg/kg (max. 2mg) daily.

Butabarbital See secbutobarbitone.

Butalbital 1–2mg/kg per dose (max. 100mg) 8–24 hourly oral.

Butobarbitone 2–4mg/kg (max. 200mg) at night oral.

Butorphanol *i.m.:* 0.02–0.1mg/kg per dose (max. 4mg) 3–4 hourly. *i.v.:* 0.01–0.05mg/kg (max. 2mg) 3–4 hourly.

Butriptyline 0.5–1.0mg/kg per dose (max. 50mg) 8 hourly oral.

Caffeine 1–5mg/kg per dose (max. 250mg) 4–8 hourly oral or p.r.

Calamine, lotion Usually applied 6–8 hourly.

Calcitonin *Hypercalcaemia:* 4iu/kg per dose 12–24 hourly i.m. or s.c., may increase up to 8iu/kg per dose 6–12 hourly. *Paget's:* 1.5–3iu/kg (max. 160mg) × 3/week i.m. or s.c.
Calcitriol See vitamin D.
Calcium (as carbonate, lactate or phosphate) NOT/kg: *<3 years:* 100mg × 2–5/day oral; *4–12 years:* 300mg × 2–3/day; *>12 years:* 1000mg × 1–2/day.
Calcium carbimide 1–2mg/kg per dose (max. 100mg) 12 hourly oral.
Calcium carbonate 840mg (NOT/kg) 8–12 hourly oral.
Calcium chloride 10% (0.7mmol/mL Ca). 0.2mL/kg (max. 10mL) slow i.v. stat. Requirement 2mL/kg per day. *Inotrope:* 0.5–2mmol/kg per day (0.03–0.12mL/kg per h).
Calcium edetate (EDTA) See sodium calciumedetate.
Calcium gluconate 10% (0.22mmol/mL Ca) 0.5mL/kg (max. 20mL) slow i.v. stat. Requirement 5mL/kg per day. *Inotrope:* 0.5–2mmol/kg per day (0.1–0.4mL/kg per h).
Canrenoate See potassium canrenoate.
Capreomycin 20mg/kg (max. 1g) i.m. on 2–7 days/week.
Captopril 0.1–1.0mg/kg per dose (max. 50mg) 8 hourly oral.
Carbachol 0.01%: max. 0.5mL in anterior chamber of eye.
Carbamazepine 2mg/kg per dose 8 hourly oral, may increase over 2 weeks to 5–10mg/kg per dose (max. 500mg) 8 hourly. Level 20–50µmol/L (× 0.24 = µg/mL) measured Mon, Wed and Fri at the Royal Children's Hospital.
Carbenicillin 25–100mg/kg per dose (max. 5g) 4–6 hourly i.m. or i.v.
Carbenoxolone *Adult:* 20–50mg (NOT/kg) 6 hourly oral. Mouth gel 2%, or 2g granules in 40mL water, apply 6 hourly.
Carbidopa See levodopa and carbidopa.
Carbimazole 0.25mg/kg per dose (max. 15mg) 8 hourly oral for 2 weeks, then 0.1mg/kg per dose 8–12 hourly.
Carbinoxamine NOT/kg: 2mg (1-3 years), 2-4mg (3-6 years), 4-8mg (>6 years) 6-8 hourly oral.
Carbocaine See mepivacaine.
Carbocisteine 10–15mg/kg per dose (max. 750mg) 8 hourly oral.
Carboplatin 300–400mg/m^2 i.v. over 60min every 4 weeks.
Carboprost (15-Me-PGF2-alpha) *Termination:* 250–500 µg per dose (NOT/kg) 1–4 hourly (max. totl 12mg) i.m. *Postpart hge:* 250 µg per dose (NOT/kg) every 15–120min i.m. (max. totl 12mg).
Carisoprodol 7mg/kg per dose (max. 350mg) 6 hourly oral.
Carmustine (BCNU) 200mg/m^2 i.v. over 2h every 6 weeks (reduce dose if nadir in leucocytes <3000/mm3 or platelets <75 000).
Carnitine. 20–35mg/kg per dose (max. 1g) 8 hourly oral or i.v.
Carob bean gum (Carobel Instant) NOT/kg: 1 scoop (1.8g) in 100mL water, give 10–20mL by spoon; or add ½ a scoop to every 100–200mL of milk.
Carteolol 0.05–0.2mg/kg (max. 10mg) daily oral.
Castor oil *Laxative:* 1mL/kg (max. 45mL) oral. *Purgative:* 2mL/kg (max. 90mL) oral.
Cefaclor (Ceclor) 10–15mg/kg per dose (max. 500mg) 8 hourly oral.
Cefadroxil 10–20mg/kg per dose (max. 1g) 12 hourly oral.

Cefamandole See cephamandole.
Cefazolin See cephazolin.
Cefixime 4mg/kg per dose (max. 200mg) 12 hourly oral.
Cefmetazole 40mg/kg per dose (max. 2g) 6–12 hourly i.v.
Cefodizime 20mg/kg per dose (max. 1g) 12 hourly i.v. or i.m.
Cefonicid 10–40mg/kg (max. 2g) i.v. over 10min or i.m. daily.
Cefoperazone 20–50mg/kg per dose (max. 3g) 6–12 hourly i.v. over 1h or i.m.
Ceforanide 10–20mg/kg per dose (max. 1g) 12 hourly i.m. or i.v.
Cefotaxime 75mg/kg per dose 12 hourly (<4 weeks), 8 hourly (4 + weeks) i.v. *Severe infection:* 50mg/kg per dose (max. 3g) i.v. 12 hourly (preterm), 8 hourly (1st week of life), 6 hourly (2–4 weeks), 4–6 hourly or constant infusion (4 + weeks).
Cefotetan 10–20mg/kg per dose (max. 1g) 12 hourly i.m., i.v. *Severe infection:* 40mg/kg per dose (max. 3g) 12 hourly or constant infusion.
Cefoxitin (Mefoxin) 20–40mg/kg per dose (max. 3g) 12 hourly (1st week of life), 8 hourly (1–4 weeks), 6 hourly (>4 weeks) i.v.
Cefpodoxime 2–4mg/kg per dose (max. 200mg) 12 hourly oral.
Cefprozil 15mg/kg per dose (max. 500mg) 12–24 hourly oral.
Cefsulodin 20–50mg/kg per dose (max. 2g) 6 hourly i.v.
Ceftazidime 30mg/kg per dose 8 hourly i.v. or i.m. *Severe infection:* 50 mg/kg per dose (max. 2g) 12 hourly (1st week of life), 8 hourly (2–4 weeks), 6 hourly or constant infusion (4 + weeks).
Ceftizoxime 20–60mg/kg per dose (max. 3g) 6–8 hourly i.v.
Ceftriaxone 30mg/kg per dose 12–24 hourly i.v., or i.m. (in 1% lignocaine). *Severe infection:* 50–75mg/kg per dose (max. 4g) daily (1st week of life), 12 hourly (2 + weeks). *Epiglottitis:* 100mg/kg stat, then 50mg/kg after 24h. *Haemophilus or meningococcus prophylaxis:* 100mg/kg i.m. in 1% lignocaine once.
Cefuroxime *Oral:* 5–10mg/kg per dose 12 hourly. *i.v.:* 15–30mg/kg per dose 8 hourly. *Severe infection:* 50mg/kg per dose (max. 2g) i.v. 12 hourly (1st week of life), 8 hourly (2nd week), 6 hourly or constant infusion (>2 weeks).
Celiprolol 4–8mg/kg (max. 400mg) daily oral.
Cellulose phosphate (Calcisorb) *Adult:* 5g per dose (NOT/kg) 8 hourly oral.
Celmoleukin (synthetic interleukin-2) See interleukin-2.
Cephalexin 10–25mg/kg per dose (max. 1g) 6–12 hourly oral. *Streptococcus:* 10mg/kg per dose (max. 500mg) 12 hourly. *Severe infection:* 20mg/kg per dose (max. 1g) i.v. 4 hourly or constant infusion.
Cephalothin 10–20mg/kg per dose 6 hourly i.v. or i.m. *Severe infection:* 50mg/kg per dose (max. 2g) i.v. 4 hourly or constant infusion. *Irrigation fluid:* 2g/L (2mg/mL).
Cephamandole 15mg/kg per dose 6 hourly i.v. over 10min or i.m. *Severe infection:* 20–40mg/kg per dose (max. 2g) i.v. over 20min 4 hourly or constant infusion.
Cephazolin (Kefzol) 20mg/kg stat, then 10mg/kg per dose 6 hourly i.v. or i.m. *Severe infection:* 20–30mg/kg per dose (max. 2g) i.v. 4 hourly or constant infusion.
Cephradine *Oral:* 5–25mg/kg per dose (max. 1g) 6 hourly. *i.m. or i.v.:* 20–40mg/kg per dose (max. 1–2g) 6 hourly.
Cerumol See dichlorobenzene + chlorbutol otic.
Cetirizine 0.2mg/kg per dose (max. 10mg) 12–24 hourly oral.

Cetylpyridinium + benzocaine, mouth wash (Cepacaine) Apply 3 hourly p.r.n. Do not swallow.
Charcoal (Activated) *Check bowel sounds present:* 0.25 g/kg per dose hourly NG. *Laxative:* sorbitol 1g/kg (1.4mL/kg of 70%) once NG, may repeat once.
Chenodeoxycholic acid 5–10mg/kg per dose 12 hourly oral.
Chloral betaine 1.7mg = 1mg chloral hydrate.
Chloral hydrate *Hypnotic:* 50mg/kg (max. 2g) stat (up to 100mg/kg, max. 5g, in ICU). *Sedative:* 6mg/kg per dose 6 hourly oral.
Chlorambucil Typically 0.1–0.2mg/kg per day oral.
Chloramphenicol *Severe infection:* 40mg/kg (max. 2g) stat, then 25mg/kg per dose (max. 1g) i.v., i.m. or oral. *1st week of life:* daily; *2–4 weeks:* 12 hourly; *5 + weeks:* 8 hourly for 5 days, then 6 hourly. Ensure serum level 20–30mg/L peak, <15mg/L trough.
Chlordiazepoxide 0.1mg/kg per dose 12 hourly oral, may increase to max. 0.5mg/kg per dose 6–8 hourly.
Chlorhexidine *0.1%:* catheterisation prep, impetigo. *0.2%:* mouthwash. *1%:* skin disinfection. *2–4%:* hand wash.
Chlorhexidine 0.5% + alcohol 70%, solution Skin disinfection.
Chlorhexidine 1.5% + cetrimide 15% *1/30 in water:* cleaning tissues or wounds, equipment before sterilisation. *140mL in 1L water:* disinfecting skin, equipment (soak 2min, rinse in sterile water).
Chlorhexidine + cetrimide, 0.05%/0.5%, 0.1%/1%, 0.15%/0.15% Wound cleaning.
Chlorhexidine 1% + hexamidine 0.15%, powder Wound cleaning.
Chlormethiazole *i.v.* (edisylate 0.8%): 1–2mL/kg (8–16 mg/kg) over 15min, then 0.5–1.0mL/kg per h (4–8mg/kg per h). *Oral* (capsule 192mg base): adult 2–4 cap stat (may repeat in 1–2h), then 1–2 cap 8 hourly.
Chlormezanone 5mg/kg per dose (max. 200mg) 6–8 hourly, or 10mg/kg (max. 400mg) at night oral.
Chlorophyllin copper complex 2mg/kg per dose 8–24 hourly oral.
Chloroprocaine Max. 11mg/kg (max. 800mg). With adrenaline (1/200 000) max. 14mg/kg (max. 1000mg).
Chloroquine *Oral:* 10mg/kg daily × 3 days. *i.m.:* 4mg/kg per dose 12 hourly for 3 days. *Prophylaxis:* 5mg/kg (max. 300mg) oral × 1/week. *Lupus, rheu arthritis:* 12mg/kg (max. 600mg) daily, reducing to 4–8mg/kg (max. 400mg) daily oral.
Chlorothiazide 5–20mg/kg per dose (max. 1g) 12–24 hourly oral, i.v.
Chlorotrianisene 0.25–0.5mg/kg (max. 25mg) daily oral.
Chloroxylenol, cream 0.3%, liquid 2.5–5% To clean skin or wounds.
Chlorphenasin, ointment 1% Apply 12 hourly.
Chlorpheniramine 0.1mg/kg per dose (max. 4mg) 6–8 hourly oral.
Chlorpheniramine 1.25mg + phenylephrine 2.5mg in 5mL syrup (Demazin) NOT/kg: 1.25–2.5mL (0–1 year), 2.5–5mL (2–5 years), 5–10mL (6–12 years), 10–15mL (>12 years) 6–8 hourly oral.
Chlorpromazine *Oral or p.r.:* 0.5–2mg/kg per dose (max. 100 mg) 6–8 hourly; up to 20mg/kg per dose 8 hourly for psychosis. *Slow i.v. or i.m.:* 0.25–1mg/kg per dose (usual max. 50mg) 6–8 hourly.
Chlorpropamide *Adult:* initially 125–250mg (NOT/kg) daily oral, max. 500mg daily.

Chlorprothixene Usually 0.5–1mg/kg per dose 6–8 hourly oral or i.m.
Chlorquinaldol, paste 5% Apply 12 hourly.
Chlortetracycline, cream or ointment 3% Apply 8–24 hourly.
Chlorthalidone 2mg/kg (max. 100mg) 3 times a week oral.
Chlorzoxazone 5–15mg/kg per dose (max. 750mg) 6–8 hourly oral.
Cholecalciferol (Vit D3) 1u = 1u ergocalcif. See vitamin D.
Cholera vaccine (CSL) Inactivated. 2 doses s.c. 7–28days apart: 0.1mL then 0.3mL (<5 years), 0.3mL then 0.5mL (5–9 years), 0.5mL then 1mL (>9 years). Boost every 6 months (use 1st dose).
Cholestyramine 50–150mg/kg per dose (max. 9g) 6–8 hourly oral.
Choline salicylate, mouth gel (Bonjela) Apply 3 hourly p.r.n.
Choline theophyllinate (200mg = theophylline 127mg) See theophylline.
Chorionic gonadotrophin Usually 100iu/kg (max. 5000iu) i.m. × 3/week for 2–8 weeks. *After FSH:* 10 000iu (NOT/kg) i.m. once. *Men:* 7000iu (NOT/kg) i.m. × 2/week, with 75iu FS hourly and 75iu L hourly i.m. × 3/week.
Chymopapain *Adult:* 2000–4000 picokatal units per disc (NOT/kg), max. 10 000 picokatal units per patient.
Cilazapril Usually 0.02–0.1mg/kg (max. 5mg) daily oral. *Renal hypertension:* 0.005–0.01mg/kg daily oral.
Cimetidine 10–15mg/kg per dose (usual max. 200mg per dose) 12 hourly (newborn), 6 hourly (>4 weeks) i.v. or oral.
Cinnarizine 0.3–0.6mg/kg per dose 8 hourly oral. *Periph vasc dis:* 1.5mg/kg per dose (max. 75mg) 8 hourly oral.
Cinchocaine Max. dose 2mg/kg (0.4mL/kg of 0.5%).
Cinoxacin 10mg/kg per dose (max. 500mg) 12 hourly oral.
Ciprofibrate 2–4mg/kg (max. 200mg) daily oral.
Ciprofloxacin 5–10mg/kg per dose (adult 250–500mg per dose) 12 hourly oral, 4–7mg/kg per dose (adult 200–300mg per dose) 12 hourly i.v. *Severe infection:* 15mg/kg per dose (max. 750mg) 12 hourly oral, 8mg/kg per dose (max. 400mg) 8 hourly i.v.; higher doses used occasionally. Reduce dose of theophylline.
Cisapride 0.2–0.6mg/kg per dose (max. 25mg) × 4/day oral before meals and at bedtime.
Cisplatin 60–100mg/m^2 i.v. over 6h every 3–4 weeks × 6 cycles.
Clarithromycin 5–10mg/kg per dose (max. 500mg) 12 hourly oral.
Clavulanic acid with amoxycillin or ticarcillin. Dose as for amoxycillin or ticarcillin.
Clemastine 0.02–0.06mg/kg per dose (max. 3mg) 12 hourly oral.
Clidinium 0.05–0.1mg/kg per dose (max. 5mg) 6–8 hourly oral.
Clindamycin 5mg/kg per dose 6 hourly oral, i.m. or i.v. over 30min. *Severe infection:* 10–20mg/kg per dose (max. 1g) 6 hourly i.v. over 1h. *Acne solution 1%:* apply 12 hourly.
Clioquinol, cream 10mg/g, powder 100% Apply 6–12 hourly.
Clobazam 0.1–0.4mg/kg per dose (max. 20mg) 8–12 hourly oral.
Clobetasone, 0.1% eye drops 1–2drops/eye 1–6 hourly.
Clofazimine 2mg/kg (max. 100mg) daily oral. *Lepra reaction:* up to 6mg/kg (max. 300mg) daily for max. 3mo.
Clofibrate 10mg/kg per dose 8–12 hourly oral.

Clomiphene citrate *Adult:* 50mg (NOT/kg) daily for 5 days oral, increase to 100mg daily for 5 days if no ovulation.
Clomipramine 0.5mg/kg per dose 8–12 hourly oral.
Clonazepam 0.02mg/kg per dose (max. 0.5mg) 12 hourly oral, slowly increase to 0.05mg/kg per dose (max. 2mg) 6–12 hourly oral. *Status* (may be repeated), NOT/kg: neonate 0.25mg, child 0.5mg, adult 1mg i.v.
Clonidine 3–5μg/kg slow i.v., 1–6μg/kg per dose (max. 300μg) 8–12 hourly oral. *Migraine:* start with 0.5μg/kg per dose 12 hourly oral.
Clorazepate 0.3–2mg/kg (max. 90mg) daily at night oral, or 0.1–0.5mg/kg per dose (max. 30mg) 8 hourly.
Clostridia antitoxin See gas gangrene antitoxin.
Clotrimazole *Topical:* 1% cream or solution 8–12 hourly. *Vaginal* (NOT/kg): 1% cream or 100mg tab daily for 6 days, or 2% cream or 500mg tab daily for 3 days.
Cloxacillin 15mg/kg per dose (max. 500mg) 6 hourly oral, i.m. or i.v. *Severe infection:* 25–50mg/kg per dose (max. 2g) i.v. 12 hourly (1st week of life), 8 hourly (2–4 weeks), 4–6 hourly (>4 weeks).
Clozapine 0.5mg/kg per dose 12 hourly oral, increase over 7–14 days to 2–5mg/kg per dose (max. 300mg) 8–12 hourly; later reducing to 2mg/kg per dose 8–12 hourly.
Coal tar, topical 0.5% increase to max. 10%, applied 6–8 hourly.
Cocaine *Topical:* 1–3mg/kg.
Codeine *Analgesic:* 0.5–1mg/kg per dose 4 hourly oral. *Antitussive:* 0.25–0.5mg/kg per dose 6 hourly.
Co–dergocrine mesylate *Adult:* usually 3.0–4.5mg (NOT/kg) daily before meal oral or sublingual. 300μg (NOT/kg) daily i.m., s.c. or i.v. infusion.
Colaspase See asparaginase.
Colchicine *Acute gout:* 0.02mg/kg per dose (max. 1mg) 2 hourly oral (max. 3 doses/day). *Chronic use* (gout, FMF): 0.01–0.04mg/kg (max. 2mg) daily oral.
Colestipol granules 0.1–0.2g/kg per dose (max. 10g) 8 hourly oral.
Colfosceril palmitate See surfactant, synthetic.
Colistimethate sodium See colistin.
Colistin (1mg = 200 000u approx) *Oral:* 1.5–3mg/kg per dose 8 hourly. *i.m. or slow i.v.:* 2mg/kg per dose (max. 100mg) 8 hourly.
Colistin 3mg/mL + neomycin 3.3mg/mL otic 4 drops 8 hourly.
Colonic lavage solution *Poisoning:* if bowel sounds present, 30mL/kg per h NG for 4–8h (until rectal effluent clear).
Coloxyl See dioctyl sodium sulphosuccinate, poloxalkol.
Corticotrophin (corticotropin) See ACTH.
Cortisone acetate *Physiological:* 0.2mg/kg per dose 8 hourly oral. Cortisone acetate 1mg = hydrocortisone 1.25mg in mineralocorticoid and glucocorticoid action.
Coryza vaccine (Neisseria, Klebsiella and Haemophilus; CSL) Inactivated. 4 doses 1 week apart: 0.25mL, 0.5mL, 0.75mL, 1mL (<12 years half dose).
Cosyntropin See tetracosactrin zinc injection.
Cotrimoxazole (trimethoprim 1mg + sulphamethoxazole 5mg). TMP 2.5mg/kg per dose 12 hourly i.v. over 1h or oral. *Pneumocystis:* TMP 250mg/m^2 stat, then 150mg/m^2 8 hourly (<11 years) or 12 hourly (>10 years) i.v. over 1h, in renal failure dose interval = serum creatinine (mmol/L) × 135 (max. 48h); peak serum TMP

5–10μg/mL, SMX 100–200μg/mL. *i.v. infusion:* TMP max. 1.6mg/mL in 5% dextrose.

Coumarin *Oral:* 1–8mg/kg (max. 400mg) daily. *Cream 100mg/g:* apply 8–12 hourly.

Cromoglycate, sodium *Inhalation* (Intal): 1 cap (20mg) 6–8 hourly, 2mL solution (20mg) 6–8 hourly, aerosol 1–10mg 6–8 hourly. *Eye drops* (2%): 1–2 drops per eye 4–6 hourly. *Oral:* 5–10mg/kg per dose (max. 200mg) 6 hourly oral. *Nasal* (Rynacrom): insufflator 5mg in each nostril 6 hourly, spray 1 puff in each nostril 6 hourly.

Cromolyn sodium See cromoglycate.

Crotamiton, cream or lotion 10% Apply ×2–3/day.

Cryoprecipitate (factor 8 about 5u/mL and 100u/bag, fibrinogen about 10mg/mL and 200mg/bag). *Low factor 8:* 1u/kg increase activity 2% (half-life 12h); usual dose 5mL/kg or 1bag/4kg 12 hourly i.v. for 1–2 infusions (muscle, joint), 3–6 infusions (hip, forearm, retroperitoneal, oropharynx), 7–14 infusions (intracranial). *Low fibrinogen:* usual dose 5mL/kg or 1bag/4kg i.v. A bag is usually 20–30mL.

Cyanocobalamin Use hydroxocobalamin.

Cyclizine 1mg/kg per dose (max. 50mg) 8 hourly oral, i.m. or i.v.

Cyclobenzaprine 0.2–0.4mg/kg per dose (max. 20mg) 8 hourly oral.

Cyclofenil *Adult:* 200mg per dose (NOT/kg) 12 hourly oral, starting 3rd day of menstruation.

Cyclopenthiazide 5–10μg/kg per dose (max. 500μg) 12–24 hourly oral.

Cyclopentolate, eye drops 0.5% or 1% 1 drop per eye, repeat after 5min. Pilocarpine 1% speeds recovery.

Cyclophosphamide A typical regimen is 600mg/m^2 i.v. over 30min daily for 3 days, then 600mg/m^2 i.v. weekly or 10mg/kg twice weekly (if leucocytes >3000/mm3).

Cycloserine 5–10mg/kg per dose (max. 500mg) 12 hourly oral. Keep plasma conc <30μg/mL.

Cyclosporin 1–3μg/kg per min i.v. for 24–48h, then 5–8mg/kg per dose 12 hourly reducing by 1mg/kg per dose each month to 3–4 mg/kg per dose oral. Trough level by Abbott TDx monoclonal specific assay (×2.5 = non-specific assay level) on whole blood (done Tues and Fri at the Royal Children's Hospital): 120–200ng/mL (marrow), 150–200ng/mL first 3mo then 100–150ng/mL (kidney), 100–400ng/mL (heart, liver).

Cyclosporine See cyclosporin.

Cyproheptadine 0.1mg/kg per dose 8–12 hourly oral.

Cyproterone acetate 25–50mg/m^2 per dose 8–12 hourly oral.

Cyproterone acetate + ethinyloestradiol (2mg/35μg) × 21 tab, + 7 inert tab *Contraception:* 1 tab daily, starting 1st day of mensturation.

Cytarabine Usually 100mg/m^2 daily for 10 days by i.v. injctn or constant infusion. *Intrathecal:* 30mg/m^2 every 4 days until CSF normal (dissolve in saline not diluent).

Cytomegalovirus immunoglobulin See immunoglobulin, CMV.

Dacarbazine 250mg/m^2 i.v. daily for 5 days every 3 weeks.

Dactinomycin Usually 400–600μg/m^2 i.v. daily for 5 days, repeat after 3–4 weeks.

Danazol 2–4mg/kg per dose (max. 200mg) 6–12 hourly oral.

Danthron 1–6 years 25mg, 7–12 years 50mg, adult 100mg stat.
Dantrolene *Hyperpyrexia:* 1mg/kg per min until improves (max. 10mg/kg), then 1–2mg/kg per dose 6 hourly for 1–3day i.v. or oral. *Spasticity:* 0.5–2mg/kg per dose (max. 100mg) 6 hourly oral.
Dapsone 1–2mg/kg (max. 100mg) daily oral. *Derm herpet:* 1–6mg/kg (max. 300mg) daily. See also pyrimethamine.
Daunorubicin 30mg/m^2 weekly slow i.v., or 60–90mg/m^2 every 3 weeks. Max. total dose 500mg/m^2.
DDAVP See desmopressin.
Debrisoquine 0.2–1mg/kg per dose (max. 60mg) 12–24 hourly oral.
Deferoxamine See desferrioxamine.
Demeclocycline *>8 years:* 3mg/kg per dose (max. 150mg) 6–12 hourly oral.
Deserpidine 0.005–0.02mg/kg (max. 1mg) daily oral.
Desferrioxamine *Antidote:* 10–15mg/kg per h i.v. for 12–24h (max. 6g/24h); some also give 5–10g (NOT/kg) once oral. *Thalassaemia* (NOT/kg): 500mg per unit blood, and 1–3g in 5mL s.c. over 10h 5–6 nights per week.
Desipramine 0.5–1.0mg/kg per dose (max. 50mg) 8–12 hourly oral.
Desmopressin (DDAVP) 5–10µg (0.05–0.1mL) per dose (NOT/kg) 12–24 hourly nasal. *Low factor VIII:* 0.3µg/kg in 1mL/kg saline i.v. over 1h 12–24 hourly.
Desogestrel + ethinyloestradiol (150µg/30µg) ×21 tab, +21 inert tab *Contraception:* 1 tab daily, starting 1st day of menstruation.
Dexamethasone 0.1–0.25mg/kg per dose 6 hourly oral or i.v. *BPD:* 0.1mg/kg per dose 6 hourly for 3 days, then 8 hourly 3 days, 12 hourly 3 days, 24 hourly 3 days, 48 hourly 7 days. *Severe croup:* 0.6mg/kg (max. 12mg) i.m. stat, then prednisolone 1mg/kg per dose 8–12 hourly oral. *Eye drops* 0.1%: 1–2 drops per eye 3–8 hourly. Dexamethasone has no mineralocorticoid action, but 1mg = 25mg hydrocortisone in glucocorticoid action.
Dexamphetamine 0.2mg/kg daily oral, increase to max. 0.6 mg/kg per dose (max. 30mg) 12 hourly.
Dexchlorpheniramine 0.04mg/kg per dose (max. 2mg) 6–8 hourly oral.
Dexfenfluramine *Adult:* 15mg (NOT/kg) 12 hourly oral.
Dextran 1 (Promit) 0.3mL/kg i.v. 1–2min before giving dextran 40 or dextran 70.
Dextran 40 *10% solution:* 10mL/kg per dose (max. 20mL/kg day 1, then 10mL/kg per day). Half life about 3h.
Dextran 70 *6% solution:* 10mL/kg per dose (max. 20mL/kg day 1, then 10mL/kg per day). Half life about 12h.
Dextroamphetamine See dexamphetamine.
Dextromethorphan 0.2–0.5mg/kg per dose 6–8 hourly oral.
Dextromoramide 0.1mg/kg per dose 8 hourly, may increase to 0.5 mg/kg per dose (max. 20mg) 8 hourly.
Dextropropoxyphene Hydrochloride 1.3mg/kg per dose (max. 65mg) or napsylate 2mg/kg per dose (max. 100mg) 6 hourly oral.
Dextrose (glucose) *Hypoglycaemia:* 1mL/kg 50% dextrose i.v., then increase infusion rate. *Hyperkalaemia:* 0.1u/kg insulin + 2mL/kg 50% dextrose i.v. *Neonates:* 6g/kg per day (about 4mg/kg per min) day 1, increase to 12 g/kg per day (up to 18 g/kg per day with hypoglycaemia). Infusion rate (mL/h) = (4.17 × wt × g/kg per day) / %dextrose. Dose (g/kg per day) = (mL/h × %dextrose) / (4.17 × wt). mg/kg per min = g/kg per day / 1.44.

Dezocine *i.m.:* usually 0.2mg/kg per dose (max. 10mg) 3–6 hourly. *i.v.:* usually 0.1mg/kg per dose 2–4 hourly.

Diazepam 0.2mg/kg per dose i.v. 0.2–0.5mg/kg per dose 8–12 hourly oral or p.r. Do not give by i.v. infusion (binds to PVC).

Diazoxide *Hypertension:* 1–3mg/kg stat by rapid i.v. injection (severe hypotension may occur) repeat once prn, then 2–5mg/kg per dose i.v. 6 hourly. *Hyperinsulinism:* 30–100 mg/m^2 per dose 8 hourly oral.

Dibromopropamidine, cream 0.15% Apply on dressing p.r.n.

Dibucaine See cinchocaine.

Dichlorobenzene 2% + chlorbutol 5% otic (Cerumol) 5 drops to ear 15min before syringing.

Dichlorphenamide 2–4mg/kg (max. 200mg) stat, then 2mg/kg per dose (max. 100mg) 12 hourly until response, then 0.5–1mg/kg per dose (max. 50mg) 8–24 hourly oral.

Diclofenac 1mg/kg per dose (max. 50mg) 8–12 hourly oral.

Dicloxacillin 3–6mg/kg per dose 6 hourly oral.

Dicobalt edetate 6mg/kg (max. 300mg) i.v. over 1–5min, repeat ×2 if no response.

Dicyclomine 0.5mg/kg per dose (max. 15mg) 6 hourly oral.

Didanosine 50–150mg/m^2 per dose 12 hourly oral.

Dideoxycytidine (ddC) See zalcitabine.

Diethylcarbamazine *Filariasis, onchocerciasis, loiasis:* 2mg/kg per dose 8 hourly oral for 3–4 weeks. *Ascariasis:* 6–10mg/kg per dose 8 hourly oral 7–10days. *Tropical eosinophilia:* 13mg/kg daily 4–7 days.

Diethylpropion *6–12 years:* 25mg (NOT/kg) 12 hourly oral. *>12 years:* 25mg (NOT/kg) 6–8 hourly oral.

Diethylstilboestrol See stilboestrol.

Difenoxin 1mg and atropine 0.025mg *Adult:* 1–2 tab (NOT/kg) 6–8 hourly oral.

Diflunisal 5–10mg/kg per dose (max. 500mg) 12 hourly oral.

Digoxin 15μg/kg stat and 5μg/kg after 6 h, then 5 μg/kg per dose (max. 200μg i.v., 250μg oral) 12 hourly slow i.v. or oral. Level 0.5–2.5 nmol/L (× 0.78 = ng/mL).

Digoxin FAB antibodies i.v. over 30min. Dose (to nearest 40mg) = serum digoxin (nmol/L) × wt (kg) × 0.3, or mg ingested × 55. Give if >0.3mg/kg ingested, or level >6.4 nmol/L.

Dihydrocodeine 0.5–1mg/kg per dose 4–6 hourly oral.

Dihydroergotamine mesylate *Adult:* 1mg (NOT/kg) i.m. or i.v., repeat hourly ×2 if needed. Max. 6mg/week.

Dihydromorphinone 0.02–0.1mg/kg per dose 3–6 hourly s.c., i.m., slow i.v., p.r. or oral.

Dihydrotachysterol See vitamin D.

Diltiazem 1mg/kg per dose 6 hourly, increase to max. 2mg/kg per dose (max. 90mg) 6 hourly oral.

Dimenhydrinate 1.0–1.5mg/kg per dose (max. 50mg) 4–6 hourly oral, i.m. or i.v.

Dimercaprol (BAL) 3mg/kg per dose (max. 150mg) i.m. 4 hourly for 2 days, then 6 hourly for 1 day, then 12 hourly for 10 days.

Dimethicone, cream 10%, 15% Barrier cream, apply p.r.n.

Dimethindene 0.02–0.04mg/kg per dose (max. 2mg) 8 hourly oral.
Dimethyl sulfoxide, 50% 50mL in bladder for 15min 2 weekly.
Dinoprost (Prostaglandin F2 alpha) *Extra-amniotic:* 1mL of 250 μg/mL stat, then 3mL 2 hourly. *Intra-amniotic:* 40mg stat, then 10–40mg after 24h if required.
Dinoprostone (Prostaglandin E2) *Labour induction:* 1mg into posterior vagina, may repeat dose 1–2mg after 6h (max. 60μg/kg over 6h). *Maintain PDA:* 25 μg/kg 1 hourly (less often after 1 week) oral; or 0.003–0.01 μg/kg per min i.v.
Dioctyl sodium sulphosuccinate See docusate sodium.
Diphemanil, powder 20mg/g (2%) Apply 8–12 hourly.
Diphenhydramine 1–2mg/kg per dose (max. 100mg) 6–8 hourly oral.
Diphenidol 0.5–1mg/kg per dose (max. 50mg) 4 hourly oral.
Diphenoxylate 2.5mg and atropine 25μg tab (Lomotil) *Adult:* 1–2 tab (NOT/kg) 6–8 hourly oral.
Diphenylmethane See bisacodyl.
Diphenylpyraline *7–12 years:* 2.5mg (NOT/kg) 8 hourly oral. *>12 years:* 2.5–5mg (NOT/kg) 8 hourly oral.
Diphtheria antitoxin (horse) *i.m. or i.v.:* 2500u (nasal), 10 000u (unilateral tonsillar), 20 000u (bilateral tonsillar), 30 000u (laryngeal), 50 000u (beyond tonsillar fossa) i.m. *Bullneck:* 150 000u. Repeat dose may be needed. See also immunoglobulin, diphtheria.
Diphtheria vaccine, adult (CSL) Inactivated. 0.5mL i.m. stat, 6 weeks later, and 6 months later. Boost every 10 years.
Diphtheria vaccine, child (CSL) Inactivated. 0.5mL i.m. stat, 6 weeks later, and 6 months later. Boost with adult vaccine.
Diphtheria + pertussis + tetanus vaccine (Triple Antigen) 0.5mL i.m. at 2 months, 4 months, 6 months, 18 months and 5 years.
Diphtheria + tetanus vaccine, adult (ADT) Inactivated. 0.5 mL i.m. stat, 6 weeks later, and 6 months later. Boost every 10.
Diphtheria + tetanus vaccine, child <8 years (CDT) Inactivated. 0.5mL i.m. stat, 6 weeks later, and 6 months later. Boost with ADT.
Dipivefrin, eye drops 0.1% 1 drop per eye 12 hourly.
Diprophylline Usually 15mg/kg per dose 6 hourly oral or i.m.
Dipyridamole 1–2mg/kg per dose (max. 100mg) 6–8 hourly oral.
Disodium edetate See trisodium edetate.
Disodium pamidronate 0.5–1.5mg/kg per dose (max. 90mg) i.v. over 24h, repeat every 2–3 weeks.
Disopyramide *Oral:* 5mg/kg stat, then 2–5mg/kg per dose (max. 200mg) 6 hourly. *i.v.:* 2mg/kg (max. 150mg) over 5min, then 0.4mg/kg per h (max. 800mg/day). Level 9–15μmol/L (× 0.3395 = μg/mL).
Distigmine *Neurogenic bladder, megacolon:* 0.01mg/kg i.m. daily, 0.1mg/kg oral daily. *Myasthenia gravis:* 0.1–0.2mg/kg per dose 12–24 hourly (max. 20mg daily) oral.
Disulfiram *Adult:* 500mg (NOT/kg) oral daily for 1–2 weeks, then 125–500mg daily.
Divalproex 5–25mg/kg per dose (max. 500mg) 8–12 hourly oral.
Dobutamine 1–20μg/kg per min i.v. See p.35.
Docusate sodium NOT/kg: 100mg (3–10 years), 120–240mg (>10 years)

daily oral. *Enema* (5mL 18% + 155mL water): 30mL (newborn), 60mL (1–12 months), 60–120mL (>12 months) p.r.

Docusate sodium 100mg + bisacodyl 10mg, suppository ½ suppos (<12 months), 1 suppos (>1 years) when required p.r.

Docusate sodium 50mg + sennoside 8mg, tab *>12 years:* 1–4 tab at night oral.

Domperidone *Oral:* 0.2–0.4mg/kg per dose (max. 20mg) 4–8 hourly. *Rectal suppos:* adult 30–60mg (NOT/kg) 4–8 hourly.

Dopamine 1–20µg/kg per min i.v. See p.35.

Dopexamine 0.5–6µg/kg per min i.v. infusion.

Dothiepin 0.5–1.0mg/kg per dose (max. 50mg) 8–12 hourly oral.

Doxacurium 50–80µg/kg stat, then 5–10µg/kg per dose i.v.

Doxapram 5mg/kg i.v. over 1h, then 0.5–1.0mg/kg per h for 1h (max. total dose 400mg).

Doxazosin Usually 0.02–0.1mg/kg (max. 4mg) daily oral.

Doxepin 0.2–2mg/kg per dose (max. 100mg) 8 hourly oral.

Doxorubicin 30mg/m^2 i.v. over 15min weekly, or 30mg/m^2 daily for 2–3days every 3–4 weeks. Max. total dose 480mg/m^2 (300mg/m^2 if mediastinal irradiation).

Doxycycline *Over 8 years:* 2mg/kg per dose (max. 100mg) 12 hourly for 2 doses, then daily.

Doxylamine 0.25–0.5mg/kg per dose (max. 25mg) 8 hourly oral. *Hypnotic:* 0.5–1mg/kg (max. 50mg).

Dronabinol Initially 5mg/m^2 per dose 2–4 hourly (max. 4–6 doses per day) oral, slow increase by 2.5mg/m^2 per dose to max. 15mg/m^2 per dose 4 hourly.

Droperidol *Oral:* 0.1–0.4mg/kg per dose (max. 20mg) 4–8 hourly. *i.m. or slow i.v.:* 0.1–0.15mg/kg per dose (max. 15mg) 4–6 hourly.

Dydrogesterone 0.2mg/kg per dose (max. 10mg) 12–24 hourly oral.

Dyphylline See diprophylline.

Econazole *Topical:* 1% cream, powder or lotion 8–12 hourly. *Vaginal:* 75mg cream or 150mg ovule twice daily.

Ecothiopate, eye drops 0.03%, 0.06%, 0.125%, 0.25% Usually 1 drop 0.125% per eye every 1–2 days nocte.

Edrophonium Test dose 20µg/kg, then 100µg/kg i.v.

EDTA See sodium calciumedetate.

Electrolyte solution See glucose electrolyte solution.

EMLA cream See lignocaine + prilocaine.

Emulsifying ointment Soap substitute or emollient for dry skin.

Enalapril 0.2–1.0mg/kg (max. 40mg) daily oral.

Enalaprilat Usually 0.025mg/kg per dose (max. 1.25mg) 6 hourly i.v., max. 0.1mg/kg per dose (max. 5mg) 6 hourly.

Enoxacin 4–8mg/kg per dose (max. 400mg) 12 hourly oral.

Enoxaparin (1mg = 100u) *Prevent DVT:* 0.4–0.8mg/kg per dose (max. 40mg) 2–12h preop, then daily s.c. *Haemodialysis:* 1mg/kg into arterial line at start 4h session.

Enoximone *i.v.:* 5–20µg/kg per min. *Oral:* 1–3mg/kg per dose (max. 150mg) 8 hourly.

Ephedrine 0.3–1mg/kg per dose (max. 60mg) 6–8 hourly oral. *Nose drops* (0.25%–1%): 1 drop each nostril 6–8 hourly for 3–4 days.

Epinephrine See adrenaline.
Epirubicin *Adult:* 75–90mg/m^2 i.v. over 10min every 3 weeks.
Epoetin See erythropoietin.
Epoprostenol (prostacyclin, PGI2) 0.01μg/kg per min i.v. Pulmonary vasodilation: 0.01μg/kg per min epoprost = 5μg/kg per min nitroglyc = 2μg/kg per min nitropr = 0.1μg/kg per min PGE1.
Epsilon aminocaproic acid See aminocaproic acid.
Ergocalciferol See vitamin D.
Ergoloid mesylates See co-dergocrine mesylate.
Ergometrine maleate *Adult:* 500μg (NOT/kg) i.m. or i.v.; 500μg per dose (NOT/kg) 8 hourly oral, sublingual or p.r.
Ergonovine maleate See ergometrine maleate.
Ergotamine tartrate *>10 years* (NOT/kg): 2mg sublingual stat, then 1mg per h (max. 6mg/episode, 10mg/week). Suppos (1–2mg): 1 stat, may repeat once after 1h.
Erythrityl tetranitrate 0.1–0.2mg/kg per dose 6–8 hourly sublingual, may increase to 0.5mg/kg per dose (max. 25mg) 6 hourly.
Erythromycin 10–25mg/kg per dose (adult 0.25–1g) 6–8 hourly oral or slow i.v. (max. 5mg/kg per h).
Erythropoietin 50u/kg ×3/week, increase to max. 200u/kg ×3/week. *Maintenance:* 150u/kg × 1–2/week.
Esmolol 0.5mg/kg over 1min, then 50μg/kg per min for 4min; if no response repeat 0.5mg/kg and give 50–200 μg/kg per min for up to 48h.
Estazolam 0.02–0.1mg/kg (max. 4mg) at night oral.
Estradiol See oestradiol.
Estramustine 200mg/m^2 per dose 8 hourly oral (avoid milk).
Estrone. See oestrone.
Estropipate *Adult:* 0.625–7.5mg (NOT/kg) daily starting 1st day of menstruation, for 3 of every 4 weeks. *Intravaginal:* 2–4g cream daily.
Ethacrynic acid *i.v.:* 0.5–1mg/kg per dose (max. 50mg) 12–24 hourly. *Oral:* 1–4mg/kg per dose (max. 200mg) 12–24 hourly.
Ethambutol 25mg/kg once daily for 8 weeks, then 15mg/kg daily oral. *Intermittent:* 35mg/kg ×3/week.
Ethamsylate 12.5mg/kg per dose (max. 500mg) 6 hourly oral, i.m., i.v.
Ethchlorvynol 10–20mg/kg (max. 1g) at night oral.
Ethinyloestradiol See desogestrel, ethynodiol, levonorgestrel, norethisterone and oestradiol.
Ethionamide *TB:* 15–20mg/kg (max. 1g) at night oral. *Leprosy:* 5–8mg/kg (max. 375mg) daily.
Ethosuximide 2.5mg/kg per dose 6 hourly oral, increase by 50% each week to max. 10mg/kg per dose (max. 500mg) 6 hourly.
Ethotoin 5mg/kg per dose 6 hourly oral after meal, increase to max. 15mg/kg per dose (max. 750mg) 6 hourly.
Ethylnoradrenaline 0.02–0.04mg/kg i.m. or s.c.
Ethylnorepinephrine See ethylnoradrenaline.
Ethyloestrenol 0.1mg/kg (max. 4mg) daily oral.

Ethynodiol diacetate + ethinyloestradiol (0.5mg/50μg or 1mg/50μg) × 21 tab, + 7 inert tab *Contraception:* 1 tab daily, starting 1st day of menstruation.

Etidocaine, 0.5–1.5% Max. 6mg/kg (0.6mL/kg of 1%) parenteral, or 8mg/kg (0.8mL/kg of 1%) with adrenaline.

Etidronate See sodium etidronate.

Etodolac 4–8mg/kg per dose (max. 400mg) 6–8 hourly oral.

Etomidate 0.3mg/kg slow i.v.

Etoposide 50–60mg/m^2 i.v. over 1h daily for 5 days, repeat after 2–4 weeks. Oral dose 2–3 times i.v. dose.

Etretinate 0.4mg/kg per dose 8–12 hourly oral for 2–4 weeks, then 0.5–1mg/kg (max. 75mg) daily for 6–8 weeks, then reducing to 0.25–0.5mg/kg daily. Teratogenic.

Factor 8 concentrate (vial 200–250u) Joint 20u/kg, psoas 30u/kg, cerebral 50u/kg.

Factor 9 complex (factor 2, 9, 10, and some 7) 40–60iu/kg, then 5–10iu/kg per dose 12 hourly i.v. *Prophylaxis:* 10–20iu/kg × 1–2/week. *Factor 8 antibodies:* 75iu/kg, repeat in 12h p.r.n.

Famotidine 0.5–1.0mg/kg per dose (max. 40mg) 12–24 hourly oral. 0.5mg/kg per dose (max. 20mg) 12 hourly slow i.v.

Fat emulsion 20% 1–3g/kg per day i.v. (mL/h = g/kg per day × wt × 0.21).

Fatty acids (Nandicelle) *Adult:* 1–2cap (NOT/kg) 8–12 hourly.

Felodipine 0.05mg/kg per dose (max. 2.5mg), increase to 0.2 mg/kg per dose (max. 10mg) 12 hourly oral.

Fenbufen 10mg/kg per dose (max. 450mg) 12 hourly oral.

Fenfluramine *Adult:* 60mg (NOT/kg) daily oral.

Fenofibrate 2mg/kg per dose (max. 100mg) 6–12 hourly oral.

Fenoprofen 4mg/kg per dose (max. 200mg) 6–8 hourly oral, may increase gradually to 12mg/kg per dose (max. 800mg).

Fenoterol *Oral:* 0.1mg/kg per dose 6 hourly. *Respiratory solution 1mg/mL:* 0.5mL per dose diluted to 2mL 3–6 hourly (mild), 1.0mL per dose diluted to 2mL 1–2 hourly (moderate), undiluted continuous (severe, in ICU). *Aerosol* (200μg/puff): 1–2 puffs 4–8 hourly.

Fentanyl 1–4μg/kg per dose (max. 200μg) i.m. or i.v.; infuse 2–4μg/kg per h. *Ventilated:* 5–10μg/kg stat or 50μg/kg i.v. over 1h; infuse 5–10μg/kg per h (amp 50μg/mL at 0.1–0.2mL/kg per h).

Ferrous salts Prophylaxis 2mg/kg per day elemental iron oral, treatment 6mg/kg per day elemental iron oral. Fumarate 1mg = 0.33mg iron. Gluconate 1mg = 0.12mg iron; so Fergon (60mg/mL gluconate) prophylaxis 0.3mL/kg daily, treatment 1mL/kg daily oral. Sulphate (dried) 1mg = 0.3mg iron; so Ferro-Gradumet (350mg dried sulphate) prophylaxis 7mg/kg (max. 350mg) daily, treatment 20mg/kg (max. 1050mg) daily oral.

Fibrinolysin 8–10u/mL and desoxyribonuclease 500–667 u/mL, ointment or solution Apply topically 6–24 h.

Filgrastim (granulocyte CSF) *Idiopathic or cyclic neutropaenia:* 5μg/kg daily s.c. or i.v. over 30min. *Congenital neutropaenia:* 12μg/kg daily s.c. or i.v. over 1h. *Marrow transplant:* 20–30μg/kg daily i.v. over 4–24h, reducing if neutrophils $>1 \times 10^9$/L.

Finasteride *Adult:* 5mg (NOT/kg) daily oral.
Flavoxate 2–4mg/kg per dose (max. 400mg) 6–8 hourly oral.
Flecainide 2mg/kg per dose (max. 100mg) 12 hourly oral or i.v. over 30min, may increase over 2 weeks to 5mg/kg per dose (max. 200mg) 12 hourly.
Flosequinan 1–3mg/kg (max. 150mg) daily oral.
Floxuridine (FUDR) 100–300μg/kg per day by constant intra-arterial infusion (400–600μg/kg per day in hepatic artery). Stop if WCC <3500/mm^3 or platelets <100 000/mm^3.
Fluclorolone, cream 0.025% Apply sparingly 12 hourly.
Flucloxacillin 10mg/kg per dose (max. 250mg) 6 hourly oral, i.m. or i.v. *Severe infection:* 25–50mg/kg per dose (max. 2g) i.v. 12 hourly (1st week of life), 8 hourly (2–4 weeks), 4–6 hourly or constant infusion (>4 weeks).
Fluconazole 4mg/kg (max. 200mg) stat, then 2mg/kg (max. 100mg) daily oral or i.v. *Severe infection:* 8mg/kg (max. 400mg) stat, then 4–8mg/kg (max. 200–400mg) daily i.v.
Flucytosine (5–fluorocytosine) 400–1200mg/m^2 per dose (max. 2g) 6 hourly i.v. over 30 min, or oral. Peak level 25–100 μg/mL, trough <20μg/mL (×7.75 = μmol/L).
Fludarabine 25mg/m^2 daily ×5 i.v. over 30min.
Fludrocortisone 0.05–0.2mg (NOT/kg) daily oral. Fludrocortisone 1mg = hydrocortisone 125mg in mineralocorticoid activity, 10mg in glucocorticoid.
Flumazenil 5μg/kg stat i.v., repeat every 60sec to max. total 40μg/kg (max. 2mg), then 2–10μg/kg per h i.v.
Flunarizine *Migraine:* 0.1–0.2mg/kg (max. 10mg) oral daily at night. *Epilepsy:* 0.4mg/kg (max. 20mg) daily at night.
Flunisolide *Asthma* (250μg/puff): 1–2 puffs 12 hourly. *Nasal* (25μg/puff): 1–2 puffs/nostril 8–24 hourly.
Flunitrazepam *Adult:* 0.5–2mg (NOT/kg) at night, oral.
Fluocinolone, cream or ointment 0.025% Apply 8–12 hourly.
Fluocortolone, cream or ointment 0.25% Apply 8–12 hourly.
Fluorescein, eye drops 1%, 2% 1–2 drops per eye.
5-Fluorocytosine See 5–flucytosine.
9-alpha-fluorohydrocortisone See fludrocortisone.
Fluorometholone, eye drops 0.1% 1–2drops/eye 6–12 hourly.
Fluorothiocarbanilide, powder 1% Apply daily.
5-Fluorouracil 15mg/kg (max. 1g) i.v. over 4h daily until side effects, then 5–10mg/kg weekly. See folinic acid.
Fluoxetine 0.5mg/kg (max. 20mg) daily, increase to max. 1.0 mg/kg per dose (max. 40mg) 12 hourly oral.
Fluoxymesterone 0.1–0.2mg/kg (max. 10mg) daily oral.
Flupenthixol *Oral:* 0.05–0.2mg/kg per dose (max. 9mg) 12 hourly. *Depot i.m.:* usually 0.4–0.8mg/kg (up to 5mg/kg, max. 300 mg) every 2–4 weeks (1mg flupenthixol deconate = 0.625mg fluphenazine decanoate = 1.25mg haloperidol).
Fluphenazine 0.02–0.2mg/kg per dose (max. 10mg) 8–12 hourly oral.
Flurazepam *Adult:* 15–30mg (NOT/kg) at night, oral.
Flurbiprofen 1–2mg/kg per dose (max. 100mg) 8 hourly oral or p.r. *Eye drops* 0.03%: 1 drop/eye every 30min.

Fluspirilene *Weekly i.m.:* 0.02mg/kg, increase to 0.05–0.2mg/kg; occasionally 0.4mg/kg (max. 20mg) weekly.
Flutamide *Adult:* 250mg (NOT/kg) 8 hourly oral.
Fluticasone *Inhaled* (NOT/kg): 50–100μg per dose (child), 100–1000μg per dose (adult) 12 hourly. *0.05% solution:* 1–4 sprays /nostril daily.
Fluvoxamine 2mg/kg per dose (max. 100mg) 8–24 hourly oral.
Folic acid *Treatment:* 0.1–0.3mg/kg (max. 15mg) daily i.v., i.m. or oral. *Pregnancy:* 0.2–0.5mg (NOT/kg) daily.
Folinic acid 5–15mg (NOT/kg) oral or 1mg i.m. or i.v. daily. *Rescue starting up to 24h after methotrexate:* 10–15 mg/m^2 per dose 6 hourly for 36–48h i.v. *Methotrexate toxicity:* 100–1000mg/m^2 per dose 6 hourly i.v. Before a fluorouracil dose of 370 mg/m^2: 200mg/m^2 i.v. daily × 5, repeat every 3–4 weeks.
Follicle stimulating hormone (FSH) Initially 75iu (NOT/kg) i.m. daily for 9–12 days (monitor urinary oestrogen and adjust dose).
Fomepizole 10mg/kg stat i.v. over 1h, then 5mg/kg per dose 12 hourly i.v. over 30min for 4 doses.
Formestane *Adult:* 250mg (NOT/kg) 2 weekly deep i.m.
Foscarnet 20mg/kg i.v. over 30min, then 200mg/kg per day by constant i.v. infusion (less if creatinine >0.11mmol/L).
Fosfestrol Adult. *Initial:* 0.5g (NOT/kg) i.v. over 1h day 1, then 1.0g × 5 days. Maintenance: 120–240mg per dose (NOT/kg) 8 hourly oral, later reducing to 120–240mg daily.
Fosinopril 0.2–0.8mg/kg (max. 40mg) daily oral.
Framycetin (Soframycin) *Subconjunctival:* 500mg in 0.5–1mL water daily × 3 days. *Bladder:* 500mg in 50mL saline 8 hourly × 10 days. *Eye/ear* 0.5%: 2–3 drops 8 hourly, ointment 8 hourly.
Framycetin 15mg/g + gramicidin 0.05mg/g, cream or ointment (Soframycin topical) Apply 8–12 hourly.
Framycetin 5mg + gramicidin 0.05mg + dexamethasone 0.5mg/mL eye/ear (Sofradex) 2–3 drops 6–8 hourly, ointment 8–12 hourly.
Fresh frozen plasma Contains all clotting factors. 10–20 mL/kg i.v. 1 bag is about 230mL.
Frusemide Usually 0.5–1.0mg/kg per dose 6–12 hourly (daily if preterm) i.m., i.v. or oral. Up to 5mg/kg per dose in resistant cases. *i.v. infusion:* 0.1–1.0mg/kg per h.
Furazolidone 2mg/kg per dose (max. 100mg) 6 hourly oral 7–10day.
Furosemide See frusemide.
Fusidic acid 10mg/kg per dose (max. 500mg) 8 hourly oral or i.v. over 2–8h. Peak level 30–200μmol/L (× 0.52 = μg/mL).
Gabapentin 5–15mg/kg per dose (max. 800mg) 8–24 hourly oral.
Galactosidase See tilactase.
Gallamine 1–2mg/kg per dose (max. 100mg) i.v.
Gallium nitrate 100–200mg/m^2 per day for 5 days by constant i.v. infusion.
Gamma benzene hexachloride See lindane.
Gamma globulin See immunoglobulin.
Gammahydroxybutyrate 40–100mg/kg i.v. stat (use the high dose for long anaesthetic or children).
Gamolenic acid 2–5mg/kg per dose (max. 240mg) 12 hourly oral.

Ganciclovir 2.5–5mg/kg per dose 8–12 hourly i.v. over 1h.

Gas gangrene (Clostridia) antitoxin *Prophylaxis:* 25 000u i.m. or i.v. *Treatment:* 75 000–150 000u i.v. over 1h, repeat ×1–2 after 8–12h. Give 100 000u i.m. as well for severe infection.

Gaviscon See alginic acid.

Gemeprost (PGE1 analogue) *Cervical dilatation:* 1 pessary (1mg) into posterior vagina 3h before surgery. *Termination:* 1 pessary (1mg) into posterior vagina 3 hourly (max. 5 pessaries).

Gemfibrozil 10mg/kg per dose (max. 600mg) 12 hourly oral.

Gentamicin *Single daily dose i.v. or i.m.:* 2.5mg/kg (<30 weeks gestation), 3.5mg/kg (30–35 weeks gestation), 5mg/kg (1st week of life), 7.5mg/kg (2 + weeks), 6mg/kg (>10 years). Trough level <1.0 mg/L, done Mon–Fri at Royal Children's Hospital.

Gestrinone *Adult:* 2.5mg (NOT/kg) ×2/week on day 1 and 4 of menstrual cycle, then on same days each week.

Gestronol *Adult:* 200–400mg (NOT/kg) every 5–7 days i.m.

Glibenclamide *Adult:* initially 2.5mg (NOT/kg) daily oral, max. 20mg daily.

Gliclazide *Adult:* initially 40mg (NOT/kg) daily oral, max. 160mg 12 hourly.

Glipizide *Adult:* initially 5mg (NOT/kg) daily oral, max. 20mg 12 hourly.

Gliquidone 0.25–1mg/kg per dose (max. 60mg) 8–12 hourly oral.

Glucagon 1u = 1mg. 0.2u/kg (max. 2mg) i.v. or i.m. stat, then 0.005–0.01 u/kg per h i.v.

Glucose See dextrose.

Glucose electrolyte solution *Not dehydrated:* 1 heaped teaspoon sucrose in a large cup of water (4% sucrose = 2% glucose); do NOT add salt. *Dehydrated:* 1 sachet of Gastrolyte in 200mL water; give frequent small sips, or infuse through a nasogastric tube.

Glutamic acid 10–20mg/kg (max. 1g) oral with meals.

Glyburide See glibenclamide.

Glyceryl trinitrate *Adult* (NOT/kg): sublingual tab 0.3–0.9 mg per dose (lasts 30–60min); sublingual aerosol 0.4–0.8 mg per dose; slow-release buccal tab 1–10mg 8–12 hourly; transdermal 0.5–5cm of 2% ointment, or 5–15mg patch 8–12 hourly. *i.v.:* see nitroglycerine.

Glycopyrrolate See glycopyrronium.

Glycopyrronium *To reduce secretions or treat bradycardia:* 4–8µg/kg per dose (max. 400µg) 6–8 hourly i.v. or i.m. *With 0.05mg/kg neostigmine:* 10–15µg/kg i.v. *Anticholinergic:* 0.02–0.04mg/kg per dose (max. 2mg) 8 hourly oral.

GM-CSF See sargramostim.

Gold sodium thiomalate See sodium aurothiomalate.

Gonadorelin (GnR hourly or LHRH) 100µg per dose (NOT/kg) i.v. See also leuprorelin.

Gonadotrophin See chorionic g, and menotrophin.

Goserelin *Adult:* 3.6mg (NOT/kg) s.c. every 28 days.

Gramicidin 25µg/mL + neomycin 2.5mg/mL + polymyxin B 5000u/mL (Neosporin) *Eye drops:* 1–2 drops/eye every 15–30min, reducing to 6–12 hourly.

Granisetron. 0.05mg/kg (max. 3mg) i.v. over 10min; up to 3 doses/day, with at least 10min between doses.

Granulocyte–macrophage colony stimulating factor (GM–CSF) See sargramostim.

Griseofulvin 10–20mg/kg (max. 1g) daily oral.

Griseofulvin (ultramicrosize) 5.5mg/kg (max. 330mg) daily oral.

Growth hormone See somatropin.

Guanabenz 0.1mg/kg per dose (max. 4mg) 12 hourly oral, increase to max. 0.6mg/kg per dose (max. 32mg) 12 hourly.

Guanadrel 0.1mg/kg per dose (max. 5mg) 12 hourly oral, increase to max. 0.5mg/kg per dose (max. 25mg) 8–12 hourly.

Guanethidene 0.2mg/kg (max. 10mg) daily oral, increase to 0.5–6mg/kg (max. 300mg) daily. *Regnl symp block* (adult): cuff 55mmHg >syst BP, 10–20mg in 10–25mL saline (arm) or 15–30mg in 15–50mL (leg) i.v., wait 10–20min, release cuff over 5min; > = 7 days between injections (max. 12 per year).

Guanfacine 0.02mg/kg (max. 1mg) daily oral, increase over several weeks to max. 0.06mg/kg (max. 3mg) daily.

Haemaccel 10–20mL/kg (may be repeated). Half life 2h.

Haemophilus influenzae type b, vaccines Inactivated. *<12 months:* give diphtheria protein conjugate (HibTITER), or tetanus protein conjugate (Act-HIB) 0.5mL i.m. at 2mo, 4mo, 6 months and 15mo; meningococcal conjugate (Pedvax HIB) 0.5mL i.m. at 2mo, 4mo and 15mo. *If 1st dose >18months:* give one dose of HibTITER or Pedvax HIB.

Halcinonide, cream 0.1% Apply sparingly 8–12 hourly.

Halofantrine 10mg/kg per dose (max. 500mg) 6 hourly for 3 doses oral, repeat after 1 week if nonimmune.

Haloperidol 0.01mg/kg (max. 0.5mg) daily, increase up to 0.1 mg/kg per dose 12 hourly i.v. or oral; up to 2mg/kg per dose (max. 100mg) 12 hourly used rarely. *Long-acting decanoate ester:* 1–6mg/kg i.m. every 4 weeks.

Hemin 1–3mg/kg per dose 12–24 hourly i.v. over 30min.

Heparin 1mg = 100u. *Low dose:* 75u/kg i.v. stat, then 10–15u/kg per h i.v. (500u/kg in 50mL at 1mL/h = 10u/kg per h). *Full dose:* 200u/kg stat, then 15–30u/kg per h. *Extracorporeal circuits:* 10–20u/kg per h prefilter, 2–5u/kg per h postfilter.

Heparin calcium *Low dose:* 75u/kg per dose s.c. 12 hourly.

Heparin, low molecular weight *Venous thrombosis:* 100u/kg per dose 12 hourly s.c., or 100u/kg i.v. over 12h. *Haemodialysis:* 5–10u/kg stat, then 4–5u/kg per h i.v. (acute renal failure, anti-Xa 0.2–0.4u/mL); 30–40u/kg stat, then 10–15u/kg per h (chronic renal failure, anti-Xa 0.5–1.0u/mL).

Hepatitis A vaccine (Havrix) Inactivated. 1mL i.m. stat, after 1mo, and after 12 months (3 doses).

Hepatitis B vaccine (Engerix–B, HB Vax II) Inactivated. Engerix-B 10μg per dose (<10 years), 20μg (>9 years); HB Vax II 2.5μg per dose (<10 years), 5μg (10–19 years), 10μg (>19 years), 40μg (dialysis) i.m. stat, after 1mo, and after 6 months (3 doses). Boost every 5 years approx.

Hetastarch, 6% 10–20mL/kg i.v.

Hexamine mandelate 15mg/kg per dose (max. 1g) 6 hourly oral.

Hexetidine *0.1% solution:* rinse/gargle 15mL (NOT/kg) 8–12 hourly.

Histrelin Usually 10μg/kg daily s.c.
Homatropine, eye drops 2% 1–2 drops 4 hourly.
Human chorionic gonadotrophin (HCG) See chorionic gonadotrophin.
Hyaluronidase *Hypodermoclysis:* add 1–1.5u/mL fluid. *Local anaesthesia:* add 50u/mL solution.
Hydralazine 0.1–0.2mg/kg (max. 10mg) stat i.v. or i.m., then 4–6μg/kg per min (max. 300μg/min) i.v. *Oral:* 0.2mg/kg per dose 12 hourly, slow increase to 1mg/kg per dose (usual max. 50mg).
Hydrochloric acid Use solution of 150mmol/L, give i.v. by central line only. Dose(mL) = BE × wt × 2.2 (give ½ this). Maximum rate = 1.33mL/kg per h.
Hydrochlorothiazide 1mg/kg per dose (max. 50mg) 12–24 hourly oral.
Hydrocodone 0.1–0.2mg/kg per dose (max. 10mg) 4–6 hourly oral.
Hydrocortisone *Cream or ointment* 0.1%, 0.5%, 1%: apply 8–24 hourly. *Eye drops* 0.5%, 1%: 1–2 drops/eye 2–4 hourly.
Hydrocortisone acetate *Cream or ointment* 0.5%: apply 6–12 hourly. *Rectal foam* 10%: 125mg per dose (Colifoam). Usually 125mg 12–24 hourly for 2–3 weeks, then 48 hourly.
Hydrocortisone 1% + clioquinol 3%, cream Apply 8–24 hourly.
Hydrocortisone sodium succinate 2–4mg/kg per dose 3–6 hourly i.m. or i.v. *Physiological:* 0.2 mg/kg per dose 8 hourly i.m. or i.v.
Hydroflumethiazide 0.5–2mg/kg per dose (max. 100mg) 12–48 hourly oral.
Hydrogen peroxide 10 volume (3%) Mouthwash 1:2 parts water. Skin or ear disinfectant 1:1 part water.
Hydromorphone See dihydromorphinone.
Hydrotalcite 20mg/kg per dose 6 hourly oral.
Hydroxocobalamin (Vit B12) 20μg/kg per dose i.m. daily for 7 days then weekly (treatment), monthly (prophylaxis). i.v. dangerous in megaloblastic anaemia.
Hydroxyapatite 20–40mg/kg per dose 8 hourly oral before meals.
Hydroxychloroquine 10mg/kg daily for 3 days oral. *Prophylaxis:* 5mg/kg (max. 300mg) once a week oral.
Hydroxyethylcellulose, eye drops 0.44% 1–2 drops per eye 6–8 hourly.
Hydroxyprogesterone *Adult:* 250–500mg/week (NOT/kg) i.m.
Hydroxyurea 20–30mg/kg daily oral.
Hydroxyzine 0.5–2.0mg/kg per dose (max. 100mg) 6–8 hourly oral.
Hyoscine 0.01mg/kg per dose (max. 0.6mg) 6 hourly, i.m. or i.v.
Hyoscine hydrobromide NOT/kg: 0.25 tab (2–7 years), 0.5 tab (7–12 years), 1–2 tab (>12 years) 6–24 hourly oral.
Hyoscine N–butylbromide 0.5mg/kg per dose (max. 40mg) 6–8 hourly i.v., i.m. or oral.
Hyoscine transdermal 1.5 mg *>10 years:* 1 patch every 72h.
Hyoscyamine (L–atropine) 2–5μg/kg per dose (max. 300 μg) 4–6 hourly oral, sublingual, i.m. or i.v.
Hypromellose, eye drops 0.5% 2–3 drops per eye p.r.n.
Hypromellose 0.3% + dextran 70 0.1%, eye drops 1–2 drops per eye p.r.n.
Ibuprofen 2.5–10mg/kg per dose (max. 600mg) 6–8 hourly oral.

Idarubicin 12 mg/m^2 i.v. over 15min daily for 3 days.
Idoxuridine *Eye drops* 0.1%: 1–2 drops every 15min for 2h, then hourly by day and 2 hourly at night. 0.1% solution or 0.5% ointment: apply hourly first 24h, then 4 hourly.
Ifosfamide Usually 1.2–2.0g/m^2 i.v. over 4h daily ×5, or 5–6g/m^2 (max. 10g) i.v. over 24h once. Repeat every 2–4 weeks.
Imipenem/cilastatin 10mg/kg per dose (max. 500mg) 6 hourly i.v. over 30min. *Severe infection:* 25mg/kg per dose i.v. over 1h (max. 1g) 12 hourly (1st week of life), 8 hourly (2–4 weeks), 6–8 hourly or constant infusion (4 + weeks).
Imipramine 0.5–1.5mg/kg per dose (max. 75mg) 8 hourly oral. *Enuresis:* 5–6 years 25mg, 7–10 years 50mg, >10 years 50–75mg nocte.
Immunoglobulin See also antivenoms.
Immunoglobulin, CMV 100–200mg/kg i.v. over 2h. *Transplant:* daily for first 3 days, weekly ×6, monthly ×6.
Immunoglobulin, diphtheria 250u i.m. once.
Immunoglobulin, hepatitis B 400u i.m. within 5 days of needle stick, repeat in 30 days; 100u i.m. within 24h birth to baby of Hep B carrier.
Immunoglobulin, lymphocyte (anti–thymocyte immunoglobulin, equine; Atgam) 10mg/kg daily for 3–5 days i.v. over 4h in saline.
Immunoglobulin, normal, human *Hypogammaglobulinaemia:* 10–15mL/kg of 6% solution (600–900mg/kg) i.v. over 4h, then 5–7.5 mL/kg (300–450mg/kg) monthly; or 0.6mL/kg of 16% solution (100mg/kg) every 2–4 weeks i.m. *Kawasaki, Guillain-Barre, ITP, myasth gravis, Still's dis:* 35mL/kg of 6% solution (2g/kg) i.v. over 10h stat, then if required 15 mL/kg (900mg/kg) i.v. over 4h each month. *Prevention hepatitis A:* 0.1mL/kg (16mg/kg) i.m. *Prevention measles:* 0.2mL/kg (32mg/kg) i.m. (repeat next day if immunocompromised).
Immunoglobulin, rabies (Hyperab, Imogam) 20iu (0.133mL)/kg i.m. once (½ infiltrated around wound), with rabies vaccine.
Immunoglobulin, Rh 1mL (625iu, 125μg) i.m. within 72h of exposure. *Large transfusion:* 0.16mL (100iu, 20μg) per mL RH positive red cells (maternal serum should be anti–D positive 24–48h after injection).
Immunoglobulin, tetanus (intramuscular, TIG) 250–500iu (1–2amp) i.m.
Immunoglobulin, tetanus (intravenous) 4000iu (100mL) given i.v. at 0.04mL/kg per min for 30min, then 0.075 mL/kg per min.
Immunoglobulin, vaccinia (16%) *To prevent vaccine complications* (NOT/kg): 4mL (<6 months), 8mL (6 months–14 years), 12mL (>14 years); double dose to treat complications.
Immunoglobulin, Zoster Prevention of chickenpox in immunocompromised, 0.4–1.2mL/kg (max. 6mL) i.m.
Indapamide *Adult:* 2.5mg (NOT/kg) daily oral.
Indomethacin *PDA:* 0.1mg/kg daily for 6 days oral or i.v. in saline over 1h (0.13mg/kg daily if >14 days old). *Arthritis:* 0.25–1mg/kg per dose (max. 50mg) 6–8 hourly oral or p.r.
Indoramin 0.5–1.5mg/kg per dose (max. 75mg) 8–12 hourly oral.
Influenza A and B vaccine (Fluvax, Vaxigrip) Inactivated. 0.125mL (<2 years), 0.25mL (2–6 years), 0.5mL (>6 years) s.c. stat and 4 weeks later (2 doses). Boost annually (1 dose).

Inosine pranobex *Herpes:* 20mg/kg per dose (max. 1g) 6–8 hourly oral. *SSPE:* 10–15mg/kg per dose 4 hourly oral.
Inosiplex See inosine pranobex.
Inositol nicotinate 20mg/kg per dose (max. 1g) 6–8 hourly oral.
Insulin *Regular insulin:* 0.05–0.2u/kg prn, or 0.1u/kg per h; later 1u/10g dextrose i.v. *Hyperkalaemia:* 0.1u/kg insulin and 2mL/kg 50% dextrose i.v. In *TPN:* 5–25u/250g dextrose. *s.c.:* regular insulin onset 30–60min, peak 4h, duration 6–8h; isophane (NPH) insulin onset 2–4h, peak 4–12h, duration 18–24h; zinc (Lente) insulin onset 2–3h, peak 7–15h, duration 24h; crystalline zinc (Ultralente) insulin onset 4–6h, peak 10–30h, duration 24–36h; protamine zinc insulin onset 4–8h, peak 15–20h, duration 24–36h.
Interferon alfa-2a, recombinant 1 700 000u/m^2 (max. 3 000 000u) s.c. or i.m. daily for 16–24 weeks, then × 3/week.
Interferon alfa-2b, recombinant *Leukaemia:* 2 000 000 u/m^2 s.c. × 3/week. *Condylomata:* 1 000 000u into each lesion (max. 5) × 3/week for 5weeks.
Interferon alpha-n3 *Adult:* 250 000u injected into base of wart (max. 10 doses per session) × 2/week for max. 8 weeks.
Interferon gamma-1b 1.5µg/kg per dose (body area $<=$ 0.5m^2) or 50µg/m^2 (area >0.5m^2) × 3/week s.c.
Interleukin-2 *Malignancy:* constant i.v. infusion less toxic than bolus injtn: 3 000 000–5 000 000u/m^2 per day for 5 days, repeat × 1–2 if tolerated (5 days between courses).
Ipecacuanha syrup 1–2mL/kg (max. 30mL) stat oral, NG.
Ipratropium *Respiratory solution* (250µg/mL): 0.25–1.0mL diluted to 4mL 4–6 hourly. *Aerosol* 20µg/puff: 2–4 puffs 6–8 hourly.
Iprindole 0.3–1mg/kg per dose (max. 60mg) 8 hourly oral.
Iron See ferrous gluconate, ferrous sulphate.
Iron dextran *Fe* 50mg/mL: dose (mL) = 0.05 × wt in kg × (15 – Hb in g%) i.m., i.v. infusion dangerous.
Isocarboxazid *Adult:* 30mg (NOT/kg) daily oral (may increase to 60mg/day after 4 weeks), reducing to 10–40mg daily.
Isoconazole *Topical:* 1% cream 12 hourly. *Vaginal:* 600mg (2 tab) once.
Isoetharine *Inhalation solution* (1%): 0.5mL diluted to 4mL 3–6 hourly (mild), 1.0mL diluted to 4mL 1–2 hourly (moderate), undiluted constant (severe, in ICU). *Aerosol* 340µg/puff: 1–2 puffs 4–6 hourly.
Isoniazid 5–10mg/kg (max. 300mg) daily oral. *TB meningitis:* 15–20mg/kg (max. 500mg) daily oral.
Isoprenaline 0.1–2.0µg/kg per min. *<33kg:* 0.3mg/kg in 50mL at 1mL/h = 0.1µg/kg per min. *>33kg:* 0.1µg/kg per min using 1/5000 (0.2 mg/mL) solution = 0.03 × wt mL/h. *Aerosol* 80–400µg/puff: 1–3puffs 4–8 hourly.
Isoproterenol See isoprenaline.
Isosorbide dinitrate *Sublingual:* 0.1–0.2mg/kg per dose (max. 10mg) 2 hourly or as needed. *Oral:* 0.5–1.0mg/kg per dose (max. 40mg) 6 hourly or as needed. *Sustained release tab:* adults 1–2 tab (NOT/kg) daily.
Isotretinoin *Adult:* 0.5–1.0mg/kg daily oral for 2–4 weeks, reducing if possible to 0.1–0.2mg/kg daily for 15–20 weeks. *Gel 0.05%:* apply sparingly at night.
Isoxsuprine 0.2–0.5mg/kg per dose (max. 20mg) 6–12 hourly oral.

Ispaghula husk *Adult:* 1–2 teaspoonfuls (NOT/kg) 6–12 hourly oral. Half this dose in child.
Isradipine 0.05mg/kg per dose 12 hourly oral, may increase after 2–4 weeks gradually to 0.1–0.2mg/kg per dose (max. 10mg) 12 hourly.
Itraconazole 2–4mg/kg per dose (max. 200mg) 12–24 hourly oral after food.
Ivermectin 0.15–0.2mg/kg (max. 12mg) oral every 6–12 months.
Josamycin 10–15mg/kg per dose (max. 750mg) 8–12 hourly oral.
Kanamycin *Single daily dose i.v. or i.m.:* 7.5mg/kg (<30 weeks gestation), 10mg/kg (30–35 weeks gestation), 15mg/kg (1st week of life), 22.5mg/kg (2 + weeks), 18mg/kg (>10 years). Trough <5mg/L.
Ketamine 1–2mg/kg i.v., 5–10mg/kg i.m. *Infusion:* anaesthesia 10–20μg/kg per min, analgesia 4μg/kg per min.
Ketoconazole 3–5mg/kg per dose (max. 400mg) 12–24 hourly oral. *Cream* 2%: apply 12–24 hourly. *Shampoo* 2%: wash hair, apply liquid for 5min, wash off.
Ketoprofen 0.5–2mg/kg per dose (max. 50–100mg) 8–12 hourly oral, p.r. *Slow release (adults):* 200mg (NOT/kg) daily.
Ketorolac *Oral:* 0.2mg/kg per dose (max. 10mg) 4–6 hourly (max. 0.8mg/kg per day or 40mg/day). *i.m.:* 0.6mg/kg (max. 30mg) stat, then 0.2–0.4mg/kg per dose (max. 20mg) 4–6 hourly for 5 days, then 0.2mg/kg per dose (max. 10mg) 6 hourly.
Ketotifen *Child >2 years:* 1mg per dose (NOT/kg) 12 hourly oral with food. *Adult:* 1–2mg per dose (NOT/kg) 12 hourly oral with food.
Labetalol 1–2mg/kg per dose (max. 100mg) 12 hourly oral, may increase weekly to max. 10mg/kg per dose (max. 600mg) 6 hourly.
Lacidipine 0.04–0.12mg/kg (max. 6mg) daily oral with food.
Lactulose 50% (Duphalac) *Laxative:* 0.5mL/kg per dose 12–24 hourly oral. *Hepatic coma:* 1mL/kg per dose hourly until bowel cleared, then 6–8 hourly.
Lamotrigine 0.5mg/kg oral daily for 2 weeks, then 1mg/kg daily 2 weeks, then 1–4mg/kg per dose (max. 200mg) 12 hourly (double dose if taking carbamazepine, phenobarbitone, phenytoin or primidone; halve dose if taking valproate).
L-asparaginase See colaspase.
Latamoxef (Moxalactam) 25–50mg/kg per dose (max. 2g) 4–6 hourly i.v., i.m.
Lenograstim (rHuG–CSF, Granocyte) 150μg/m^2 daily s.c. or i.v. over 30min. Keep WCC 5 000–10 000/mm^3.
Leucovorin See folinic acid.
Leuprolide See leuprorelin.
Leuprorelin (GnR hourly or LHRH) *Adult:* 7.5 mg (NOT/kg) depot injection monthly i.m.
Levamisole *Anthelmintic:* 3mg/kg (max. 150mg) oral once (ascaris), repeat in 1 week (hookworm). Adenocarcinoma colon (with 5-fluorouracil 450mg/m^2 i.v. weekly): 1mg/kg (max. 50mg) 8 hourly oral for 3 days every 2 weeks.
Levobunolol *0.5% solution:* 1drop/eye 12–24 hourly.
Levocarnitine See carnitine.
Levodopa and benserazide (4:1) *Adult:* initially levodopa 100mg per dose (NOT/kg) 8 hourly oral; if not controlled, increase weekly by 100mg/day to max. 250mg per dose (NOT/kg) 6 hourly.

Levodopa and carbidopa (250mg/25mg and 100mg/10mg tabs) *Adult* (NOT/kg): initially one 100/10 tab 8 hourly oral; if not controlled, substitute one 250/25 tab for one 100/25 tab every 2nd day; if not controlled on 250/25 8 hourly, increase by one 250/25 tab every 2nd day to max. 6–8 tab/day.

Levonorgestrel. *Contraception:* 30μg daily oral, starting 1st day of menstruation.

Levonorgestrel + ethinyloestradiol (150μg/30μg or 125μg/ 50μg) × 21 tab, + 7 inert tab *Contraception:* 1 tab daily, starting 1st day of menstruation.

Levorphanol 0.03–0.1mg/kg per dose 12–24 hourly oral or s.c.

Levothyroxine sodium See thyroxine.

Lidocaine See lignocaine.

Lignocaine *i.v.:* 1mg/kg stat (0.1mL/kg of 1%), then 15–50μg/kg per min (see p.35). *Nerve block:* without adrenaline max. 4mg/kg (0.4mL/kg of 1%), with adrenaline 7mg/kg (0.7mL/kg of 1%). *Topical spray:* max. 3–4mg/kg (Xylocaine 10% spray pack: about 10mg/puff). Topical gel 2%, solution 2% and 4%, ointment 5%, dental ointment 10%: apply p.r.n.

Lignocaine 2.5% compound, mouth paint/gel (SM–33) Apply 3 hourly p.r.n.

Lignocaine 2.5% + prilocaine 2.5%, cream (EMLA) 1.5g/10cm^2 under occlusive dressing for 1–3h.

Lincomycin 10mg/kg per dose (max. 600mg) 8 hourly oral, i.m. or i.v. over 1h. *Severe infection:* up to 20mg/kg per dose (max. 1.2g) i.v. over 2h 6 hourly.

Lindane, cream or lotion 1% *Scabies:* apply from neck down, wash off after 8–12h. *Lice:* rub into hair for 4min, then wash off; repeat after 24h (max. × 2/week).

Linoleic acid See fatty acids.

Liothyronine (T3) *Oral:* 0.2μg/kg per dose (max. 10μg) 8 hourly, may increase to 0.4μg/kg per dose (max. 20μg) 8 hourly. *i.v.:* 0.1–0.4μg/kg per dose (max. 20μg) 8–12 hourly.

Liotrix Liothyronine (T3) plus thyroxine (T4) mixture.

Lipid emulsion 20% 1–3g/kg per day i.v. (mL/h = g/kg per day × wt × 0.21).

Lipolytic enzymes See pancreatic enzymes.

Lisinopril 0.1mg/kg daily oral, may increase over 4–6 weeks to 0.2–0.4mg/kg (max. 20mg) daily.

Lithium carbonate 5–20mg/kg per dose 12–24 hourly to maintain trough serum level 0.8–1.6mmol/L (>2mmol/L toxic).

Lodoxamide *0.1% solution:* 1–2drops/eye 6 hourly.

Lofepramide *Adult* (NOT/kg): 70mg morning, 70–140mg night oral.

Lofexidine 2–8μg/kg per dose (max. 400μg) 6–12 hourly oral.

Lomefloxacin 8mg/kg (max. 400mg) daily oral.

Lomustine (CCNU) 100–130mg/m^2 oral every 6 weeks.

Loperamide 0.05–0.1mg/kg per dose (max. 2mg) 8–12 hourly oral.

Loracarbef 4–8mg/kg (max. 400mg) 12 hourly oral.

Loratadine 0.2mg/kg (max. 10mg) daily oral.

Lorazepam *Acute:* 0.05–0.2mg/kg (max. 10mg) i.v. over 2min. *Chronic:* 0.02–0.06mg/kg per dose 8–24 hourly oral.

Lovastatin 0.4–0.8mg/kg per dose (max. 40mg) 12–24 hourly oral.

Loxapine 0.2–1mg/kg per dose (max. 60mg) 6–12 hourly oral or i.m.
Lymecycline 408mg = 300mg tetracycline base.
Lymphocyte immune globulin See immunoglobulin, lymphocyte immune.
Lypressin (lysine-8-vasopressin) 1 spray (2.5iu) into 1 nostril 4–8 hourly, may increase to 1 spray both nostrils 4–8 hourly.
Lysuride *Migraine:* 0.5μg/kg per dose (max. 25μg) 8 hourly oral. *Parkinson's, adults* (NOT/kg): 0.2mg daily, increase by 0.2 mg daily each week to max. 1.6mg per dose 8 hourly oral.
Magaldrate 5–30mg/kg per dose (max. 1.6g) 6 hourly oral.
Magnesium chloride 0.48g/5mL (1mmol/mL Mg). 0.4mmol (0.4mL)/kg per dose 12 hourly slow i.v. *Myoc infarct* (NOT/kg): 5mmol per h i.v. for 6h, then 1mmol per h for 24–48h.
Magnesium hydroxide *Antacid:* 10–40mg/kg per dose (max. 2g) 6 hourly oral. *Laxative:* 50–100mg/kg (max. 5g) oral.
Magnesium sulphate *Deficiency:* 50% mag sulph (2 mmol/mL) 0.2mL/kg per dose (max. 10mL) 12 hourly i.m., slow i.v. *Myoc infarct* (NOT/kg): 5mmol per h i.v. for 6h, then 1.0 mmol per h for 24–48h. *Digoxin tachyarrhythmia:* 50% mag sulph 0.1 mL/kg (max. 5mL) i.v. over 10min, then infuse 0.4mL/kg (max. 20mL) over 6h, then 0.8mL/kg (max. 40mL) over 18h (keep serum Mg 1.5–2.0 mmol/L). *Pul ht newborn:* aim for 3–4mmol/l. *Laxative:* 0.5g/kg per dose (max. 15g) as 10% solution 8 hourly for 2 days oral. *Asthma:* 25mg/kg (max. 1.2g) i.v. over 30min once.
Malathion See maldison.
Maldison, liquid 0.5% 20mL to hair, wash off after 12h.
Mannitol 0.25–0.5g/kg per dose i.v. (2–4mL/kg of 12.5%, 1.25–2.5mL/kg of 20%, 1–2mL/kg of 25%) 2 hourly prn, provided serum osmolality < 330mmol/L.
Maprotiline 0.15–1mg/kg per dose (max. 50mg) 8–24 hourly oral.
Mazindol. *Adult:* 0.5mg (NOT/kg) daily oral, may increase to 1–3mg daily.
Measles accine (Attenuvax) Live. *>12 months:* 0.5mL s.c. once.
Measles + mumps vaccine (Rimparix) Live. *>12 months:* 0.5mL s.c. once.
Measles + mumps + rubella vaccine (MMRII) Live. *>12 months:* 0.5mL s.c.
Mebendazole 100mg per dose (NOT/kg) 12 hourly ×3 days. *Enterobiasis:* 100mg once (NOT/kg), repeat after 2–4 weeks.
Mebeverine (135mg tab) *Adult:* 1–3 tab (NOT/kg) daily oral.
Mebhydrolin 1–2mg/kg per dose (max. 100mg) 8–12 hourly oral.
Mecamylamine 0.05mg/kg per dose (max. 2.5mg) 12 hourly oral; may increase to max. 0.5mg/kg per dose (max. 25mg) 6 hourly oral.
Mechlorethamine See mustine HCl.
Meclizine See meclozine.
Meclocycline sulfosalicylate, 1% cream Apply 12 hourly.
Meclofenamate 1–2mg/kg per dose (max. 100mg) 6–8 hourly oral.
Meclozine 0.5–1.0mg/kg per dose (max. 50mg) 12–24 hourly oral.
Medazepam 0.05–0.2mg/kg per dose (max. 10mg) 6–8 hourly oral.
Medroxyprogesterone *Adult* (NOT/kg): 5mg daily for 5–10 days per month oral; malignancy 0.5g daily i.m. or oral for 4 weeks, then 1g weekly.

Medroxyprogesterone (MP) + conjugated oestrogens (CO) *MP* (NOT/kg): 10mg (up to 20mg) daily oral for last 10–14 days of 28 day cycle. *CO* (NOT/kg): 0.625mg (0.3–1.25mg) daily continuously.
Medroxyprogesterone 10mg tab + oestradiol 4mg patch NOT/kg: 10mg tab daily oral for first 10–14 days of each 28 day cycle, and 4mg patch × 2/week continuously.
Medrysone, eye drops 1% 1 drop/eye 6–12 hourly.
Mefenamic acid 10mg/kg per dose (max. 500mg) 8 hourly oral.
Mefloquine 15mg/kg (max. 750mg) stat, then 10mg/kg (max. 500mg) after 6–8h. *Prophylaxis:* 5mg/kg (max. 250mg) once a week.
Mefruside 0.5–1mg/kg (up to 2mg/kg for 3 days) daily for 10–14 days, then 0.5–1mg/kg (max. 50mg) every 2–3 days.
Megestrol acetate 80mg per dose (NOT/kg) 12 hourly oral.
Melphalan Typically 6mg/m^2 daily for 4–6days, repeat every 6 weeks.
Menadione, menadiol See menaphthone sod bisulphate.
Menaphthone sodium bisulphate 0.6mg/kg (max. 30mg) daily oral.
Meningococcus gp A, C, W135 and Y vaccine (Mencevax ACWY) Inactivated. *>2 years:* 0.5mL s.c. Boost 1–3 yearly.
Menotrophin (FSH + LH activity) *Females:* 75 + 75iu or 150 + 150iu (NOT/kg) i.m. daily for 9–12 days until oestrogen levels rise, then give HCG. *Males:* 75 + 75iu (NOT/kg) i.m. × 2–3/week with HCG 7000iu i.m. × 2/week.
Mepacrine *Giardia:* 2mg/kg per dose (max. 100mg) 8 hourly oral 5–7 days.
Mepenzolate 0.5–1mg/kg per dose (max. 50mg) 6–8 hourly oral.
Meperidine See pethidine.
Mephenytoin See methoin.
Mephobarbital See methylphenobarbitone.
Mepivacaine Max. dose 5–7mg/kg.
Meprobamate 5–10mg/kg per dose (max. 800mg) 8–12 hourly oral.
Meptazinol 4mg/kg per dose (max. 200mg) 3–6 hourly oral.
Mepyramine 2–4mg/kg per dose (max. 200mg) 8 hourly oral.
Mequitazine 0.1mg/kg per dose (max. 5mg) 12 hourly oral.
Mercaptopurine (6MP) 75–100mg/m^2 daily oral
Mesalamine See mesalazine.
Mesalazine Initially 15–30mg/kg per dose (max. 1.6g) 8 hourly oral, reducing to 10–15mg/kg per dose (max. 750mg) 8 hourly. *Suppos:* 5–10mg/kg (max. 500mg) 8 hourly. *Enema:* 20mg/kg (max. 1g) nocte.
Mesna 20% (up to 40%) of the cyclophosphamide or ifosfamide dose i.v. over 30min 4 hourly for 3 doses (at 0, 4 and 8 h). *Nebuliser:* 0.6–1.2g per dose (NOT/kg) 4–6 hourly.
Mesoridazine 0.25–3mg/kg per dose (max. 150mg) 8 hourly oral. 0.5mg/kg per dose (max. 75mg) 8 hourly i.m.
Mesterolone 0.5mg/kg per dose (max. 25mg) 6–12 hourly oral.
Mestranol See norethisterone.
Metaproterenol See orciprenaline.
Metaraminol *i.v.:* 0.01mg/kg stat (repeat prn), then 0.1–1.0 μg/kg per min and titrate dose against BP. *s.c.:* 0.1mg/kg.
Metaxalone 15mg/kg per dose (max. 800mg) 6–8 hourly oral.

Metformin *Adult:* initially 500mg (NOT/kg) 8–24 hourly oral, max. 1g per dose 8 hourly.
Methacycline *Over 8 years:* 150mg (NOT/kg) 12 hourly oral. *Adult:* 300mg (NOT/kg) 12 hourly oral.
Methadone Usually 0.1–0.2mg/kg per dose (max. 10mg) 6–12 hourly oral, s.c. or i.m.
Methamphetamine See methylamphetamine.
Methazolamide 1–2mg/kg per dose (max. 100mg) 8–12 hourly oral.
Methdilazine 0.1–0.3mg/kg per dose (max. 16mg) 12–24 hourly oral.
Methenamine mandelate See hexamine mandelate.
Methicillin 20–50mg/kg per dose (max. 2g) 4–6 hourly i.v. or i.m.
Methimazole 0.3–1mg/kg (max. 60mg) daily oral, reducing when euthyroid to 0.1–0.5mg/kg (max. 30mg) daily.
Methionine 50mg/kg per dose (max. 2.5g) oral 4 hourly for 4 doses.
Methixene 0.05–0.4mg/kg per dose (max. 20mg) 8 hourly oral.
Methocarbamol *Oral:* 30mg/kg per dose (max. 1.5g) 6 hourly for 3 days, then 15–20mg/kg per dose (max. 1g) 6–8 hourly. *i.v. over 5–10 min or i.m.:* 15 mg/kg per dose (max. 750mg) 6 hourly.
Methohexital See methohexitone.
Methohexitone 1.5–2.0mg/kg per dose (max. 120mg) slow i.v.
Methoin. 1mg/kg daily oral, may increase by 1mg/kg each week to max. 10mg/kg (max. 600mg) daily.
Methoserpidine 0.2–0.4mg/kg per dose (max. 20mg) 8 hourly oral.
Methotrexate *Leukaemia:* typically 3.3mg/m^2 i.v. daily for 4–6 weeks; then 2.5mg/kg i.v. every 2 weeks, or 30mg/m^2 oral or i.m. ×2/week; much higher doses with folinic acid rescue. *Intrathecal:* 12 mg/m^2 weekly for 2 weeks, then monthly. *Adult psoriasis:* 0.2–0.5mg/kg weekly oral, i.v. or i.m. until response, then reduce.
Methotrimeprazine *Psychosis:* 0.5–4mg/kg (max. 200mg) daily oral. *Pain:* 0.25–1mg/kg per dose (max. 50mg) 4–8 hourly.
Methoxamine 0.1–0.4mg/kg (max. 20mg) i.m., or 0.1–0.2 mg/kg (max. 10mg) i.v. over 5–10min (at least 15min between doses). *Nose drop* 0.25%: 1–3drop/nostril 6–12 hourly.
Methoxsalen *Adult:* 20mg (NOT/kg) 2h before UV exposure. *Lotion* 1%: weekly before 1min of UV light.
Methscopolamine See hyoscine.
Methsuximide 5mg/kg daily, may increase to max. 10mg/kg per dose (max. 400mg) 8–12 hourly oral.
Methyclothiazide 0.05–0.2mg/kg (max. 10mg) daily oral.
Methylamphetamine *>5 years* (NOT/kg): 2.5–5.0mg per dose 12–24 hourly oral, increase to about 10–15mg per dose 12 hourly.
Methylcellulose *Constipation:* 30–60mg/kg per dose (max. 3g) with at least 300mL fluid 12 hourly oral.
Methylcysteine 4mg/kg per dose (max. 200mg) 6–12 hourly oral.
Methyldopa. 3mg/kg per dose 8 hourly oral, may increase to max. 15 mg/kg per dose (max. 750mg).
Methyldopate 5–20mg/kg per dose (max. 1g) 6 hourly i.v. over 1h.
Methylene blue 1–4mg/kg per dose i.v.

Methylergometrine *Adult:* 200μg (NOT/kg) i.m., i.v. over 5min, or oral; may repeat in 2h, then 4–6 hourly.
Methylergonovine See methylergometrine.
Methylphenidate *Hyperactivity:* 0.25mg/kg daily oral, may increase to max. 2mg/kg daily. *Narcolepsy:* 0.1–0.4mg/kg per dose (max. 20mg) 8 hourly oral.
Methylphenobarbitone 4–12mg/kg (max. 600mg) daily.
Methylphenylsuccinimide See phensuximide.
Methylprednisolone *Asthma:* 0.5–1.0mg/kg per dose 6 hourly oral, i.v. or i.m. day 1, 12 hourly day 2, then 1.0 mg/kg daily, reducing to minimum effective dose. *Severe croup:* 4mg/kg i.v. stat, then 1mg/kg per dose 12 hourly. *Spinal cord injury* (within 8h): 30mg/kg stat, then 5mg/kg per h 2 days. *Lotion* 0.25%: apply sparingly 12–24 hourly. Methylpred 1mg = hydrocortisone 5mg in glucocorticoid activity, 0.5mg in mineralocorticoid.
4–Methylpyrazole See fomepizole.
Methyltestosterone 2.5–12.5mg/day (NOT/kg) buccal.
Methysergide 0.02mg/kg per dose (max. 1mg) 12 hourly oral, increase to max. 0.04mg/kg per dose (max. 2mg) 8 hourly oral for 3–6 months.
Metirosine. 5–20mg/kg per dose (max. 1g) 6 hourly oral.
Metoclopramide 0.12mg/kg per dose (max. 15mg) 6 hourly i.v., i.m. or oral. 0.2–0.4mg/kg per dose (max. 20mg) 8 hourly p.r.
Metocurine iodide *ICU:* 0.4mg/kg i.v. p.r.n. *Theatre:* 0.1–0.4mg/kg stat, then 0.01–0.02 mg/kg per dose.
Metolazone 0.1–0.2mg/kg (max. 10mg) daily oral. Up to 0.5mg/kg (max. 30mg) daily short term.
Metoprolol *i.v.:* 0.1mg/kg (max. 5mg) over 5 min, repeat every 5 min to max. 3 doses, then 1–5μg/kg per min. *Oral:* 1–2mg/kg per dose (max. 100mg) 6–12 hourly.
Metronidazole 15mg/kg stat, then 7.5mg/kg per dose (max. 800mg) 12 hourly in neonate (1st maintenance dose 48h after load in preterm, 24h in term baby), 8 hourly (4 + weeks) i.v., p.r. or oral. *Topical gel* 0.5%: apply daily. Level 60–300μmol/mL (× 0.17μg/mL).
Metyrapone *Diagnosis:* 15mg/kg per dose (minimum 250mg) 4 hourly × 6 dose oral. *Cushing:* 1–20mg/kg per dose (max. 1g) 4 hourly.
Metyrosine See metirosine.
Mexiletine *i.v. infusion:* 2–5mg/kg (max. 250mg) over 15 min, then 5–20μg/kg per min (max. 250mg per h). *Oral:* 8mg/kg (max. 400mg) stat, then 4–8mg/kg per dose (max. 400mg) 8 hourly starting 2h after loading dose.
Mezlocillin 50mg/kg per dose 6–8 hourly (1st week of life), 4–6 hourly (2 + weeks) i.m. or i.v. *Serious infection:* 60mg/kg per dose (max. 3g) 4 hourly.
Mianserin 0.2–0.5mg/kg per dose (max. 40mg) 8 hourly oral.
Miconazole 7.5–15mg/kg per dose (max. 1.2g) 8 hourly i.v. over 1h. *Topical:* 2% cream, powder, lotion, tincture or gel 12–24 hourly. *Vaginal:* 2% cream or 100mg ovule daily.
Microlax enema <12 months 1.25mL, 1–2 years 2.5mL, >2 years 5mL.
Midazolam *Sedation:* usually 0.1–0.2mg/kg i.v. or i.m.; up to 0.5mg/kg used safely in children. *Anaesthesia:* 0.5 mg/kg, then 2μg/kg per min (3mg/kg in 50mL at 2mL/h) i.v.

Mifepristone *Termination:* 600mg (NOT/kg) oral once, then gemeprost 1mg p.v. in 36–48h if abortn incomplete.
Milrinone 50μg/kg i.v. over 10min, then 0.375–0.75 μg/kg per min (max. 1.13mg/kg per day).
Mineral mixture (Aminogram) *<5.5kg:* 1.5g/kg daily oral, mixed with feed. *>5.5kg:* 8g daily (NOT/kg).
Mineral oil See paraffin liquid.
Minocycline *Over 8 years:* 4mg/kg (max. 200mg) stat, then 2mg/kg per dose (max. 100mg) 12 hourly oral or i.v. over 1h.
Minoxidil 0.1mg/kg (max. 5mg) daily, increase to max. 0.5mg/kg per dose (max. 25mg) 12–24 hourly oral. *Male baldness:* 2% solution 1mL 12 hourly to dry scalp.
Misoprostol (PGE1 analogue) 5μg/kg per dose (max. 200μg) 4–6 hourly oral.
Mitomycin C, crystalline 2mg/m^2 i.v. daily × 10 days, repeat only if leucocytes >3000/mm^3 + platelets >75 000/mm^3.
Mitotane 10–80mg/kg per dose (max. 4g) 6 hourly oral.
Mitoxanthrone See mitozanthrone.
Mitozantrone *Breast cancer or lymphoma:* 10–14mg/m^2 i.v. over 10min every 3 weeks. *Leukaemia:* 10–12mg/m^2 i.v. over 10min daily for 3–5 days.
Mivacurium 150μg/kg stat, then 100μg/kg per dose i.v. *Infusion:* 5–15μg/kg per min.
Moclobemide 2–3mg/kg per dose (max. 150mg) 6–12 hourly oral.
Molgramostim See sargramostim.
Molidone 0.1–1.5mg/kg per dose (max. 75mg) 8 hourly oral.
Mometasone furoate *0.1% cream or ointment:* apply daily.
Moracizine 4–6mg/kg per dose (max. 300mg) 8 hourly oral.
Moricizine See moracizine.
Morphine 0.1–0.2mg/kg per dose i.v., 0.2mg/kg per dose i.m. (half-life 2–4h). *Infusion:* 0.5mg/kg in 50mL 5%D at 1–5mL/h (10–50μg/kg per h).
Morrhuate sodium *Adult:* 50–250mg per injtn (NOT/kg).
Moxalactam See latamoxef.
Mumps vaccine (Mumpsvax) Live. *>12 months:* 0.5mL s.c. once. See also measles + mumps + rubella vaccine.
Mupirocin, ointment 2% Apply 8–12 hourly.
Muromonab-CD3 (Orthoclone OKT3) 0.1mg/kg (max. 5mg) daily for 10–14 days i.v. over 1min.
Mustine HCl (nitrogen mustard) 0.1mg/kg i.v. daily for 3–4 days. *Hodgkins:* 6mg/m^2 i.v.
Nabilone 0.02–0.04mg/kg per dose (max. 2mg) 12 hourly oral.
Nabumentone 10–20mg/kg per dose (max. 1g) 12–24 hourly oral.
Nadolol 1–5mg/kg (max. 240mg) daily oral.
Nafarelin *Adult:* 200μg (NOT/kg) spray to 1 nostril 12 hourly.
Nafcillin *Oral:* 15–30mg/kg per dose 6 hourly. *Severe infection* (slow i.v., i.m.): 40mg/kg per dose (max. 2g) 12 hourly (1st week of life), 8 hourly (2nd week), 6 hourly or constant infusion (>2 weeks).
Naftidrofuryl 2–4mg/kg per dose (max. 200mg) 8 hourly (oral) or 12 hourly (i.m., or i.v. or IA infusion over 2h).

Nalbuphine 0.2–0.5mg/kg per dose (max. 20–30mg) 3–6 hourly s.c., i.m. or i.v. *Anaesthesia:* 0.3–1.0mg/kg i.v. over 15min, then 0.2–0.5mg/kg every 30min.
Nalidixic acid 15mg/kg per dose (max. 1g) 6 hourly oral, reducing to 7.5mg/kg per dose 6 hourly after 2 weeks.
Nalorphine 0.1–0.2mg/kg stat, repeat every 10–15min to max. 0.8mg/kg (max. 40mg).
Naloxone *Opiate intoxication* (including newborn): 0.1 mg/kg (max. 2mg) stat i.v. or intratracheal, then 0.01 mg/kg per h i.v. *Postoperative sedation:* 0.002mg/kg per dose repeat every 2min, then 0.01 mg/kg per h (0.2μg/kg per min) i.v.
Naltrexone 1mg/kg (max. 50mg) daily oral.
Nandrolone in oil 0.5–4mg/kg (max. 0.4g) each 1–3 weeks i.m.
Naphazoline 0.025–0.1%: 1–2drops each nostril or eye 3 hourly.
Naproxen 5–7.5mg/kg per dose (max. 500mg) 12–24 hourly oral.
Nedocromil *Inhalation:* 4mg per dose (NOT/kg) 6–12 hourly.
Nefopam *Oral:* 0.5–2mg/kg per dose (max. 90mg) 8 hourly. *i.m.:* 0.4 mg/kg (max. 20mg) stat, may repeat in 6h.
Neomycin 12.5–25mg/kg per dose (max. 1g) 6 hourly oral. *Bladder washout:* 40–2000mg/L.
Neostigmine *Oral:* 0.3–0.6mg/kg per dose 3–4 hourly (max. 400mg /day). *i.v., i.m.:* 0.01–0.05mg/kg per dose 3–4 hourly (max. 20mg /day). *Reverse relaxants:* 0.05–0.07 mg/kg per dose i.v.; *suggested dilution:* neostigmine (2.5mg/mL) 0.5mL + atropine (0.6mg/mL) 0.5mL + saline 0.5mL, give 0.1mL/kg i.v.
Netilmicin *Single daily dose i.v. or i.m.:* 2.5mg/kg (<30 weeks gestation), 3.5mg/kg (30–35 weeks gestation), 5mg/kg (1st week of life), 7.5mg/kg (2 + weeks), 6mg/kg (>10 years). Trough <1.0mg/L.
Nicardipine 0.4–0.8mg/kg per dose (max. 40mg) 8 hourly oral.
Niclosamide 40mg/kg (max. 2g) oral.
Nicofuranose 10–20mg/kg per dose (max. 1g) 8 hourly oral.
Nicotine resin chewing gum NOT/kg: 2–4mg chewed over 30min when inclined to smoke; usually need 16–24 mg/day, max. 60mg/day.
Nicotine transdermal patches (Nicabate 7mg, 14mg, 21mg; Nicotinell 10 = 17.5mg, 20 = 35mg, 30 = 52.5mg) *Adult:* if smoked >20cig/day apply strongest patch daily 3–4 weeks, then medium patch daily 3–4 weeks (initial dose if smoked < = 20cig/day), then weakest patch daily 3–4 weeks.
Nicotinic acid *Hypercholesterolaemia and hypertriglycerideaemia:* 5mg/kg per dose (max. 200mg) 8 hourly, gradually increase to 20–30 mg/kg per dose (max. 2g) 8 hourly oral.
Nicoumalone 0.1–0.25mg/kg (max. 12mg) daily oral. INR usually 2–2.5 for prophylaxis, 2–3 for treatment.
Nifedipine Caps 0.25–0.5mg/kg (max. 20mg) 6–8 hourly, tabs 0.5–1.0mg/kg per dose (max. 40mg) 12 hourly oral or sublingual.
Nimodipine 10–15μg/kg per h (max. 1mg per h) i.v. for 2h, then 10–45μg/kg per h.
Nitrazepam NOT/kg: 1–5mg per dose 12 hourly. *Hypnotic:* 2–5mg.
Nitric oxide 5–10ppm (up to 80ppm used occasionally). [NO] = Cylinder [NO] × (1 – (Patient FiO2 / Supply FiO2)).
Nitrofurantoin 1.5mg/kg per dose (max. 100mg) 6 hourly oral. *Prophylaxis:* 1–2.5mg/kg at night.

Nitrofurazone *0.2% cream, solution:* apply every 1–3 days.
Nitrogen mustard See mustine HCl.
Nitroglycerine 1–10μg/kg per min i.v. (see p.35). Use polyethylene-lined syringe and tubing (not PVC). *Pulmonary vasodilation:* 5μg/kg per min nitroglyc = 2μg/kg per min nitropr = 0.1 μg/kg per min PGE1.
Nitroprusside 0.5–10μg/kg per min (see p.35); used for >24h, max. 4μg/kg per min. Max. total 70mg/kg with normal renal function (or sodium thiocyanate <1725 μmol/L, ×0.058 = mg/L). *Pulmonary vasodilation:* 5μg/kg per min nitroglyc = 2 μg/kg per min nitropr = 0.1 μg/kg per min PGE1 approx.
Nizatidine 3mg/kg per dose (max. 150mg) 12 hourly oral for max. 8 weeks, then 3mg/kg (max. 150mg) daily.
Nonoxynol *Cream* 2% (Ortho) or 5% (Delfen): 1 applicatorful just before intercourse. *Foam* 12.5% (Delfen): 1 applicatorful <60min before intercourse.
Noradrenaline *i.v. infusion:* 0.05–0.5μg/kg per min. See p.35.
Norepinephrine See noradrenaline.
Norethindrone See norethisterone.
Norethisterone *Contraception:* 350μg daily, starting 1st day of menstruation. *Menorrhagia:* 10mg 3 hourly until bleeding stops, then 5mg 6 hourly for 1 week, then 5mg 8 hourly for 2 weeks.
Norethisterone + ethinyloestradiol (0.5mg/35μg or 1mg/35μg) × 21 tab, + 7 inert tab *Contraception:* 1 tab daily, starting 1st day of menstruation.
Norethisterone 1mg + mestranol 50μg *Contraception:* 1 tab daily from 5th to 25th day of menstrual cycle.
Norfloxacin 7.5mg/kg per dose (max. 400mg) 12 hourly oral.
Norgestrel See levonorgestrel.
Normacol granules 6 months–5 years ½ teasp 12 hourly, 6–10 years 1 teasp 12 hourly, over 10 years 1 teasp 8 hourly.
Nortriptyline 0.5–1.5mg/kg per dose (max. 75mg) 8 hourly oral.
Noxythiolin 1–2.5% solution into body cavity 12–24hourly, left at least 30min. Max. daily dose 200mg/kg (max. 10g).
Nystatin 500 000u (1 tab) 6–8 hourly NG or oral. *Neonates:* 100 000u (1mL) 8 hourly, prophylaxis 50 000u (0.5mL) 12 hourly. *Topical:* 100 000u/g gel, cream or ointment 12 hourly. *Vaginal:* 100 000u 12–24 hourly.
Octoxinol (octoxynol) *Jelly* 1% (Ortho-Gynol): 1 teaspoonful on diaphragm before intercourse.
Octreotide 1μg/kg per dose 12–24 hourly s.c., may increase to 4 μg/kg per dose (max. 250μg) 8 hourly. *i.v.:* 3–5μg/kg per h.
Oestradiol, vaginal tab 25μg 1 tab daily for 2 weeks, then 1 tab ×2/week.
Oestradiol 2mg or 4mg (×12 tab), oestradiol 1mg (×6 tab), oestradiol 2mg or 4mg + norethisterone 1mg (×10 tab) 1 tab daily, starting 5th day of menstruation.
Oestriol *Vaginal:* 0.5mg daily, reducing to twice a week.
Oestrogen See ethinyloestradiol.
Oestrone *Vaginal:* 0.1–1mg daily, decrease to 1mg ×2–3/week.
Ofloxacin 4–8mg/kg per dose (max. 400mg) 12–24 hourly oral or i.v. over 1h.
OKT3 See muromonab-CD3.
Olsalazine *250mg cap:* 1–3 cap (NOT/kg) 6–12 hourly oral.

Omeprazole Usually 0.4–0.8mg/kg (max. 40mg) daily oral. *ZE synd:* 0.4–1.0mg/kg (max. 60mg) 12–24 hourly oral. *i.v.:* 2 mg/kg (max. 80mg) stat, then 1mg/kg (max. 40mg) 8–12 hourly. *H. pylori:* 0.4 mg/kg per dose (max. 20mg) 12 hourly with amoxycillin 10mg/kg per dose 6 hourly oral for 2 weeks.
Ondansetron *i.v.:* 0.1–0.2mg/kg (usual max. 8mg) over 15 min, then 0.25–0.5μg/kg per min. *Oral:* 0.1–0.2 mg/kg per dose (usual max. 8mg) 8–12 hourly.
Oral rehydratn solution (ORS) See glucose electrolyte solution.
Orciprenaline *Oral:* 0.25–0.5mg/kg per dose (max. 20mg) 6 hourly. *Respiratory solution* (2%): 0.5mL per dose diltd to 4mL 3–6 hourly (mild), 1.0 mL per dose diltd to 4mL (moderate), undiluted continuously (severe, in ICU). *Aerosol* 750μg per dose: 2 puffs 4–6 hourly.
Ornipressin (POR 8) *i.v.:* 0.1u/kg per h (max. 6u per h) for max. 4h, then 0.03u/kg per h (max. 1.5u per h). *s.c.:* 5u in 30mL saline, max. total dose 0.1u/kg.
Orphenadrine 2–5mg/kg per dose (max. 150mg) 8–12 hourly oral.
Oxacillin *Oral:* 15–30mg/kg per dose 6 hourly. *Severe infection* (i.v.,i.m.): 40mg/kg per dose (max. 2g) 12 hourly (1st week of life), 8 hourly (2nd week), 6 hourly or constant infusion (>2 weeks).
Oxandrolone 0.05–0.1mg/kg per dose (max. 5mg) 6–12 hourly oral.
Oxatomide 0.6–1.2mg/kg per dose (max. 60mg) 12–24 hourly oral.
Oxazepam 0.2–0.5mg/kg per dose 6–8 hourly oral.
Oxerutin 10mg/kg per dose (max. 500mg) 12 hourly oral.
Oxitropium *Inhalation:* 200μg per dose (NOT/kg) 8–12 hourly.
Oxpentifylline *Sustained release tab:* 8mg/kg per dose (max. 400mg) 8–12 hourly oral.
Oxprenolol 0.5–2mg/kg per dose (max. 120mg) 8–12 hourly oral.
Oxtriphylline See choline theophyllinate.
Oxybutynin NOT/kg: 5–12 years 5mg per dose 8–12 hourly oral, >12 years 5mg per dose 6–8 hourly.
Oxycodone 0.1–0.2mg/kg per dose (max. 10mg) 4–6 hourly oral.
Oxymetazoline, nasal 0.25mg/mL (<6 years), 0.5mg/mL (>6 years): 2–3 drops or sprays in each nostril 8–12 hourly.
Oxymetholone 1–2mg/kg per dose 12–24 hourly oral.
Oxymorphone Usually 0.02–0.03mg/kg per dose (max. 1.5mg) 4–6 hourly i.m. or s.c. *Slow i.v.:* 0.01mg/kg per dose (max. 0.5mg) 4–6 hourly. *p.r.:* 0.1mg/kg (max. 5mg) 4–6 hourly.
Oxypentifylline 8mg/kg per dose (max. 400mg) 8–12 hourly oral.
Oxyphenbutazone, 10% ointment Apply × 2–5 times/day.
Oxytetracycline *>8 years:* 250–500mg per dose (NOT/kg) 6 hourly oral, or 250–500mg per dose (NOT/kg) 6–12 hourly slow i.v.
Oxytocin *Labour:* 1–4mU/min (NOT/kg) i.v., may increase to 20 mU/min max. *Lactation:* 1 spray (4iu) into each nostril 5min before infant feeds.
Packed cells 4mL/kg raises Hb 1g%. 1 bag is about 300mL.
Paclitaxel 100–250mg/m^2 i.v. over 24h each 3 weeks, total of 3–6 doses.
Pamidronate See disodium pamidronate.
Pancreatic enzymes *With meals* (NOT/kg): 1–3 Cotazyme-S Forte cap, 1–5 Pancrease cap oral.
Pancuronium *ICU:* 0.1–0.15mg/kg i.v. p.r.n. *Theatre:* 0.1mg/kg i.v., then 0.02mg/kg p.r.n. *Infusion:* 0.25–0.75μg/kg per min.

Papaveretum (Omnopon) 0.2mg/kg per dose i.v., 0.4 mg/ kg per dose i.m. (half life 2–4h). *ICU:* 0.3mg/kg per dose i.v., 0.6 mg/kg per dose i.m.

Papaveretum (20mg/mL) and hyoscine (0.4mg/mL) 0.4 mg/kg (P) + 0.008mg/kg (H) = 0.02mL/kg per dose i.m.

Papaverine *Adult* (NOT/kg): 150–300mg 12 hourly oral, 12–40 mg × 1–2/week intracavernosal. *IA lines:* 0.12mg/mL.

Paracetamol 20mg/kg stat, then max. 15mg/kg per dose 4 hourly (max. 4g/day) oral or p.r. *Overdose:* see acetylcysteine.

Paraffin *Liquid:* 1mL/kg (max. 45mL) daily oral. *Liquid 50% + white soft 50%, ointment:* apply 6–12 hourly.

Paraffin 65% + agar NOT/kg: 6 months–2 years 5mL, 3–5 years 5–10mL, >5 years 10mL 8–24 hourly oral.

Paraffin, phenolphthalein and agar (Agarol) NOT/kg: 6 months–2 years 2.5mL, 3–5 years 2.5–5mL, >5 years 5mL 8–24 hourly oral.

Paramethadione 5–10mg/kg per dose (max. 600mg) 6–8 hourly oral.

Paraldehyde *i.m.:* 0.2mL/kg (max. 10mL) stat, then 0.1 mL/kg per dose 4–6 hourly. *i.v.:* 0.2mL/kg (max. 10mL) over 15 min, then 0.02mL/kg per h (max. 1.5mL/h). *Rectal or NG:* 0.3 mL/kg per dose diluted 1:10.

Paromomycin 10mg/kg per dose 8 hourly for 5–10 days oral.

Paroxetine 0.4–1.0mg/kg (max. 50mg) daily oral.

Pegademase 10u/kg i.m. weekly, increase to 20u/kg weekly.

Pemoline *>6 years:* 20–120mg (NOT/kg) daily oral.

Penbutolol 0.5–1.5mg/kg (max. 80mg) daily oral.

Penicillamine 5–7.5mg/kg per dose 8 hourly (max. 2g/day) oral.

Penicillin, benzathine 25 000–50 000u(20–40mg)/kg (max. 1.8g) i.m. once. Strep proph: 25 000u(20mg)/kg (max. 900mg) i.m. 3–4 weeksly, or 12,500(10mg)/kg i.m. 2 weeksly.

Penicillin, benzathine co (Bicillin 1 200 000u) 0–2 years ½ vial, 3–6 years 3/4 vial, >6 years 1 vial i.m. once.

Penicillin G (benzyl) 50 000u(30mg)/kg per dose 4–6 hourly. *Severe infection:* 100 000u (60mg)/kg per dose (max. 3g) i.v. 12 hourly (1st week of life), 6 hourly (2–4 weeks), 4 hourly or constant infusion (>4 weeks).

Penicillin, procaine 25 000–50 000u(25–50mg)/kg (max. 1.2–2.4g) 12–24 hourly i.m. *Single dose:* 100mg/kg (max. 4.8g).

Penicillin V (phenoxymethylpenicillin) 7.5–15mg/kg per dose (max. 500mg) 6 hourly oral. *Proph:* 12.5mg/kg per dose 12 hourly oral.

Penicilloyl polylysine (Prepen, 0.00006 molar) *Scratch:* 1 drop. *Intradermal:* 0.01–0.02mL (NOT/kg).

Pentaerythritol tetranitrate 0.2–1.0mg/kg per dose (max. 60mg) 6–8 hourly oral.

Pentagastrin 6μg/kg s.c., or 0.6μg/kg per h i.v.

Pentastarch *10% solution:* 10–40mg/kg i.v.

Pentamidine isethionate 4mg/kg of base i.v. over 2h or i.m. daily for 10–14 days (1mg base = 1.5mg mesylate = 1.74 mg isethionate).

Pentazocine *Oral:* 0.5–2.0mg/kg per dose (max. 100mg) 3–4 hourly. *s.c., i.m. or slow i.v.:* 0.5–1.0mg/kg per dose (max. 60mg) 3–4 hourly. *p.r.:* 1.0 mg/kg per dose (max. 50mg) 6–12 hourly.

Pentobarbital See pentobarbitone.

Pentobarbitone 0.5–1.0mg/kg per dose (max. 60mg) 6–8 hourly oral, i.m., slow i.v. *Hypnotic:* 2–4mg/kg (max. 200mg).
Pentostatin 4mg/m^2 i.v. weekly.
Pentoxifylline See oxypentifylline.
Pergolide *Parkinson's:* 1μg/kg (max. 50μg) daily, increase to max. 25μg/kg per dose (max. 2mg) 8 hourly oral. *Hyperprolactinaemia:* 0.5–3μg/kg daily.
Pericyazine 0.15–1mg/kg per dose (max. 150mg) 12 hourly oral.
Perindopril 0.05–0.15mg/kg (max. 8mg) daily oral.
Permethrin *Creme rinse* 1% (head lice): wash hair, apply creme for 10min, wash off; may repeat in 2 weeks. *Cream* 5% (scabies): apply to whole body except face, wash off after 12–24h.
Perphenazine 0.1–0.3mg/kg per dose (max. 20mg) 8–12 hourly oral.
Pertussis See diphtheria + tetanus + pertussis vaccine.
Pethidine 0.5–1.0mg/kg per dose i.v., 1–1.5mg/kg per dose i.m. (half-life 2–4h). *Infusion:* 5mg/kg in 50mL heparin–5%D at 1–3mL/h (100–300μg/kg per h).
Phenacemide 10–20mg/kg per dose (max. 1g) 8 hourly oral.
Phenazone 5.4% + benzocaine 1.4% otic (Auralgin) 3 drops 6–8 hourly.
Phenazocine 0.1–0.4mg/kg per dose (max. 20mg) 4–6 hourly oral or sub-lingual.
Phenazopyridine 4mg/kg per dose (max. 200mg) 6 hourly oral for 2 days.
Phendimetrazine 0.4–1.4mg/kg per dose (max. 70mg) 8 hourly oral.
Phenelzine 0.3–2mg/kg per dose (max. 90mg) 8 hourly oral.
Phenethicillin 5–10mg/kg per dose (max. 500mg) 6 hourly oral.
Phenindamine 0.5–1.0mg/kg per dose (max. 50mg) 8–12 hourly oral.
Phenindione Usually 0.25–1.0mg/kg per dose (max. 50mg) 12 hourly oral.
Pheniramine 0.5–1mg/kg per dose (max. 50mg) 6 hourly oral.
Phenobarbital See phenobarbitone.
Phenobarbitone *Loading dose in emergency:* 20–30mg/kg i.m. or i.v. over 30min stat. *Ventilated:* repeat doses of 10–15mg/kg up to 100mg/kg in 24h (beware hypotension). *Usual maintenance:* 5mg/kg (max. 300mg) daily i.v., i.m. or oral. *Infant colic:* 1mg/kg per dose 4–8 hourly oral. Level 80–120μmol/L (× 0.23 = μg/mL) done Mo, We and Fr at Royal Children's Hospital.
Phenolphthalein 0.5–5mg/kg (max. 270mg) at night oral.
Phenoperidine 0.03–0.05mg/kg per dose (max. 1mg) every 40–60min. *Ventilated:* 0.1–0.15mg/kg per dose (max. 5mg) every 40–60min.
Phenoxybenzamine 0.2–1mg/kg 12–24 hourly oral. *Cardiac surgery:* 1mg/kg i.v. over 1h stat, then 0.5mg/kg per dose 6–12 hourly i.v. over 1h or oral.
Phenoxymethylpenicillin See penicillin V.
Phensuximide 10–20mg/kg per dose (max. 1g) 8–12 hourly oral.
Phentermine *Adult* (NOT/kg): 30–40mg daily oral, reducing to 15–40mg daily.
Phentolamine 0.1mg/kg stat, then 5–50μg/kg per min i.v.
Phenylacetate See sodium phenylacetate.
Phenylbutazone Initially 2mg/kg per dose (max. 100mg) 4hourly, reducing to 1–2mg/kg per dose (max. 100mg) 6–8 hourly oral.
Phenylephrine *i.v.:* 2–10μg/kg stat (max. 500μg), then 1–5μg/kg per min. *s.c. or i.m.:* 0.1–0.2mg/kg (max. 10mg). *Eye drops* (0.12%, 10%): 1–2 drops/eye 6–8 hourly. *Nose drops* (0.25%, 0.5%): 1–3 drops/sprays per nostril 6–8 hourly.

Phenylpropanolamine 0.5mg/kg per dose (max. 25mg) 6–8 hourly oral.
Phenyltoloxamine 1mg/kg per dose (max. 50mg) 8 hourly oral.
Phenytoin *Loading dose in emergency:* 15–20mg/kg (max. 1.5g) i.v. over 1 h. *Maintenance:* oral or i.v. 4mg/kg per dose 12 hourly (1st week of life; ½ dose if preterm), 8 hourly (2nd week), 6 hourly (3 weeks–5 years), 8 hourly (5–9 years); 2 mg/kg per dose (usual max. 100mg) 6–12 hourly >12 years. Level 40–80 μmol/L (× 0.25 = μg/mL), done Mo, We and Fr morning at Royal Children's Hospital.
Pholcodine 0.1–0.2mg/kg per dose (max. 10mg) 6–12 hourly oral.
Phosphate, potassium (1mmol/mL) 0.1–1mmol/kg per day (max. 20mmol/day) i.v. infusion.
Phosphate, sodium (500mg tab) 0.5–1g (NOT/kg) 8 hourly oral.
Physostigmine 0.02mg/kg (max. 1mg) i.v. every 5 min till response (max. 0.1mg/kg), then 0.5–2.0μg/kg per min.
Phytomenadione 0.3mg/kg (max. 10mg), i.m. or i.v. over 1h. *Prophylaxis in neonates* (NOT/kg): 1mg i.m. at birth; or 1mg oral or 0.1mg i.m. at birth, at 4–7 days, and 3–4 weeks (give ½ dose if weight <1500g).
Phytonadione See phytomenadione.
Pilocarpine, eye drops 0.5%, 1%, 2%, 3%, 4% 1–2 drops 2–4 times a day.
Pimozide 0.04–0.4mg/kg (max. 20mg) daily oral.
Pindolol 0.3mg/kg per dose (max. 15mg) 8–24 hourly oral.
Pine tar, gel, solution 5mL to baby bath, 15–30mL to adult bath; soak for 10min.
Pipenzolate 0.1mg/kg per dose (max. 5mg) 6 hourly oral.
Piperacillin 50mg/kg per dose (max. 4g) i.v. 4–8 hourly (1st week of life), 4–6 hourly or constant infusion (2 + weeks).
Piperazine 75mg/kg (max. 4g) oral daily for 2 days (ascaris), 7 days (pinworm).
Pipothiazine *Oily injection:* initially 0.5mg/kg (max. 25mg), then 1–4mg/kg (max. 200mg) every 4 weeks i.m.
Piracetam 15mg/kg per dose (max. 800mg) 8 hourly oral, i.m. or i.v.
Pirbuterol *Oral:* 0.2–0.3mg/kg per dose (max. 15mg) 6–8 hourly. *Inhalation:* 0.2–0.4mg per dose (NOT/kg) 4–6 hourly (max. 2.4mg/day).
Pirenzepine 1mg/kg per dose (max. 50mg) 12 hourly oral.
Piretanide *Sust relse tab:* 0.1–0.2mg/kg (max. 12mg) daily.
Piroxicam 0.2–0.4mg/kg (max. 20mg) daily oral.
Pivampicillin 20mg/kg per dose (max. 500mg) 8–12 hourly oral.
Pivampicillin 1.25mg + pivmecillinam 1mg. 5–10mg/kg per dose (max. 250mg) of pivampicillin 12 hourly oral.
Pizotifen NOT/kg: 1–3mg daily oral, usually 0.5mg morning, 1mg night.
Plague vaccine (CSL) Inactivated. *Adult* (>11 years): 0.5mL s.c. stat, and 1–4 weeks later (2 doses); boost every 6 months. *Child:* 0.1mL (6 months–2 years), 0.2mL (3–6 years), 0.3mL (7–11 years) s.c. stat, 1–4 weeks later, and 1–4 weeks later (3 doses); boost every 6 months.
Platelets 10mL/kg i.v. stat, then daily if necessary. 1 unit is about 60mL.
Plicamycin *Testicular tumours:* 25–30μg/kg daily for 8–10 days i.v. over 6h, repeat monthly if response. *Hypercalcaemia:* 25μg/kg daily for 3–4 days, then × 1–3/week.

Pneumococcus vaccine (Pneumovax 23) Inactivated. >2 years: 0.5mL s.c. or i.m. once.
Podofilox See podophyllotoxin.
Podophyllotoxin, paint 0.5% Apply 12 hourly for 3 days, then none for 4 days; 4 weeks course.
Podophyllum, solution or ointment 15–25% Apply to wart × 2/day.
Poldine 0.1mg/kg per dose (max. 4mg) 6 hourly oral.
Polio vaccine, oral (Sabin) Live. 2 drops oral at 2months, 4month and 6 months. Boost at 5 years, and if going to epidemic area.
Polio vaccine, s.c. (Enpovax HDC) Inactivated. 0.5mL s.c. stat, 8 weeks later, and 8 weeks later (3 doses). Boost 12 months later, and at school entry.
Poloxalkol *10% solution:* 1 drop per month of age (max. 25 drops) 8 hourly oral.
Polyestradiol *Adult:* 40–80mg (NOT/kg) i.m. every 2–4 weeks.
Polyethylene glycol See colonic lavage solution.
Polymyxin B See bacitracin + neomycin + polymyxin.
Polynoxylin, gel 10% Apply 12 hourly.
Polycarbophil Ca 20mg/kg per dose (max. 1g) 4–24 hourly oral.
Polystyrene sulphonate (Resonium) 0.3–0.6g/kg per dose (max. 30g) 6 hourly NG (give lactulose) or p.r.
Polythiazide 0.02–0.1mg/kg per dose (max. 4mg) daily oral.
Polyvinyl alcohol, eye drops 1.4%, 3% 1–2 drops per eye p.r.n.
POR 8. See ornipressin.
Potassium Max. i.v. 0.4mmol/kg per h. Max. oral 1mmol/kg per dose (<5 years), 0.5mmol/kg per dose (>5 years). Need 2–4mmol/kg /day. 1g KCl = 13.3mmol K, 7.5% KCl = 1mmol/mL.
Potassium canrenoate 3–8mg/kg (max. 400mg) daily i.v.
Potassium guaiacolsulfonate 1–3mg/kg per dose (max. 160 mg) 4–6 hourly oral.
Povidone-iodine, cream, ointment, paint, solution Apply 6–12 hourly.
Pralidoxime 25–50mg/kg (max. 2g) over 30min, then up to 10mg/kg per h (max. 12g/day).
Pravastatin 0.2–0.4mg/kg (max. 20mg) at bedtime oral.
Prazepam 0.2–1mg/kg (max. 60mg) at night oral.
Praziquantel 20mg/kg per dose 4 hourly for 3 doses oral.
Prazosin 0.005mg/kg (max. 0.25mg) test dose, then 0.025–0.1 mg/kg per dose (max. 5mg) 6 hourly oral.
Prednisolone *Asthma:* 0.5–1.0mg/kg per dose 6 hourly for 24h, 12 hourly for the next 24h, then 1.0mg/kg daily. *Severe croup:* 4mg/kg stat, then 1mg/kg per dose 8–12 hourly oral. Prednisolone 1mg = hydrocortisone 0.8mg in mineralocorticoid action, 4mg in glucocorticoid. See also methylprednisolone.
Prednisolone acetate 1% + phenylephrine 0.12%, eye drops 1–2 drops per eye 6–12 hourly.
Prednisolone sodium phosphate, ear/eye drops 0.5% 1–3 drops per eye 2–6 hourly.
Prednisone Action equivalent to prednisolone.
Prilocaine Max. dose 6mg/kg (0.6mL/kg of 1%). With adrenaline max. dose 9mg/kg (0.9mL/kg of 1%).

Primaquine Usually 0.3mg/kg (max. 15mg) daily for 14–21 days oral. *Gameteocyte:* 0.7mg/kg (max. 45mg) once.
Primidone 5–15mg/kg per dose (max. 750mg) 12 hourly oral.
Probenicid 25mg/kg (max. 1g) stat, then 10mg/kg per dose (max. 500mg) 6 hourly oral.
Probucol 10mg/kg per dose (max. 500mg) 12 hourly oral.
Procainamide 3–6mg/kg (max. 100mg) i.v. over 15 min, then 20–80 μg/kg per min (max. 80mg per h). 2.5–7.5mg/kg 4 hourly oral.
Procaine Max. dose 20mg/kg (1mL/kg of 2%).
Procarbazine 1mg/kg daily oral, increase over 4–6 days to 4–6mg/kg (max. 300mg) daily until remission, then 1–2mg/kg daily. Suspend if leucocytes <3000/mm^3 or platelets <80 000/mm^3.
Prochlorperazine (1mg base = approx 1.5mg edisylate, maleate or mesylate) Only use if >10kg. *i.m. or slow i.v.:* 0.1–0.2mg/kg (max. 15mg salt) 6–8 hourly. *Oral or p.r.:* 0.1–0.4mg/kg per dose (max. 25mg salt) 6–8 hourly, slow increase to max. 0.6mg/kg per dose (max. 35mg) 6 hourly in psychosis. *Buccal:* 0.05–0.1mg/kg (max. 6mg salt) 12–24 hourly.
Procyclidine 0.05–0.2mg/kg per dose (max. 10mg) 6–8 hourly oral.
Progesterone Adult. *Premenst syn:* 200–400mg per dose (NOT/kg) p.v. or p.r. 12–24 hourly (last ½ cycle). *Dysf ut hge:* 5–10mg/day (NOT/kg) i.m. for 5–10 days before menses. *Prevent abtn:* 25–100mg (NOT/kg) i.m. every 2–4 days.
Proguanil 4mg/kg (max. 200mg) daily oral after food.
Promazine *Oral:* 2–4mg/kg per dose (max. 200mg) 6 hourly. i.m. 0.7 mg/kg per dose (max. 50mg) 6–8 hourly.
Promethazine *Antihist, antiemetic:* 0.2–0.5mg/kg per dose (max. 25mg) 6–8 hourly i.v., i.m. or oral. *Sedative, hypnotic:* 0.5–1.5mg/kg per dose (max. 100mg).
Propafenone *Oral:* 3–5mg/kg per dose (max. 300mg) 8 hourly. *i.v.:* 1–2mg/kg over 15min, then 10–20μg/kg per min.
Propantheline bromide 0.3–0.6mg/kg per dose (max. 30mg) 6 hourly oral.
Propofol. 1–3mg/kg stat, then 4–12mg/kg per h i.v. Beware acidosis and myocardial depression.
Propoxyphene See dextropropoxyphene.
Propranolol *i.v.:* 0.02mg/kg test dose then 0.1mg/kg (max. 5mg) over 10 min (repeat × 1–3 p.r.n.), then 0.1–0.3mg/kg per dose 3 hourly. *Oral:* 0.2–0.5mg/kg per dose 6–12 hourly, slow increase to max. 1.5 mg/kg per dose (max. 80mg) 6–12 hourly if required.
Propylthiouracil 50mg/m^2 per dose 8 hourly oral, reduce according to response.
Prostaglandin See alprostadil (PGE1), carboprost (15-Me-PGF2-alpha), dinoprost (PGF2-alpha), dinoprostone (PGE2), epoprostenol (PGI2), gemeprost (PGE1 analogue), and misoprostol (PGE1 analogue).
Protamine i.v. 1mg/100u heparin (or 1mg per 25mL pump blood) i.v. stat; subsequent doses of protamine 1mg/kg (max. 50mg). Heparin 1mg = 100u (half-life 1–2h).
Prothionamide *TB:* 15–20mg/kg (max. 1g) at night oral. *Leprosy:* 5–8mg/kg (max. 375mg) daily.
Prothrombinex (factors 2, 9 and 10; 250u/10mL) 1mL/kg slow i.v. daily. Risk of thrombosis in acute liver failure.

Protionamide See prothionamide.
Protirelin 200μg (NOT/kg) i.v. stat.
Protriptyline 0.1–0.2mg/kg per dose (max. 20mg) 6–8 hourly oral.
Proxymetacaine, eye drops 0.5% 1–2 drops stat, then 1 drop every 10min.
Pseudoephedrine 1mg/kg per dose (max. 60mg) 6 hourly oral.
Psyllium Usually 0.1–0.2g/kg (max. 10g) at night oral.
Pyrantel embonate 10mg/kg once oral. *Necator:* 20mg/kg daily × 2 doses. *Enterobius:* 10mg/kg each 2 weeks × 3 doses.
Pyrazinamide 20–35mg/kg per dose (max. 3g) daily oral.
Pyridostigmine 1–3mg/kg per dose (usual max. 200mg) 4–12 hourly oral. *180mg slow rel tab* (Timespan): adult 1–3 tab (NOT/kg) 12–24 hourly. 1mg i.v., i.m. or s.c. = 30mg oral.
Pyridoxine *With isoniazid:* 5–10mg daily (NOT/kg) i.v. or oral. *Neonatal fitting:* 50–100mg daily (NOT/kg) i.v. or oral. *Siderobl anaem:* 2–8mg/kg (max. 400mg) daily i.v. or oral.
Pyrilamine See mepyramine.
Pyrimethamine 12.5mg and dapsone 100mg (Maloprim) 1–4 years quarter tab weekly, 5–10 years ½ tab, >10 years 1tab.
Pyrimethamine 25mg and sulphadoxine 500mg (Fansidar) <4 years ½ tab once, 4–8 years 1 tab, 9–14 years 2 tab, >14 years 3 tab. *Prophylaxis:* <4 years ¼ tab weekly, 4–8 years ½ tab, 9–14 years 3/4 tab, >14 years 1 tab.
Q fever vaccine (Q–Vax) Inactivated. 0.5mL s.c. once.
Quazepam 0.15–0.6mg/kg (max. 30mg) at night oral.
Quinacrine See mepacrine.
Quinalbarbitone Sedative 5mg/kg. Premed 10mg/kg.
Quinapril 0.2–0.8mg/kg (max. 40mg) daily oral.
Quinestrol *Adult* (NOT/kg): 100μg daily for 7 days, then 100–200μg weekly oral.
Quinethazone 1–3mg/kg (max. 200mg) daily oral.
Quinidine sulphate 12mg/kg stat, then 6mg/kg per dose (max. 400mg) 4–6 hourly oral. *i.v.:* 7.5mg/kg i.v. over 2h, then 15 μg/kg per min. *i.m.:* 15mg/kg stat, then 7.5mg/kg per dose (max. 400mg) 8 hourly.
Quinine sulphate *Oral:* 10mg/kg per dose (max. 600mg) 8 hourly for 7–10 days. *Parenteral:* 20mg/kg i.v. over 4h or i.m., then 7.5 mg/kg per dose 8 hourly i.v. over 1h or i.m. for 2–3 days, then 10mg/kg per dose 8 hourly oral for 5 days.
Rabies vaccine, inactivated (HDCV, Merieux) 1mL i.m. stat, 7 days later, and 28 days later (3 doses). Boost every 2 years. *Postexposure:* if immune, 1mL i.m. day 0 and day 3; if non–immune, give 1mL i.m. on days 0,3,7,14,30 and 90, with immunoglobulin.
Ramipril 0.05mg/kg (max. 2.5mg) oral daily, may increase over 4–6 weeks to 0.1–0.2mg/kg (max. 10mg) daily.
Ranitidine *i.v.:* 1mg/kg per dose slowly 6–8 hourly, or 2μg/kg per min. *Oral:* 2–4mg/kg per dose (max. 300mg) 12 hourly.
Razoxone 2mg/kg per dose (max. 125mg) 8–24 hourly oral; or 7.5–15mg/kg (max. 750mg) daily for 2–3 days every 1–4 weeks. *Kaposi sarc, leukaemia:* max. 0.33g/m^2 per dose 8 hourly oral.

Remoxipride 1.5–6mg/kg per dose (max. 300mg) 12 hourly oral.
Renatonium, solution 2mg/mL Apply 8 hourly and after washing hands.
Reproterol *Aerosol* 0.5mg/puff: 1–2 puffs 3–8 hourly.
Reserpine 0.005–0.01mg/kg per dose (max. 0.5mg) 12–24 hourly oral.
Resonium See polystyrene sulphonate.
Retinol A See vitamin A.
Ribavirin *Inhalation* (Viratek nebulizer): 20mg/mL at 25mL/h (190μg/L of gas) for 12–18h/day for 3–7 days.
Riboflavine 5–10mg daily (NOT/kg) oral.
Rifabutin 3–12mg/kg (max. 600mg) daily oral.
Rifampicin 10–15mg/kg (max. 600mg) daily oral fasting, or i.v. over 3h (monitor AST). *Prophylaxis* (meningococcus, haemophilus): 10mg/kg daily (newborn), 20mg/kg (max. 600mg) daily (>4 weeks old) oral for 4 days.
Rifampin See rifampicin.
Rimipril Initially 0.05mg/kg (max. 2.5mg) oral daily, increase over 4–6 weeks to max. 0.2mg/kg (max. 10mg) daily if needed.
Rimiterol *Aerosol* 0.2mg/puff: 1–3puffs 3–8 hourly.
Risperidone 0.02mg/kg per dose (max. 1mg) 12 hourly, increase to 0.02–0.15mg/kg per dose (max. 8mg, usually 2–4mg) 12 hourly oral.
Ritodrine. *Premature labour:* 0.05–0.45mg/min (NOT/kg) i.v.; 10–20mg per dose (NOT/kg) 4–6 hourly oral.
Rolitetracyline (Reverin) *>8 years:* 10mg/kg per dose (max. 275 mg) daily slow i.v.
Roxithromycin 2.5mg/kg per dose (max. 150mg) 12 hourly oral before meals.
Rubella vaccine (Ervevax, Meruvax II) Live. *>12 months:* 0.5mL s.c. once. See also measles + mumps + rubella vaccine.
Salbutamol 0.1–0.15mg/kg per dose (max. 8mg) 6 hourly oral. Inhalation *mild:* respiratory solution (5mg/mL, 0.5%) 0.5mL per dose diluted to 4mL, or nebule 2.5mg/2.5mL 3–6 hourly; *moderate:* 0.5% solution 1mL per dose diluted to 4mL, or nebule 5mg/2.5mL 1–2hourly; *severe* (in ICU): 0.5% solution undiluted continuous. *Aerosol* 100μg/puff: 1–2 puff 4–6 hourly. *Rotahaler:* 200–400 μg 6–8 hourly. *i.m. or s.c.:* 8μg/kg. *i.v.:* child 5μg/kg over 10 min, then 1–5μg/kg per min (1μg/kg per min using 1mg/mL solution = 0.06 × wt mL/h); adult 4μg/kg over 10min, then (NOT/kg) 10–50μg/min (0.6mL/h of 1mg/mL solution = 10 μg/min).
Salcatonin *Hypercalcaemia:* 4u/kg per dose 12 hourly i.m. or s.c., may increase to 8u/kg per dose 6–12 hourly.
Salicylic acid *Cradle cap:* 6% solution (Egocappol) 12 hourly 3–5 days. *Plantar warts:* 15% solution × 1–2/day, 40% medicated disc 24–48 hourly.
Salicylsalicylic acid See salsalate.
Salmeterol. *Aerosol or diskhaler* (NOT/kg): 50–100mg 12 hourly.
Salmonella typhi vaccine See typhoid vaccine.
Salsalate 10–20mg/kg per dose (max. 1g) 6 hourly oral.
Sargramostim (GM–CSF, Leucomax.) 3–5μg/kg daily s.c., or i.v. over 6h. Keep WCC 5 000–10 000/mm^3.
Scopolamine See hyoscine.
Secbutobarbitone 0.3–0.6mg/kg per dose (max. 30mg) 6–8 hourly, or 1–4mg/kg (max. 200mg) nocte oral.
Secobarbital sodium See quinalbarbitone.

Secretin (1cu = 4chr units) 1-2cu/kg slow i.v.
Selegiline *Adult* (NOT/kg): 10mg each morning, oral.
Selenium sulphide, 2.5% Shampoo × 2/week for 2 weeks.
Sennoside *Tab* 7.5mg daily (NOT/kg): 6 months–2 years 0.5–1 tab, 3–10 years 1–2 tab, >10 years 2–4 tab. *Granules* 22.5mg/teasp, 12–24 hourly (NOT/kg): <6 months 0.25–0.5teasp, 6 months–2 years 0.5–1teasp, 3–10 years 1–2teasp.
Sermorelin (GHRH) 1μg/kg fasting in morning i.v.
Sertraline 1–2mg/kg (max. 100mg) daily oral; may give 3–4mg/kg (max. 200mg) daily for up to 8 weeks.
Silver nitrate, stick Apply daily to affected area only.
Silver sulfadiazine 1% + chlorhexidine 0.2%, cream Apply in 3–5mm layer.
Simethicone See aluminium hydroxide compound.
Simvastatin Initially 0.2mg/kg (max. 10mg) daily, may increase every 4 weeks to max. 1mg/kg (max. 40mg) daily oral.
Sodium *Deficit:* mL of 20% NaCl = weight × 0.2 × (140 − serum Na); do not increase serum Na faster than 2 mmol/L per h. Need 2–6 mmol/kg per day. NaCl MW = 58.45, 1g NaCl = 17.1mmol Na, NaCl 20% = 3.4mmol/mL.
Sodium alginate See alginic acid.
Sodium aurothiomalate 0.25mg/kg weekly i.m., increase to 1 mg/kg (max. 50mg) weekly for 10 weeks, then every 2–6 weeks. i.m., then every 1–4 weeks.
Sodium benzoate *Neonate:* 250mg/kg over 2h stat, then 10–20mg/kg per h i.v.
Sodium bicarbonate See bicarbonate.
Sodium calciumedetate (EDTA) 30–40mg/kg per dose 12 hourly i.m. or i.v. over 1h for 5 days.
Sodium chloride See sodium.
Sodium citrotartrate 40–80mg/kg per dose (max. 4g) in 50mL water 8–12 hourly oral.
Sodium clodronate 6mg/kg (max. 300mg) i.v. over 2h daily for 7 days, then 15–30/mg/kg per dose (max. 1.6g) 12 hourly oral.
Sodium cromoglycate (Intal) See cromoglycate.
Sodium etidronate 5–20mg/kg daily oral (no food for 2h before and after dose) for max. 6 months.
Sodium fluoride NOT/kg: <2 years 0.55mg oral daily, 2–4 years 1.1 mg, >4 years 2.2mg. *Osteoporosis, Paget's, bone secondaries in adult:* 20–40mg per dose (NOT/kg) 8–12 hourly.
Sodium nitrite *3% solution:* 0.2mL/kg (max. 10mL) i.v. over 5min.
Sodium nitroprusside See nitroprusside.
Sodium phenylacetate *Neonate:* 250mg/kg i.v. over 2h, then 10mg/kg per h.
Sodium picosulphate 0.1–0.3mg/kg (max. 15mL) at night oral.
Sodium tetradecyl sulphate 0.25–1mL per vein (NOT/kg) as 1% (max. 10 small veins) or 3% (max. 4 large veins).
Sodium thiosulphate 1mL/kg (max. 50mL) 25% solution i.v. over 10min.
Sofradex, Soframycin See framycetin.
Somatostatin See octreotide.
Somatrem 4u/m^2 3 days a week i.m.

Somatropin Usually 2–3iu/m^2 on 5–7 days a week s.c., or 4–6iu/m^2 on 3 days a week i.m.
Sorbitol 70% 0.2–0.5mL/kg per dose (max. 30mL) 8 hourly oral. *With activated charcoal:* 1g/kg (1.4mL/kg) NG, may repeat × 1.
Sorbolene cream; pure, with 10% glycerin, or with 5% or 10% olive oil or peanut oil Skin moisturiser, apply p.r.n.
Sotalol *i.v.:* 0.5–2mg/kg per dose (max. 100mg) over 10min 6 hourly. *Oral:* 1–4 mg/kg per dose (max. 200mg) 8 hourly.
Spectinomycin 40–80mg/kg (max. 4g) i.m. once.
Spironolactone *Oral:* 0–10kg 6.25mg per dose (NOT/kg) 12 hourly, 11–20kg 12.5 mg per dose (NOT/kg) 12 hourly, 21–40kg 25 mg per dose (NOT/kg) 12 hourly, over 40kg 25mg per dose (NOT/kg) 8 hourly. *i.v.:* see potassium canrenoate.
Stanozolol 0.05–0.2mg/kg oral (max. 10mg) daily at first, then every 2–3 days.
Sterculia 3.5–7g per dose (NOT/kg) 12–24 hourly oral.
Stilboestrol *Ca breast:* 10–20mg (NOT/kg) daily oral. *Ca prostate:* 1–3mg (NOT/kg) daily oral or i.v.
Streptokinase (SK) *Short term* (myoc infarct): 30 000u/kg (max. 1 500 000u) i.v. over 60min, repeat if occlusion recurs <5 days. *Long term* (DVT, pul emb, art thrombosis): 5 000u/kg (max. 250 000u) i.v. over 30min, then 2000 u/kg per h (max. 100 000u per h); stop heparin and aspirin, if PTT < × 2 normal at 4h give extra 10 000u/kg (max. 500 000u) i.v. over 30min, stop SK if PTT > × 5 normal then give 1000u/kg per h. *Local infusion:* 50 u/kg per h (continue heparin 10–15u/kg per h). *Blocked i.v. cannula:* 5000u/kg in 2mL in cannula for 2h then remove, may repeat × 1.
Streptomycin 20–30mg/kg (max. 1g) i.m. daily.
Streptozocin 1.0–1.5g/m^2 weekly i.v.
Succinyl choline See suxamethonium.
Sucralfate 1g tab NOT/kg: 0–2 years quarter tab 6 hourly, 3–12 years ½ tab 6 hourly, >12 years 1 tab 6 hourly oral.
Sufentanil 2–50µg/kg slow i.v.; may then infuse so that total dose is 1µg/kg per h of expected surgical time.
Sulbactam See ampicillin + sulbactam.
Sulfacetamide See sulphacetamide.
Sulfadiazine 50mg/kg per dose (max. 2g) 6 hourly slow i.v.
Sulfadoxine See pyrimethamine and sulfadoxine.
Sulfamethizole See sulphamethizole.
Sulfamethoxazole See cotrimoxazole.
Sulfametopyrazine 40mg/kg (max. 2g) weekly oral.
Sulfasalazine See sulphasalazine.
Sulfinpyrazone See sulphinpyrazone.
Sulfisoxazole See sulphafurazole.
Sulindac 4mg/kg per dose (max. 200mg) 12 hourly oral.
Sulphacetamide 10% + prednisolone 0.2% + phenyl-ephrine 0.12%, eye drops 1 drop per eye 6–12 hourly.
Sulphafurazole 75mg/kg (max. 4g) stat, then 35mg/kg per dose (max. 1.5g) 4–6 hourly oral.
Sulphamethizole 15mg/kg per dose (max. 1g) 8 hourly oral.

Sulphamethoxazole See cotrimoxazole.
Sulphasalazine *Active disease:* 10–15mg/kg per dose (max. 1g) 6 hourly oral. *Remission:* 5–7.5mg/kg per dose (max. 0.5g) 6 hourly.
Sulphinpyrazone 2–3mg/kg per dose (max. 200mg) 6–12 hourly oral.
Sulpiride 4mg/kg per dose (max. 200mg) 12 hourly, slow increase to 4–24mg/kg per dose (max. 1.2g) 12 hourly oral.
Sulthiame 1mg/kg per dose 8–12 hourly oral, may increase to 5mg/kg per dose (max. 200mg) 8 hourly.
Sumatriptan *Oral:* 2mg/kg (max. 100mg) stat, may repeat twice. *s.c.:* 0.12mg/kg (max. 6mg) stat, may repeat once after 1h.
Surfactant, bovine (Survanta) See beractant.
Surfactant, synthetic (Exosurf Neonatal) *Prophylaxis:* 5 mL/kg intratracheal over 5min immediately after birth, and at 12h and 24h if still ventilated. *Rescue:* 5mL/kg intratracheal over 5min, repeat in 12h if still ventilated.
Suxamethonium *i.v.:* neonate 3mg/kg per dose, child 2mg/kg per dose, adult 1mg/kg per dose. *i.m.:* double i.v. dose.
Tacrine (THA) 0.5–2mg/kg per dose (max. 120mg) 3 hourly i.v.
Talampicillin 5–10mg/kg per dose (max. 500mg) 8 hourly oral.
Tamoxifen. *Adult:* 20mg daily (NOT/kg), increase to 40mg daily if no response after 1month.
Tar. See coal tar.
Teceleukin (synthetic interleukin–2) See interleukin–2.
Teicoplanin 250mg/m^2 i.v. over 30min stat, then 125 mg/m^2 i.v. or i.m. daily. *Severe infection:* 250mg/m^2 12 hourly × 3 doses, then 250mg/m^2 i.v. or i.m. daily.
Temazepam *Adult:* 10–30mg (NOT/kg) at night, oral.
Temocillin 20–50mg/kg per dose (max. 2g) 12 hourly i.v. or i.m.
Teniposide 100–150mg/m^2 i.v. over 1h weekly.
Tenoxicam 0.2–0.4mg/kg (max. 20mg) daily oral.
Terazosin 0.02mg/kg test, then 0.04–0.4mg/kg (max. 20 mg) daily oral.
Terbinafine 5mg/kg (max. 250mg) daily oral.
Terbutaline *Oral:* 0.05–0.1mg/kg per dose (max. 5mg) 6 hourly. *s.c.:* 5–10μg/kg per dose (max. 500μg). *i.v.:* 5μg/kg stat over 10min, then 1–10μg/kg per h. Inhalation *mild:* respiratory solution (1%, 10mg/mL) 0.25mL per dose diluted to 4mL 3–6 hourly; *moderate:* 0.5mL of 1% diluted to 4mL, or respule 5mg/2mL 1–2hourly; *severe* (in ICU): undiluted continuous. *Aerosol* 250μg /puff: 1–2 puffs 4–6 hourly.
Terfenadine 1mg/kg per dose (max. 60mg) 12 hourly oral.
Testolactone 5–10mg/kg per dose (max. 250mg) 6 hourly oral.
Testosterone *Esters:* 100–500mg (NOT/kg) i.m. every 2–4 weeks. *Implant:* 8mg/kg (to nearest 100mg). *Undecanoate:* 40–120mg (NOT/kg) daily oral. *Testosterone level:* <16 years 5–10nmol/L, >16 years 10–30nmol/L.
Tetanus toxoid (CSL) 0.5mL i.m. stat, 6 weeks later, and 6 months later. Boost every 10 years, or if contaminated wound. See also diphtheria (+ pertussis) + tetanus vaccines.
Tetrabenazine 0.5–2mg/kg per dose (max. 100mg) 12 hourly oral.
Tetracaine See amethocaine.
Tetracosactrin zinc injection (Synacthen Depot) 600 μg/m^2 (max. 1mg) i.m. every 1–7 days.

Tetracycline *Over 8 years:* 250–500mg per dose (NOT/kg) 6 hourly oral. See also rolitetracycline.
Tetrahydrozoline, eye drops 0.5% 1–2 drops/eye 8–12 hourly.
Tetrahydrozoline 0.05% + macrogol 400 (polyethylene glycol) 1%, eye drops 1–2 drops/eye 8–12 hourly.
THAM See tromethamine.
Theophylline (80mg theophylline = 100mg aminophylline) *Loading dose:* 8mg/kg (max. 500mg) oral. *Maintenance:* 1st week of life 2mg/kg per dose 12 hourly; 2nd week of life 3mg/kg per dose 12 hourly; 3 weeks–12 months (0.1 × age in weeks) + 3mg/kg per dose 8 hourly; 1–9 years 4mg/kg per dose 4–6 hourly, or 10mg/kg per dose slow rel 12 hourly; 10–16 years or adult smoker 3mg/kg per dose 4–6 hourly, or 7mg/kg per dose 12 hourly slow rel; adult non-smoker 3 mg/kg per dose 6–8 hourly; elderly 2mg/kg per dose 6–8 hourly. *Monitor serum level:* neonate 60–80μmol/L, asthma 60–110 (× 0.18 = μg/mL).
Thiabendazole 25mg/kg per dose (max. 1.5g) 12 hourly oral for 3 days.
Thiamine *Beriberi:* 1–2mg/kg i.v., i.m. or oral daily.
Thiamylal 0.05–0.1mL/kg of 2.5% solution i.v. over 1min; may then infuse 0.3% solution.
Thiethylperazine maleate *>10kg:* 0.2mg/kg per dose (max. 10mg) 8–24 hourly oral, i.m., or p.r.
Thioguanine 100mg/m^2 daily oral; or 100mg/m^2 per dose 12 hourly for 5–7 days.
Thiopental See thiopentone.
Thiopentone 3–5mg/kg slowly stat (beware hypoten-sion), then 1–5mg/kg per h i.v. Level 150–200μmol/L (× 0.24 = μg/mL).
Thioridazine 0.5–3mg/kg per dose (max. 150mg) 6–8 hourly oral, i.m.
Thiosulphate See sodium thiosulphate.
Thiotepa 10–14mg/m^2 i.v. every 1–4 weeks.
Thiotepa, eye drops 1 in 2000 2 drops/eye 4–6 hourly for 6 weeks.
Thiothixene *>12 years:* initially 2mg per dose (NOT/kg) 8 hourly oral, slow increase to 2–20mg per dose.
Thrombin, topical 100–2000u/mL onto bleeding surface.
Thymoxamine *Adult:* 40–80mg per dose (NOT/kg) 6 hourly oral.
Thyroxine *Infants:* 25μg daily (NOT/kg), gradually increase to 3–5μg/kg per day oral. *Adult:* 100–200μg daily (NOT/kg).
Tiaprofenic acid 2–4mg/kg per dose (max. 200mg) 8 hourly oral.
Tibolone *Adult:* 2.5mg (NOT/kg) daily oral.
Ticarcillin 50mg/kg per dose (max. 3g) i.v. 6–8 hourly (1st week of life), 4–6 hourly or constant infusion (2 + weeks).
Ticarcillin and clavulanic acid Dose as for ticarcillin.
Ticlopidine 5mg/kg per dose (max. 250mg) 12 hourly oral.
Tilactase *200u/drop:* 5–15 drops/L milk 24h before use. *3300u/tab:* 1–3tabs with meals.
Timolol 0.1mg/kg per dose (max. 5mg) 8–12 hourly, increase to max. 0.3 mg/kg per dose (max. 15mg) 8 hourly. *Eye drops* (0.25%, 0.5%): 1 drop/eye 12 hourly.
Tinidazole *Giardia:* 50mg/kg (max. 2g) stat, repeat after 48h. *Amoebic dys:* 50mg/kg (max. 2g) daily for 3 days.
Tinzaparin (1mg = 75 anti–Xa IU) 50u/kg s.c. 2h before surgery, then daily for 7–10 days.

Tioconazole, 280mg/mL Apply to nails 12 hourly for 6–12 months.
Tissue plasminogen activator See alteplase.
Tobramycin *Single daily dose i.v. or i.m.:* 2.5mg/kg (<30 weeks gestation), 3.5mg/kg (30–35 weeks gestation), 5mg/kg (1st week of life), 7.5mg/kg (2 + weeks), 6mg/kg (>10 years). Trough level <1.0 mg/L, done Mon–Fri at Royal Children's Hospital.
Tocainide 5–10mg/kg per dose (max. 400–800mg) 8–12 hourly i.v. over 30min or oral.
Tocopherol See vitamin E.
Tolazamide 2–5mg/kg per dose (max. 250mg) 6–24 hourly oral.
Tolazoline *Newborn:* 1–2mg/kg slowly stat (beware hypotension), then 2–6μg/kg per min (0.12–0.36mg/kg per h) i.v. *Note:* 1–2mg/kg per h too much (*Pediatrics* 1986;**77:**307).
Tolbutamide *Adult:* initially 1g (NOT/kg) 12 hourly oral, often reducing to 0.5–1g daily.
Tolmetin 5–10mg/kg per dose (max. 400–600mg) 8 hourly oral.
Tolnaftate, cream, ointmnt, powdr, solution 1% Apply 8–12 hourly.
Tramazoline 120μg + dexamethasone 20μg per dose, nasal *Aerosol:* 1 puff in each nostril 4–8 hourly.
Trandolapril 0.01–0.1mg/kg (max. 4mg) daily oral.
Tranexamic acid 15–20mg/kg per dose (max. 1g) 8 hourly oral.
Tranylcypromine 0.2mg/kg per dose (max. 10mg) 8–12 hourly oral.
Trazodone 1–4mg/kg per dose (max. 200mg) 8 hourly oral.
Tretinoin, cream or lotion 0.05%, gel 0.01% Apply daily.
Triacetyloleandomycin 6–12mg/kg per dose (max. 250–500 mg) 6 hourly oral.
Triamcinolone *Joint, tendon:* 2.5–15mg (NOT/kg) stat. *i.m.:* 0.05–0.2mg/kg every 1–7 days. *Cream or ointment* 0.02%, 0.05%: apply sparingly 6–8 hourly. Triamcinolone has no mineralcorticoid action, 1mg = 5mg hydrocortisone in glucocorticoid action.
Triamcinolone 0.1% + neomycin 0.25% + gramicidin 0.025% + nystatin 100 000u/g *Kenacomb cream, ointment:* apply 8–12 hourly. *Kenacomb otic cream, ointment, drops:* apply 8–12 hourly (2–3 drops).
Triamterene 2mg/kg per dose (max. 100mg) 8–24 hourly oral.
Triazolam *Adult:* 0.125–0.5mg (NOT/kg) at night, oral.
Tribavirin See ribavirin.
Triclosan, emulsion 2% 2mL to wet skin for 20sec, rinse and repeat.
Trientine 10mg/kg per dose (max. 500mg) 6–12 hourly oral.
Triethylenethiophosphoramide See thiotepa.
Trifluoperazine 0.02–0.2mg/kg per dose (max. 10mg, occasionally 20mg) 12 hourly oral.
Trifluridine *1% solution:* 1 drop/eye 2 hourly (max. 9 drops/day) until epithelialised, then 4 hourly (max. 5 drops/day) for 7 days.
Trihexyphenidyl See benzhexol.
Triiodothyronine (T3) See liothyronine.
Trilostane 0.5–4mg/kg per dose (max. 240mg) 6 hourly oral.
Trimeprazine (Vallergan) *Antihist:* 0.1–0.5mg/kg per dose (max. 25mg) 6 hourly oral. *Sedation:* 0.5–1mg/kg per dose i.m., 2–4 mg/kg per dose oral.

Trimetaphan 0.04–0.1mg/kg per min (max. 4mg/min) i.v.
Trimethadione See troxidone.
Trimethobenzamide 5mg/kg per dose (max. 250mg) 6–8 hourly oral, i.m. or p.r.
Trimethoprim 3–4mg/kg per dose (usual max. 150mg) 12 hourly, or 6–8mg/kg (usual max. 300mg) daily oral or i.v.
Trimethoprim-sulphamethoxazole See cotrimoxazole.
Trimipramine 1–2mg/kg per dose (max. 100mg) 8–24 hourly oral.
Trioxsalen See trioxysalen.
Trioxysalen *Adult:* 5–10mg (NOT/kg) daily 2h before UV exposure.
Tripelennamine 1.25mg/kg per dose (max. 75mg) 6 hourly oral.
Tripotassium dicitratobismuthate (bismuth subcitrate) 50 mg/kg per dose (max. 240mg) 12 hourly oral 30min before meal. *H. pylori* (>5 years old): 25mg/kg per dose 6 hourly oral for 2–4 weeks, with metronidazole and (if >7 years) tetracycline. Avoid milk.
Triprolidine 2.5mg + pseudoephedrine 60mg (Actifed) 10mL elixir = 1tab. NOT/kg: 2.5mL (<2 years), 2.5–5mL (2–5 years), 0.5tab (6–12 years), 1tab (>12 years) 6–8 hourly oral.
Trisodium edetate 40–70mg/kg (max. 3g) i.v. over 6h daily for 5 days; max. 3 courses each 2 days apart.
Troleandomycin See triacetyloleandomycin.
Tromethamine (THAM) mL of 0.3 molar (18g/500mL) solution = wt × BE (give ½ this) i.v. over 30–60min.
Tropicamide, eye drops 0.5%, 1% 1–2 drops/eye, repeat after 5min.
Tropisetron 0.1mg/kg (max. 5mg) slow i.v. just before chemotherapy, then oral 1h before breakfast for 5 days.
Troxidone. 10–15mg/kg per dose (max. 800mg) 8 hourly oral.
Tubocurarine. *ICU:* 0.6mg/kg i.v. p.r.n. *Theatre:* 0.3–0.6mg/kg i.v. stat, then 0.15mg/kg per dose.
Tulobuterol. 0.04mg/kg per dose (max. 2mg) 8–12 hourly oral.
Typhoid vaccine, oral (Typh–Vax). Live. 1 cap oral days 1, 3, 5 and (for better immunity) 7. Boost yearly.
Typhoid vaccine, parenteral (CSL). Inactivated. 0.1mL (<6 years), 0.25mL (6–12 years), 0.5mL (>12 years) s.c. stat, and 4 weeks later. Boost every 3 years.
Typhoid vaccine, parenteral, polysaccharide (Typhim Vi). Inactivated. *>5 years:* 0.5mL i.m. once. Protects 3 years or more.
Urea, cream 10%. Apply 8–12 hourly.
Urofollitrophin. As for menotrophin.
Urokinase. 4000u/kg i.v. over 10min, then 4000u/kg per h for 12h (start heparin 3–4h later). *Blocked cannula:* instill 5000–25000u (NOT/kg) in 2–3mL saline for 2–4h.
Ursodeoxycholic acid. 4–8mg/kg per dose 12 hourly oral.
Ursodiol. See ursodeoxycholic acid.
Valproate. 5–25mg/kg per dose (max. 500mg) 8–12 hourly oral. Level 0.3–0.7mmol/L (× 144 = μg/mL), done Fri at Royal Children's Hospital.
Vancomycin. 15mg/kg per dose (max. 500mg) *i.v. over 2h:* daily (preterm), 12 hourly (1st week of life), 8 hourly (2 + weeks). *Oral:* 5–10mg/kg per dose 6 hourly. *Intraventric:* 10mg per dose (NOT/kg) 48 hourly. Peak 25–40mg/L, trough <10mg/L; done Mon–Fri at Royal Children's Hospital.
Vasopressin. *Aqueous:* put 1–2u in 1L fluid, and replace urine output + 10%

i.v.; or 2–10u i.m. or s.c. 8 hourly. *Brain death:* 0.0003u/kg per min (1u/kg in 50mL at 1mL/h) + adrenaline 0.1–0.2μg/kg per min. Oily: 2.5–5u (NOT/kg) i.m. every 2–4 days. *GI hge* (aqueous solution): 0.4u/min i.v. in adult; 0.1 u/min local IA in adult. See desmopressin and lypressin.

Vecuronium. *ICU:* 0.1mg/kg p.r.n. *Theatre:* 0.1mg/kg stat, then 1–10μg/kg per min i.v.

Verapamil. *i.v.:* 0.1–0.2mg/kg (max. 10mg) over 10min, then 5μg/kg per min. *Oral:* 1–3mg/kg per dose (max. 120mg) 8–12 hourly.

Vidarabine. Eye *ointment:* × 5/day until epithelialised, then 12 hourly 7 days. *i.v. infusion:* 10mg/kg per day 5–10 days (varicella-zoster), 15mg/kg per day 10 days (herpes encephalitis).

Vigabatrin. Initially 40mg/kg (max. 2g) daily oral, may increase to 80–100mg/kg (max. 4g) daily (given in 1–2 doses).

Viloxazine 1–4mg/kg (max. 250mg) morning, and 1–2mg/kg (max. 150mg) noon oral.

Vinblastine 6.5mg/m^2 i.v. over 1 min every 1–4 weeks.

Vincristine 1.5mg/m^2 weekly i.v. over 1 min.

Vindesine 3–4mg/m^2 i.v. every 7–10day if WCC >2500/mm^3.

Vitamin A *High risk:* 200 000iu (NOT/kg) oral every 4–6 months.

Vitamin A, B, C, D compound (Pentavite) Neonate 12drop, 0–6 years 2.5–5mL, >6 years 5mL (NOT/kg) daily oral.

Vitamin A + D (Royal Children's Hospital 12 000u A, 2 000u D/mL) 1mL/day.

Vitamin B group *Amp:* i.v. over 30 min. *Tab:* 1–2/day.

Vitamin B1 See thiamine.

Vitamin B12 See hydroxycobalamin.

Vitamin C See ascorbic acid.

Vitamin D *Nutritional rickets:* ergocalciferol (D2) 10 000u daily (NOT/kg) for 30 days, oral. *Renal rickets or hypoparathyroidism:* calcitriol (1,25-OH D3) start 0.01μg/kg daily; dihydrotachysterol (1-OH D2) 20μg/kg per day; *ergocalciferol* (D2): 50 000–300 000u/day (NOT/kg).

Vitamin E (Copherol E) *Preterm babies:* 40u (2 drops) daily (NOT/kg) oral. 1u = 1mg.

Vitamin K1 See phytomenadione.

Vitamins, parenteral *MVI-12* (for adult): 5mL in 1 litre i.v. fluid. *MVI Paediatric, added to i.v. fluid:* 65% of a vial (<3kg), 1 vial (3kg to 11 years).

Vitaprem (RCH) (Pentavite, folate, B12, C) 1mL daily oral.

Warfarin Usually 0.2mg/kg (max. 10mg) stat, 0.2mg/kg (max. 10mg) next day providing INR <1.3, then 0.05–0.2mg/kg (max. 10mg) daily oral. INR usually 2–2.5 for prophylaxis, 2–3 for treatment. Beware of drug interactions.

Whole blood 8mL/kg increase Hb 1g%. 1bag = 400mL approx.

Xamoterol 4mg/kg per dose (max. 200mg) 12–24 hourly oral.

Xipamide 0.5–1.5mg/kg (max. 80mg) every morning oral.

Xylometazoline *<6 years:* 0.05% 1 drop or spray 8–12 hourly. *6–12 years:* 0.05% 2–3 drops or sprays 8–12 hourly. *>12 years:* 0.1% 2–3 drops or sprays 6–12 hourly.

Yellow fever vaccine (CSL) *>12 months:* 0.5mL s.c. once. Boost every 10 years.

Yohimbine 0.05–0.1mg/kg per dose (max. 5.4mg) 8 hourly oral.
Zalcitabine 0.015mg/kg per dose (max. 0.75mg) 8 hourly oral.
Zidovudine (AZT) *Oral:* usually 180 mg/m^2 per dose (max. 200 mg) 6 hourly oral, adjusted to 75–240 mg/m^2 per dose 6–8 hourly. *i.v.:* 50–150 mg/m^2 per dose 6–8 hourly.
Zinc sulphate *Adult:* 50–220mg (NOT/kg) 8–24 hourly oral.
Zopiclone 0.1–0.3mg/kg (max. 15mg) at bedtime oral.
Zuclopenthixol 0.4–3mg/kg (max. 150mg) daily oral.

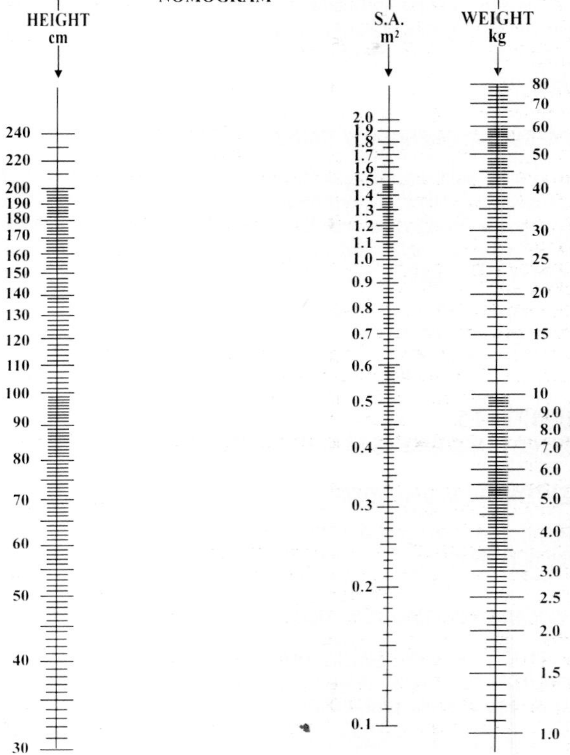

Figure 35.1 Nomogram

CHAPTER 1
CRITICAL CARE

OBTAINING HELP

Help within the Royal Children's Hospital (RCH) can be obtained by dialling **777**. The switchboard operator will notify the Intensive Care Unit (ICU) and other medical personnel (see Emergency Instructions, pp. 000). A registrar and nurse from the ICU will attend the scene bringing an ECG-defibrillator. Other emergency resuscitation equipment and medications are provided in mobile trolleys in every ward and department.

PAEDIATRIC EMERGENCY TRANSPORT SERVICE (PETS)

In Victoria, southern New South Wales and Tasmania, transport of critically ill or injured children may be undertaken by the Paediatric Emergency Transport Service. This service is located in the ICU at the RCH, and is also accessible for telephone advice about the management of such patients.

Tel: (03) 9345 5211
(03) 9345 5212
(03) 9345 5213

CHAPTER 5
INFECTIOUS DISEASES AND MICROBIOLOGY

ENTEROVIRUS DIAGNOSIS

Polymerase chain reaction of CSF for enterovirus can be undertaken by the RCH laboratory.

ISOLATION PRECAUTION POLICY OF THE RCH

Within the RCH, patients who have a communicable disease or nosocomial (hospital acquired) infection caused by virulent pathogenic organisms, require 'isolation precautions' to prevent spread of infection.

The isolation policy should be followed as closely as possible for the protection of patients or staff. However, other arrangements may be required if an isolation room is not available, there are insufficient nursing staff available or the patient's clinical condition is such that isolation may jeopardize his/her management.

NOTIFIABLE DISEASES IN VICTORIA

Notifiable infectious diseases in Victoria are divided into four groups on the basis of the method of notification and the information required. Special notification forms are used and these are available from:

- Medical Records Department (RCH)
- Health and Community Services, tel: (03) 9616 7777

Completed forms are taken to the discharge clerk in Medical Records who will send them to:

The Chief Health Officer
Statewide Services
Health and Community Services
PO Box 4003
Melbourne, Victoria 3001

Details should also be entered on the back of the yellow case divider.

Numbers for notification of disease:

Tel: (03) 9616 7482
(03) 9616 7132
(03) 9616 7127
(008) 034 280
Fax: (03) 9616 7147 (Attention: Chief Health Officer)

After hours, contact the Duty Medical Officer. Ring the paging service on (03) 9614 4600 and give pager no. 46870.

GROUP A DISEASES

The Health and Community Services should be notified of a case of any of the following diseases by telephone or fax upon initial diagnosis (presumptive or confirmed) with written notification to follow within 7 days.

- Australian arbo encephalitis
- Anthrax
- Botulism
- Cholera
- Food-borne and water-borne illness (two or more related cases)
- Legionellosis
- Measles

- Meningitis or epiglottitis due to *H. influenzae*
- Meningococcal infection (meningitis or meningococcaemia)
- Plague
- Poliomyelitis
- Primary amoebic meningo-encephalitis
- Rabies
- Typhoid and paratyphoid fevers
- Typhus
- Viral haemorrhagic fevers
- Yellow fever

GROUP B DISEASES

For the following diseases, written notification only is sufficient, within 7 days of confirmation of diagnosis.

- Amoebiasis
- Arbovirus infections (except for Australian arbo encephalitis)
- Brucellosis
- *Campylobacter* infection
- Giardiasis
- Hepatitis, viral – all forms including: hepatitis A, B, C and non-A non-B, hepatitis (viral, unspecified)
- Hydatid disease
- Leprosy
- Leptospirosis
- Listeriosis
- Malaria
- Mumps
- Pertussis
- Psittacosis (ornithosis)
- Q fever
- Rubella (including congenital rubella)
- Salmonellosis
- Shigellosis
- Taeniasis (tapeworm infections)
- Tetanus
- Tuberculosis
- Yersiniosis

GROUP C DISEASES

Notification of the following sexually transmitted diseases should be made using the same notification form, but, to preclude identification of the patient, only the first two letters of the given name and surname of the patient are required.

- Chancroid
- Donovanosis
- Gonorrhoea (all forms)
- Lymphogranuloma venereum
- Other chlamydial infections
- Syphilis (all forms)

GROUP D DISEASES

AIDS

Written notification is required within 7 days of confirmation of diagnosis. A separate form is used for this purpose due to the need to have national uniformity in collection of data. To preclude identification of the patient, only the first two letters of the given name and surname of the patient are required.

Cancer

Does not include any type of skin cancer other than melanoma. Notifications are to be made by hospitals and pathology laboratories only, direct to:

ANTI-CANCER COUNCIL OF VICTORIA
1 Rathdowne Street
Carlton South 3052
Tel: (03) 9279 1111

NEEDLESTICK INJURIES: RCH POLICY

Reporting Incident and Medical Advice

The incident should be reported immediately to the department Head or the person in charge of the area at the time, and a non-patient incident form completed and signed.

Within normal working hours, staff are to report immediately to Staff Clinic, who will be responsible for initial advice and for ensuring that a record is kept of action taken. If there is any concern that the patient's blood may carry HIV, the staff member will be referred immediately to the Infection Control Officer (outside normal working hours — Emergency, under the direction of the Admitting Officer).

The Staff Clinic will also:

- Facilitate the taking of blood and vaccination if necessary (during normal working hours – Staff Clinic)
- Maintain contact with the staff member to monitor any further action required beyond the initial response, maintain a confidential record of the injury and action taken and, when action is completed, give the record to the human resources department.

Queries

Any queries should be referred to the Infection Control Officer (Pager no. 8–6341) or Staff Clinic (ext. 5971).

CHAPTER 7 GASTROINTESTINAL CONDITIONS

ENCOPRESIS

Special 'Fitness Training Diaries' are available through the Child Health Information Centre at the RCH.

CHAPTER 11 HAEMATOLOGIC CONDITIONS AND ONCOLOGY

TRANSFUSION SERVICES FOR THALASSAEMIA MAJOR PATIENTS

This is now performed for most patients on an outpatient basis at Monash Medical Centre and at the RCH.

HYPERIMMUNE γ-GLOBULINS

These products are available from either the Red Cross Blood Transfusion Services (anti-Rh(D) and zoster immune globulin) or from the Commonwealth Serum Laboratories.

ONCOLOGY SERVICES

In Victoria, the Departments of Haematology and Oncology at the RCH and Monash Medical Centre provide consultation on children with a malignancy who require medical attention. The therapeutic effects of modern chemotherapy involve multiple systems and are complex. These departments provide liaison both within the hospital and outside.

CHAPTER 12
NEUROLOGIC CONDITIONS

HEAD INJURIES

Within the RCH, skull X-rays may only be ordered for children with head injuries by the neurosurgery registrar or neurosurgery consultant if the child has been or is to be admitted.

HEAD INJURY INSTRUCTIONS TO PARENTS

A h*ead injury information sheet* is available in the emergency department at the RCH for issue to parents.

CHAPTER 14
ENDOCRINE CONDITIONS

Referral of Short Children

The following short children should be referred to the paediatric endocrine clinic:

- Those in whom the cause of the short stature has not been found
- Those requiring pituitary function testing
- Those needing GH or androgen therapy
- Those with emotional and behavioural problems attributed to the growth problem

'Growth Groups' run by the Endocrine Social Worker provide short pre-adolescent children with coping strategies.

CHAPTER 15
DISORDERS OF GLUCOSE METABOLISM

HYPOGLYCAEMIA KIT

Available in the RCH Emergency Department refrigerator or from Biochemistry.

Lactate/Glucose

- 0.5 mL blood in glucose/lactate pot (white top), *or*
- Heparin fluoride tube (yellow top)

Free Fatty Acids/Ketones

One mL of blood in a BLF (butyrate–lactate–fluoride) tube on wet ice.

Cortisol/Growth Hormone

Two to 3 mL of blood in a serum (plain) tube.

Insulin/C-peptide Amino Acids

Four to 5 mL of blood in heparin tube (orange top) on wet ice.

LACTATE COLLECTION

Venous stasis and muscular exertion markedly increase blood lactate concentrations which can invalidate interpretation of any result. Add 0.5 mL of whole blood, collected without venous stasis to lactate tube. **Mix well** (invert tube at least five times), label and place on wet ice or chill pack and transport *ASAP* to Biochemistry Department (*routine hours* – 9th Floor routine laboratory; *after hours* – 2nd Floor ICU laboratory). **Label each tube and fill in a request card for each tube clearly indicating tests required and time at which sample was taken.**

CHAPTER 23
BURNS

BURNS CONSULTATION SERVICE

Within the RCH, the burns surgeon on duty is available for consultation regarding the resuscitation and transfer of any child with a burn injury.

Tel: (03) 9345 5946; Fax: (03) 9345 6668.

FOLLOW-UP

Within Victoria, the District Nursing Service provides care in the home between outpatient consultations.

CHAPTER 24
DENTAL CONDITIONS

Within the RCH, the department of dentistry provides separate consultative service for more difficult *paediatric dental problems* and for *traumatic injuries*. It provides ongoing routine clinic care for patients of the hospital covering all aspects of dentistry

EMERGENCIES

The dentist and oral surgeon on call can be contacted via the switchboard. During normal hospital hours simple emergency department problems (such as non-urgent toothache in a normal child or minor tooth fractures) should be referred to the Royal Dental Hospital of Melbourne or the local dentist.

After hours emergencies:

Royal Dental Hospital of Melbourne, tel: (03) 9341 0222 (weekends, tel: (03) 341 0325)
Weekdays: 1800–2115 h
Saturdays: 0900–2115 h
Sundays and public holidays: 0900–2115 h or the local dentist.

SUSPECTED FRACTURES OF THE MANDIBLE AND MAXILLA

Within the RCH, notify the dental consultant or the oral and maxillofacial registrar, who will then notify the oral surgeon on call immediately. This should be done on presentation and before any radiological investigations are undertaken, even if other injuries are the main problem. The registrar will order the appropriate radiograph.

OTHER DENTAL PROBLEMS

Patients presenting to the RCH with such non-emergency dental problems should be advised to ring their own dentist or the department of dentistry (if already attending here) for an appointment at the earliest opportunity.

CHAPTER 26
DEVELOPMENTAL DELAY AND DISABILITY

SERVICES FOR CHILDREN WITH DEVELOPMENTAL DELAYS AND DISABILITIES AND THEIR FAMILIES

Health and Community Services Victoria regional teams provide early intervention and information about local government and non-government early intervention programmes, family support agencies, respite care options and parent-to-parent support groups. Telephone liaison is advisable to identify the appropriate referral.

Metropolitan

Eastern: 883 Whitehorse Road, Box Hill 3128, tel: (03) 9248 7248 7 John Street, Lilydale 3140, tel: (03) 9735 5911
Northern: 145 Smith Street, Fitzroy 3065, tel: (03) 9412 5333
Southern: 122 Thomas St, Dandenong 3175, tel: (03) 9213 2111
Western: 71 Moreland Street, Footscray 3011, tel: (03) 9275 7000

Country

Barwon/South Western: Fenwick Street, Geelong 3222, tel (052) 26 4540
Gippsland: 64 Church Street, Traralgon 3844, tel: (051) 76 2500
Grampians: Mar Street, Ballarat 3350, tel: (053) 33 6669
Loddon Mallee: Lister House, 37 Rowan Street, Bendigo 3550, tel: (054) 34 5555

Noah's Ark Toy Library and Family Resource Centre

28 The Avenue, Windsor 3181, tel: (03) 9529 1466
Cnr Dundas and Newcastle Streets, Thornbury 3071, tel: (03) 9484 4318
16 Thomson St, Maidstone 3012, tel: (03) 9317 9512

Spastic Society of Victoria

135 Inkerman Street, St Kilda 3182, tel: (03) 9537 2611

Yooralla Society of Victoria

52 Thistlethwaite St, South Melbourne 3205, tel: (03) 9254 5666

Royal Victorian Institute For The Blind

Burwood Highway, Burwood 3125, tel: (03) 9808 6422

CONSUMER GROUPS

Down Syndrome Association of Victoria

55 Victoria Parade, Collingwood 3066, tel: (03) 9419 1653

STAR: Victorian Action on Intellectual Disability

247 Flinders Lane, Melbourne 3000, tel: (03) 9650 2730

Action Group for Children with a Disability

19B William Street, Richmond 3121, tel: (03) 9427 0827

Epilepsy Foundation of Victoria

818 Burke Road, Camberwell 3124, tel: (03) 9813 2866

A.D.E.C. Action on Disability within Ethnic Communities

123 Sydney Road, Brunswick 3056, tel: (03) 9388 1613

Autism Victoria

35 High Street, Glen Iris 3146, tel: (03) 9885 0533

FAMILY SUPPORT

In Australia, families with a significantly disabled child are eligible to receive the Child Disability Allowance from the Department of Social Security.

CHAPTER 27
ADOLESCENT HEALTH

CONFIDENTIALITY

It is a legal requirement in Victoria for confidentiality to be maintained when treating adolescents who are 16 years of age or above.

REFERRALS

The Centre for Adolescent Health at the RCH provides specialist services using an interdisciplinary approach to the delivery of comprehensive health care to young people.

CHAPTER 30
CHILD ABUSE AND NEGLECT

MANDATORY REPORTING

In accordance with Victorian legislation, professionals are mandated to notify Child Protection Services of Health and Community Services (H&CS), Victoria, if they believe on reasonable grounds that a child has suffered, or is likely to suffer, significant harm as a result of physical injury or sexual abuse, and that the child's parents have not protected or are unlikely to protect the child from such harm.

CONSULTATIONS AND MEDICAL ADVICE

Consultation and advice regarding abused children is available from the Gatehouse Centre for the Assessment and Treatment of Child Abuse, tel: (03) 9345 6391; after hours via RCH switchboard, tel: (03) 9345 5522.

NOTIFICATION TO PROTECTIVE SERVICES (HEALTH AND COMMUNITY SERVICES)

During working hours notify the regional team (according to the child's address). Telephone numbers under H for Health and Community Services – Protective Services Teams in A–K White Pages.
After hours: 24 h crisis line, tel: (03) 9131 278

COURT APPEARANCES

Advice is available from the Gatehouse Centre for the Assessment and Treatment of Child Abuse regarding court procedures and preparations for appearing in court.

CHAPTER 31
THE DEATH OF A CHILD

SUPPORT SERVICES

RCH Parent Bereavement Support Group

Social Work Department, RCH
Tel: (03) 9345 6111
Monthly meetings.

Stillbirth and Neonatal Death Support Group (S.A.N.D.S.)

19 Canterbury Rd, Camberwell 3124
Tel: (03) 9882 1590
Parent support group for miscarriage, stillbirth or neonatal death.

Sudden Infant Death Research Foundation (S.I.D.R.F.)

1227 Malvern Rd, Malvern 3144
Tel: (03) 9822 9611
Crisis intervention, counselling and support

The Compassionate Friends

300 Camberwell Rd, Camberwell 3124
Tel: (03) 9882 3355
Self-help organization for parents who have suffered the death of a child.

Barwon Paediatric Bereavement Program

P.O. Box 281, Geelong 3220
Tel: (052) 26 7525 during business hours.
(008) 811 522 after hours and 24 hour crisis counselling.
Community-based support and education for all those affected by the death of a child. Crisis intervention, counselling and support.

CHAPTER 33
INFANT AND CHILD NUTRITION

BREAST FEEDING ADVICE

If in doubt of appropriate advice to give, refer to *Breastfeeding Information & Guidelines. A Manual for Breastmilk Feeding Support in Paediatric & Neonatal Units* by Suzanne Murray, available from the Child Health Information Centre, RCH.

BREAST PUMPS

These can be purchased from any chemist (KANESON, CANNON or MEDELA) or hired from the Nursing Mothers' Association. Telephone (03) 9877 5011 for name of local branch.

MEDELA Lactina Electric pumps are available for hire also from Nursing Mothers' Association or from many local chemists. Contact Fisher &

Paykel (who manufacture MEDELA Pumps, tel: (03) 9879 5022) for name of local chemist or a list of chemists for your reference.

NURTURE III: a small portable electric pump is available on order, tel: (03) 9885 0226.

MATERNAL DRUGS

Check with Drug Advisory Services if further reassurance is needed.

Royal Women's Hospital Drug Information Centre	(03) 9344 2277
Monash Medical Centre Drug Information Service	(03) 9550 2361
Royal Children's Hospital Drug Information Centre	(03) 9345 5208

Drugs & Breastfeeding, compiled by Ron Batagol, Drug Information Service, Royal Women's Hospital, is a small handy reference available from RCH Child Health Information Centre or Royal Women's Hospital.

BREAST FEEDING SUPPORT

Maternal and Child Health Centres

Check the Child Health Record for the name and telphone number.

Nursing Mothers Association of Australia (NMAA)

General enquiries (03) 9877 5011
Australia-wide 24 hour counselling:

VIC	(03) 9878 3304
QLD	(07) 3844 8977
NSW	(02) 639 8686
WA	(09) 309 5393
ACT	(06) 258 8928
NT	(089) 32 2838
SA	(08) 339 6783
TAS	(002) 232 609

Australian Lactation Consultants' Association

Lactation consultants are people (mostly but not necessarily with a health background) with an interest and expertise in breast feeding matters. They may be midwives, maternal and child health nurses, medical practitioners or NMAA counsellors. Lactation consultants work in a variety of settings. Some are hospital based, others community based. Those who work as fee-for-service private practitioners visit the mother's home to assess and advise on breast feeding problems.

Names of lactation consultants available in a particular area can be obtained from: Lactation Resource Centre, PO Box 1129, Carlton, Vic 3053, tel: (03) 9877 5011

Mother and Baby Units in Melbourne

Queen Elizabeth Centre, Carlton, tel: (03) 9347 2777
Tweddle Child & Family Centre, Footscray, tel: (03) 9689 1577
O'Connell Family Centre, Canterbury, tel: (03) 9882 2327

HOME ENTERAL FEEDING

The Equipment Distribution Centre provides enteral feeding pumps and consumables for RCH patients. These are provided at a reduced cost. Formulas are dispensed by the hospital pharmacy at a set cost per week depending on the age of the child.

Support Service for Families

The Home Nutrition Service is a service provided by Abbott Australia and can be contacted via Ms P. Montgomery [Pager (03) 9483 8558]. The Gastrostomy Information and Support Society is a self-help group for families and can be contacted on (03) 9537 2611.

PARENTERAL NUTRITION SOLUTIONS

At the RCH, two nutrient solutions are available: *Vamin* (Vamin N with Glucose 7%) is recommended for infants <5 kg while *Synthamin* (Synthamin 17 : 10%) is recommended for patients >5 kg.

PRESCRIBING PARENTERAL NUTRITION

Prior to commencing a patient on parenteral nutrition, the Nutrition Support Service should be contacted (via switchboard). This service provides advice on all aspects of parenteral and enteral nutrition delivery and monitors all patients receiving parenteral nutrition. The Service consists of a Physician (Dr Julie Bines: Gastroenterologist), Nutrition Support Co-ordinator (Mrs Gabrielle Curwood), Gastroenterology Fellow, Pharmacist (Ms Thirza Titchen) and Dietitian (Ms Ruth Tulip).

APPENDIX 1
LABORATORY REFERENCE RANGES
BIOCHEMISTRY

URGENT REQUESTS

When a test requires immediate or special attention, the registrar or resident responsible must contact the senior biochemist on duty and be prepared to justify the need for urgent work. The word 'urgent' on a request form is not sufficient to justify diverting staff from existing work.

OUTPATIENTS

An outpatient blood collection centre is located on the ground floor and patients for biochemistry collections should be referred to this facility. The outpatient collection centre is open 0900–1700 h on weekdays.

INPATIENTS

Monday–Friday, 0900–1700 h

Capillary blood collection rounds occur at 0900, 1100 and 1400 h. A request card may be sent to the outpatient blood collection centre or retained in the ward and a telephone message given. Telephone 5821 (answering service available before 0830 h).

Monday–Friday, 1700–0900 h

Minimum staff are on duty at all times for tests requiring immediate attention.

Saturdays, Sundays and Public Holidays

Mornings

Capillary blood collection rounds occur at 0900 and 1100 h. Because of reduced staffing, requests for capillary blood collections should reach the laboratory by 0900 h if possible. Requests accompanied by venous or arterial specimens should reach the laboratory by 1030 h.

Other times

Minimum staff are on duty at all times for tests requiring immediate attention.

TESTS ROUTINELY AVAILABLE OUT OF HOURS (MONDAY–FRIDAY, 0900-1700 H)

- Acid–base/blood gases
- Electrolytes, urea, creatinine
- Calcium (total, ionized), magnesium
- Glucose
- Albumin/total protein, γ-glutamyl transpeptidase (GGT), alanine-aminotransferase (ALT), alkaline phosphatase (ALP), aspartate aminotransferase (AST), bilirubin (conj., unconj.)
- Ammonia
- Lactate
- Lipase
- Osmolality
- Pregnancy test
- Theophylline
- Creatine Kinase (CK)
- Digoxin (Saturday morning only)
- Uric acid
- Galactoscreen

Antibiotics are assayed once daily, Monday to Sunday. All other tests require the approval of the senior biochemist on duty.

EMERGENCY DEPARTMENT REQUESTS

All emergency department samples should be sent to the second floor of the Intensive Care Unit laboratory. Anticonvulsant drugs, paracetamol, salicylate and ethanol will be analysed as soon as possible following arrival. The laboratory should be notified (ext 5217) but approval by the duty biochemist is not required.

SPECIMEN REQUIREMENTS

Blood tests

Arterial po_2

Collect blood using a pre-heparinized syringe stored on the ward. Remove all bubbles, label and place in a cold pack (at 4°C, not frozen). Transport to the second floor ICU laboratory immediately. Arterial blood may also be used for other biochemical analyses.

Capillary collections

Collection of capillary specimens by Pathology collection staff is restricted to patients less than 3 years of age, except by special arrangement with the duty biochemist. Capillary collections at specific times (e.g. for drug levels) cannot be guaranteed. In such cases, the responsible medical staff should make alternative arrangements. Capillary blood is unsuitable for po_2, ammonia and lactate.

Venous Collections

For inpatients, it is the responsibility of medical staff to collect venous specimens. Outpatients may have venous specimens taken in the ground floor outpatient collection centre.

In general:

- For urea and electrolytes analysis, 1.0 ml of blood is required
- For additional tests, a total of 2–3 mL of blood is required
- Contact the laboratory or consult the Biochemistry Reference Range Handbook for details on more specialized tests.

Heparinized blood is preferred for most tests, and is always required for:

- Ammonia
- Galactose-1-phosphate
- Enzymes related to metabolic disease
- Lead
- Galactoscreen
- Porphyrins
- Galactose
- Vitamin D

EDTA blood should only be used for :

- Adrenocorticotrophic hormone
- Haemoglobin A1c
- Cyclosporine
- Parathormone

Blood tests requiring consultation before specimen collection :

- ACTH
- Lactate
- Ammonia
- Paracetamol
- Cortisol
- Parathormone
- Drug screen
- Plasma renin activity

- Enzymes related to metabolic disease
- Provocation tests (e.g. GTT, loading studies.)
- Ethanol
- 17-Hydroxyprogesterone
- PTHRP
- Insulin
- Pyruvate
- Isoenzymes
- Vitamin D

Urine Tests

Random urine specimens

All random urine specimens should be delivered to the laboratory immediately after collection. For some this is essential, namely :

- Cystine
- Homocystine
- Metabolic screen (amino acids, organic acids)
- pH
- Porphobilinogen: must reach the laboratory within 30 min wrapped in foil
- Porphyrins (screen): must be wrapped in foil

24 h urine collections

Collection bottles are available on presentation of the request slip to the Biochemistry department or ground floor Pathology collection centre. Bottles for acidified collections are available only from the Biochemistry department. During collection, the specimen must be stored at 4°C in a refrigerator.

Clearance studies

Creatinine Clearance, Phosphate Excretion Index: an accurately timed urine collection is required, plus a specimen of blood obtained during this period. **Height and weight of the patient must be stated on the request card**.

Metabolic screen

See also Metabolic Conditions, p. 207.

- Urine screen: 10 mL of fresh random specimen is required. Details of

current medication and clinical notes must be provided. Investigations include chemical tests for pH, protein, reducing substances, glucose, blood and ketones plus amino acid profile and screen for methylmalonic acid. Organic acid or other profiles are performed if clinical notes or other laboratory findings indicate the need for such studies
- Blood screen (only required in special circumstances). For amino acids only — 1 ml heparinized blood.

Urgent metabolic screening requires consultation with the clinical staff of the Genetics Department and the senior biochemist on duty.

Drug Screen

Requires urine (20 mL) and occasionally serum or plasma (2 mL). Clinical notes, with details regarding suspected toxic medications and drugs given therapeutically, must be provided. Requests for urgent drug screens from Emergency must be approved by the on-duty Emergency consultant and the on-duty senior biochemist and notification made to the screening laboratory (ext. 5923, Monday–Friday, 0900–1700 h).

DISTRIBUTION OF RESULTS

Ward Enquiry Terminals

Following analysis and validation, all results are immediately available via the hospital computer network. If a result is listed as 'to follow' this indicates that the analysis is in progress and therefore the result is not available by telephone.

Ward Interim Reports

These summaries of all the most recent results from any given area are generated and delivered by couriers at 0800 and 1400 h, Monday–Friday, and once daily at 1300 h on Saturdays, Sundays and public holidays.

Patient Cumulative Reports

These reports, which are intended for insertion into the patient's medical record, are generated at 1400 h on all weekdays. They include all confirmed test results to that time and are distributed at 0800 h, Monday–Friday.

Patient Advance Reports

- Automatic. Printers linked to the Pathology computer are situated in the Intensive Care Unit and the Neonatal Unit. In these areas, all results are printed as soon as they have been validated
- On request. Printed advance reports can be obtained on request at any time

Telephone enquiries

Results are available by telephone on ext. 5902 between 0900 and 1700 h, Monday to Friday, and on ext. 5217 outside these times. However, enquiry via the computer network is preferred as transcription errors and distraction of laboratory staff from analytical duties are thus avoided.

HAEMATOLOGY

Telephone inquiries 5822, 5824; Front Desk 5824; Lab. Manager 5823; Director 5827. The department is situated on the 8th floor of the main block. It provides a wide range of haematology, coagulation and blood bank services.

HOURS

A 24 h service is provided for 5 nights a week. On Friday and Saturday nights, after midnight, the department is on call for home for *urgent* coagulation tests and cross-matching *only*. (FBE parameters are available from the Intensive Care Unit laboratory, 2nd floor, 52/7.)

Tests Available During Non-Routine Hours

The following tests can be provided by the after hours service. Any other test will only be done during these times by special arrangement.

- FBE and differential
- Blood grouping and cross-matching
- Coombs' test
- G6PD screen
- PT, APTT, XDP, fibrinogen

BLOOD COLLECTION

A combined pathology service is available for collection of capillary blood specimens from both inpatients and outpatients. The collection area is situated on the ground floor. Requests for ward collections should reach there before the rounds at 0900, 1100 and 1400 h. A request card may be sent to the collection rooms or retained in the ward and a phone message given. Phone 5821 (answering service available before 0830 h).

Venous blood collection by ward staff is required for some specimens and is preferred from children over 3 years of age. Venous blood collection from outpatients is performed in the pathology outpatient rooms.

SPECIMEN REQUIREMENTS

Capillary Blood

Capillary blood collections can be made for the tests listed below. For children 3 years of age and over, venous specimens are preferable.

- FBE (parameters), differential count and film report
- Reticulocyte count
- IM screen
- G6PD screen
- Thrombotest

RESULTS

Reports are issued routinely at 1200 and 1800 h. If a test is required to be performed urgently the laboratory must be phoned to indicate this need. Results for urgent FBE are usually available within 2 h of receipt of the specimen.

Phone calls regarding results frequently interrupt staff carrying out the tests and should be avoided if possible.

LABORATORY REFERENCE RANGES

BIOCHEMISTRY

Reference ranges for a selected list of more commonly ordered biochemistry tests are included below. For ranges for other tests, consult printed reports or the booklet, *Reference Ranges in Clinical Biochemistry and Notes on Therapeutic Drug Monitoring.*

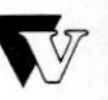

Reference ranges are derived from experience with patients of the Royal Children's Hospital, supplemented by values from normal children and from the literature. Results within these ranges can be considered to be 'within normal limits'. Where possible, results are expressed in SI units. **These ranges may not apply to results obtained using different methodologies and instrumentation.**

Because of changes in laboratory methods, reference ranges are subject to revision. Therefore, if in doubt about the significance of a result, consult the laboratory. Where possible up-to-date reference ranges are quoted on reports.

Table A1 Blood, serum and plasma

Test	*Arterial or venous specimens: volume required (mL)*	*Age*	*Reference range(s)*	*Comments*
Acid/base (P)	0.5			Arterial or capillary samples only are suitable for pH, $P\text{CO}_2$
pH		1 d	7.30–7.46	
		2 d–1 m	7.23–7.46	
		> 1 m	7.34–7.43	
$P\text{CO}_2$			32–45 mmHg	Higher values seen in newborn
Base excess			– 4 – + 3 mmol/L	Lower values seen in newborn
Actual bicarbonate			18–25 mmol/L	
Alkaline phosphatase–ALP (S,P)	0.5	0–2 y	100–350 U/L	Higher values may be seen during periods of rapid growth
		2–10 y	100–300 U/L	
		10–16 y	100–350 U/L	
		Adult	30–120 U/L	
Aspartate amino-transferase – AST (S,P)	0.5	< 1 y	20–80 U/L	Formerly SGOT. Upper limit of reference range, particularly in infancy, not well-defined
		1–3 y	15–60 U/L	
		3–16 y	10–45 U/L	
		> 16 y	0–40 U/L	

Table A1 (*Continued*)

Bilirubin – unconjugated (S,P)	0.5	Full-term		Higher values in newborn due to increase in indirect (unconjugated) fraction. Even higher values in premature infants
		0–24 h	< 65 µmol/L	
		24–48 h	< 115 µmol/L	
		3–5 d	< 155 µmol/L	
		1 m	< 10 µmol/L	
Bilirubin – conjugated (S,P)	< 1 m	< 10 µmol/L		Positive interference by sulphasalazine, nitrofurantoin
	> 1 m			
Calcium – ionized (P)	0.5	Adult	1.19–1.29 mmol/L	Whole blood specimen needed. Must be collected anaerobically, in special syringe. Consult laboratory for details
Calcium – total (S,P)	0.5	< 2 w	1.90–2.70 mmol/L	Lower limit of normal range in neonates not well-defined
		2 w–1 y	2.10–2.70 mmol/L	
		> 1 y	2.10–2.60 mmol/L	
Chloride			98–110 mmol/L	
Cholesterol – total (S,P)	0.5	6 m	2.3–4.9 mmol/L	Reference ranges based on USA data. Australian National Heart Foundation recommends adult cholesterol levels < 5.5 mmol/L and children cholesterol levels < 4.5 mmol/L.
		1 y	2.5–4.9 mmol/L	
		2–14 y	3.1–5.4 mmol/L	

h, hour; d, day; w, week; m, month; y, year; f, fasting; P, plasma; S, serum; U, urine.

(*Continued*)

Table A1 (*Continued*)

Test	*Arterial or venous specimens: volume required (mL)*	*Age*	*Reference range(s)*	*Comments*
Creatine kinase – CK (S,P)	0.5		40–240 units/L	Higher values in newborn. Specimens on three separate occasions recommended when testing for carriers of Duchenne muscular dystrophy
Creatinine (S,P)	0.5	1 m–1 y 1–4 y 4–10 y 10–16 y > 16 y	0.01–0.03 mmol/L 0.01–0.05 mmol/L 0.02–0.06 mmol/L 0.03–0.08 mmol/L 0.05–0.11 mmol/L	Reference range related to muscle mass. Higher values seen in newborns
Glucose f (S,P)	0.5	2 d–1 m > 1 m	2.2–5.0 mmol/L 3.6–5.4 mmol/L	Lower values may be seen on day 1 and in premature infants. Therapy for hypoglycaemia should aim to keep glucose level greater than 3 mmol/L. Whole blood glucose approximately 10% lower than plasma
γ-Glutamyltransferase – GGT (S,P)	0.5	0–1 m > 3 m	< 225 U/L < 40 U/L	Newborns have very high levels of GGT which rapidly decrease to adult levels by about three months. Higher levels of GGT may be seen if on anticonvulsants or alcohol

Table A1 (*Continued*)

Iron (S,P)	0.5		9–27 μmol/L	
Magnesium (S,P)	0.5		0.7–1.0 mmol/L	
Osmolality (S,P)	1		265–295 mmol/kg	
Phosphorus – inorganic (S,P)	0.5	< 2 w	1.7–3.0 mmol/L	
		2 w–2 y	1.3–2.3 mmol/L	
		2–16 y	1.1–1.8 mmol/L	
Po_2 **(P)**	0.5 Arterial only	< 2 w	55–100 mmHg	
		> 2 w	80–100 mmHg	
Potassium		2 d–2 w	3.7–6.0 mmol/L	Ranges quoted are based on artrial/venous specimens. Capillary samples have higher potassium concentrations (up to 0.6 mmol/L higher)
		2 w–3 m	3.7–5.7 mmol/L	
		3 m–1 y	3.5–5.1 mmol/L	
		1–16 y	3.5–5.0 mmol/L	
		> 16 y	3.5–5.0 mmol/L	
Proteins (s)	0.5			
Total protein		< 1 m	45–70 g/L	
		1 m–1 y	50–71 g/L	
		1–4 y	55–74 g/L	
		4–16 y	57–80 g/L	
		> 16 y	60–80 g/L	

h, hour; d, day; w, week; m, month; y, year; f, fasting; P, plasma; S, serum; U, urine.

(*Continued*)

Table A1 (*Continued*)

Test	*Arterial or venous specimens: volume required (mL)*	*Age*	*Reference range(s)*	*Comments*
Albumin		< 1 m	23–43 g/L	
		1 m–1 y	29–45 g/L	
		1–16 y	33–47 g/L	
		> 16 y	35–50 g/L	
Total globulins		< 1 m	10–31 g/L	Consult with immunology laboratory regarding specific globulin fractions
		1 m–1 y	12–27 g/L	
		1–4 y	14–37 g/L	
		4–16 y	17–38 g/L	
Sodium			135–145 mmol/L	
Thyroid function (S,P)	3			
Thyroxine total (TT4)		1–3 d	130–270 nmol/L	
		1–2 w	125–215 nmol/L	
		2–4 w	105–215 nmol/L	
		1–4 m	90–190 nmol/L	
		4 m–1 y	70–175 nmol/L	
		> 1 y	70–155 nmol/L	
free (FT4)		Adult	9–26 pmol/L	Higher values in infants
T3 Resin uptake (T3 RU)	< 1 m	70–115%		
	1–4 m	70–110%		
	4 m–1 y	70–110%		
	> 1 y	75–115%		

Table A1 (*Continued*)

Free thyroxine index (FTI)	< 1 m	80–210%		
	1–4 m	70–180%		
	4 m–1 y	60–160%		
	> 1 y	60–155%		
Triiodothyronine (T3)		Adult	1.0–2.7 nmol/L	Higher values in infants and children
Thyroxine binding globulin (TBG)		Adult	12–28 mg/L	Higher values in infants
Thyroid stimulating hormone (TSH)		1–3 d	< 40 mU/L	
		3–7 d	< 25 mU/L	
		7–14 d	< 10 mU/L	
		> 14 d	< 5 mU/L	
Triglycerides f (P)	0.5	Adult	0.9–2.0 mmol/L	*Note:* fasting essential
Urea (S,P)	0.5	< 1 m	1.3–5.7 mmol/L	Related to protein intake. Lower values in breast fed infants and newborns
		1 m–4 y	1.3–6.6 mmol/L	
		> 4 y	2.1–6.5 mmol/L	
Uric acid (S,P)	0.5	Prepubertal	0.13–0.39 mmol/L	Higher values may be seen in first 2 years and following onset of puberty
		Adult male	0.18–0.48 mmol/L	
		Adult female	0.11–0.42 mmol/L	
Zinc (S,P)	2		11–22 µmol/L	

h, hour; d, day; w, week; m, month; y, year; f, fasting; P, plasma; S, serum; U, urine.

(*Continued*)

Table A2 Urine

Test	*Specimens: Volume required (mL)*	*Age*	*Reference range(s)*	*Comments*
Calcium	24 h		< 0.12 mmol/kg per day	Include weight of patient on request card. Specimen must be collected into special bottle containing acid.
Calcium/creatinine ratio	Random	> 2 y	< 0.7 mmol/day	
Creatinine clearance	24 h		1.4–2.4 mL/s per 1.73 m^2	Plasma sample for creatinine required during urine collection period. Height and weight must be recorded on request card. See special note in general instructions.
Drug screen	Random (20 mL)			
Potassium	Random		Variable (mmol/L)	Many factors determine excretion rates, e.g. intake, renal function, hormonal influences and drug therapy.
Protein	Timed collection overnight		$mg/h/m^2 < 4$	Height and weight of patient must be recorded on request card
Protein/creatinine ratio	Random (early morning)		mg/mmol < 30	Consult laboratory
Sodium	Random		Variable (mmol/L)	Many factors influence urinary sodium concentration. This test is of value in differentiating causes of hyponatraemia

h, hour; y, year.

Table A3 Sweat

Test	*Specimens: volume required (mL)*	*Age*	*Reference range(s)*	*Comments*
Sodium chloride	–	Prepubertal	< 40 mmol/L < 40 mmol/L	Contact gastroenterology department. At least 100 mg of sweat must be collected. If sodium is > 50 mmol/L and chloride is > 60 mmol/L, result is definitely abnormal. All other results outside reference ranges are doubtful. Higher values may be seen in normal adolescents and adults

Table A4 Serum drug levels

Test	*Arterial or venous specimens: volume required (mL)*	*Reference range(s)*	*Comments*
Carbamazepine (S,P)	1	20–50 μmol/L (therapeutic)	
Chloramphenicol (S,P)	0.5	Peak 20–30 mg/L (therapeutic)	
Clonazepam	1	60–150 nmol/L (therapeutic)	Therapeutic range not well-defined.
Cyclosporin (B)	1	μg/L	Collect sample in EDTA. Consult laboratory regarding therapeutic range
Digoxin (S,P)	1	Low < 0.6 nmol/L Borderline low 0.6–1.0 nmol/L Therapeutic 1.0–2.5 nmol/L Borderline high 2.5–3.0 nmol/L High > 3.0 nmol/L	
Ethosuximide (S,P)	1	0.30–0.70 mmol/L (therapeutic)	Therapeutic range not well-defined.
Gentamicin (S,P)	0.5	Peak 5–10 mg/L Trough < 2 mg/L (therapeutic)	For thrice daily dosing only
Nitrazepam (S,P)	1		Consult with laboratory regarding therapeutic range

Table A4 (*Continued*)

Paracetamol (S,P)		0.5		Only measured in suspected overdose — consult laboratory
Phenobarbitone (S,P)	1		80–120 µmol/L (therapeutic)	
Phenytoin (S,P)	1		40–80 µmol/L (therapeutic)	
Primidone (S,P)	1			Only the phenobarbitone metabolite measured as this usually gives sufficient information for therapeutic monitoring
Salicylate (S,P)	0.5		0.7–2.00 mmol/L (therapeutic)	
Theophylline (S,P)	0.5		Neonatal apnoea 40–80 µmol/L (therapeutic) Asthma 55–110 µmol/L (therapeutic-peak)	
Thiopentone (S,P)		0.5	150–200 µmol/L (for anaesthesia)	
Tobramycin (S,P)		0.5	Peak 5–10 mg/L Trough < 2 mg/L (therapeutic)	For thrice daily dosing only
Valproate (S,P)	0.5		0.30–0.70 mmol/L (therapeutic)	
Vancomycin (S,P)		0.5	Peak 25–40 mg/L Trough < 10 mg/L (therapeutic)	

B, blood (whole); P, plasma; S, serum.

HAEMATOLOGY

Table A5 Haematology reference ranges

	Haemoglobin (g/L)	*Haematocrit (L/L)*	*Reticulocytes $\times 10^9$/L (%)*
Birth	110–170	0/30–0/40	
28 weeks gestation	120–180	0.35–0.50	
34 weeks gestation	140–200	0.40–0.55	
38 weeks gestation	135–195	0.42–0.60	200–300 (2.6)
40 weeks gestation			
1 week	135–205	0.42–0.62	< 5 (0)
2 weeks	125–205	0.40–0.62	< 5 (0)
1 month	100–180	0.31–0.55	
2 months	90–135	0.27–0.40	
3 months	95–140	0.29–0.41	5–250
6–24 months	105–140	0.33–0.42	10–100 (0.5–1.5)
2–5 years	115–140	0.35–0.42	10–100 (0.5–1.5)
6–11 years	115–155	0.35–0.48	10–100 (0.5–1.5)
12–18 years (male)	130–160	0.37–0.48	10–100 (0.5–1.5)
12–18 years (female)	120–160	0.36–0.48	10–100 (0.5–1.5)

Table A6 Red cell indices

	MCV (fL)	*MCH (pg)*	*MCHC (g/L)*
Birth			
28–37 weeks gestation	120		320–360
38–40 weeks gestation	110		320–360
1 week	110		320–360
1 month	90	24–34	320–360
2 months	80	24–34	320–360
3–12 months	70	24–31	320–360
Older	84–94	24–31	320–360

Table A7 Normal white cell levels

Age	*Total* ($\times 10^9$/L)	*Neutrophils* ($\times 10^9$/L) (%)	*Lymphocytes* ($\times 10^9$/L) (%)	*Monocytes* ($\times 10^9$/L) (%)	*Platelets* ($\times 10^9$/L)
Birth	9.0–30	6.0–26 (60)	2.0–11.0 (30)	1.1 (7)	150–400
1 week	5–21	1.5–10 (45)	2.0–17.0 (40)	1.1 (9)	150–400
6 months	6–17.5	1.0–8.5 (30)	4.0–13.5 (60)	0.6 (5)	150–400
2 years	6–17.5	1.5–8.5 (33)	3.0–9.5 (60)	0.5 (5)	150–400
6 years	6–14.5	1.5–8.0 (50)	1.5–7.0 (42)	0.4 (5)	150–400
10 years	4.5–13.5	1.8–8.0 (54)	1.5–6.5 (38)	0.4 (4)	150–400
16 years	4.5–13.5	1.8–8.0 (60)	1.0–4.8 (33)	0.3 (4)	150–400

ESRO-6 mm in 1 h (micro Westergren)

Table A8 Haemoglobin electrophoresis

Age	*Percentage*
Hb F Birth (40 week gestation)	60–90
2 months	30–55
3 months	15–30
4 months	5–15
6 months	2–5.0
1 year	0.2–2.0
Hb A_2 > 1 year	1.5–3.5

Table A9 Erythropoietic factors

Test	*Reference range*
Serum iron	9–27 μmol/L
Total iron binding capacity	45–72 μmol/L
Percentage saturation	16–33%
Serum ferritin	
< 1 year	10–300 μg/L
> 1 year	16–300 μg/L
Folate	
Serum	> 4 μmol/L
Red cell	> 270 μmol/L
Whole blood	> 110 μmol/L
Vitamin B_{12}	150–590 pmol/L

Table A10 Coagulation

Test	*Reference range*
Bleeding time	1.6–7.0 min
Prothrombin time (International Normalized Ratio)	0.8–1.3 s
Activated partial thromboplastin time	22.0–39.0 s
D – Dimers	< 0.25 μg/mL
Fibrinogen < 6 months	1.5–4.0 g/L
> 6 months	1.9–5.0 g/L

A

APPENDIX 2

GROWTH CHARTS AND PUBERTAL STAGING

GIRLS IN UTERO 24–42 WKS POST NATAL 0–3 YEARS

Reproduced with permission of the Pharmacia Growth Service

INTRAUTERINE GROWTH CURVES (COMPOSITE MALE/FEMALE)

Measuring techniques: (as for ages 0–36 months – see over page)

Additional Notes: Gestational ages are recorded in completed weeks from the first day of the mother's last menstrual period. Foetal growth is influenced by many factors including age, body weight, height, parity, ethnic origin of the mother and sex of the foetus. Corrections for some of these factors are found in the quoted reference.

Data Source: W.H. Kitchen et al *Revised intrauterine growth curves for an Australian hospital population.* Aust. Paediatr. J. *(1983) 19:157–161.*

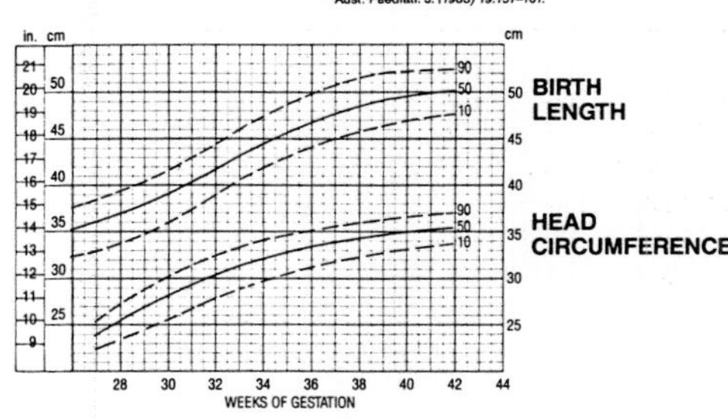

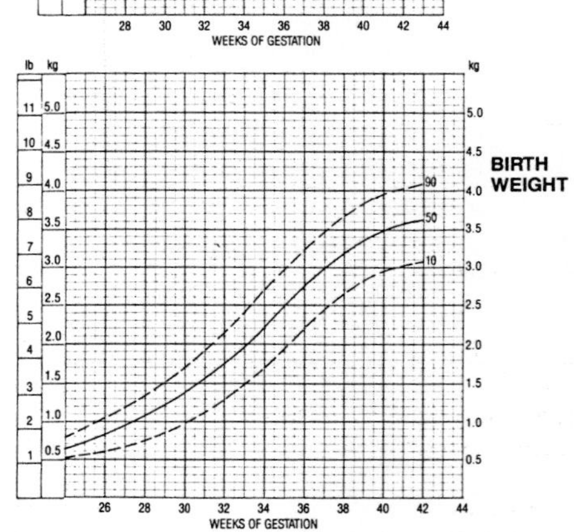

Designed by the Department of Endocrinology, The Adelaide Children's Hospital, 1989.

GIRLS 0–3 YEARS
LENGTH PERCENTILE CHART

Reproduced with permission of the Pharmacia Growth Service

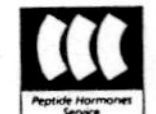

cm MOTHER'S HEIGHT________ FATHER'S HEIGHT________ cm in

Supine length (recommended up to the age of 3 so that there is overlap with standing height at 2 to 3) is taken on a flat surface, with the child lying on her back. One observer holds her head in contact with a board at the top of the table and another straightens the legs and turns the feet upward to be at right angles to the legs and brings a sliding board in contact with the child's heels.

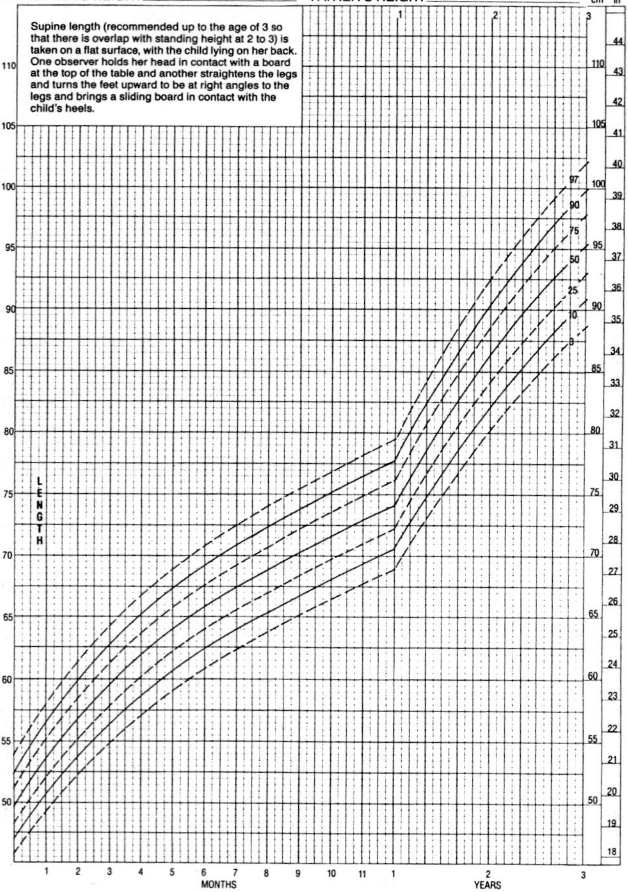

Data Source: Hamill P.V.V.: NCHS growth curves for children. DHEW publication (PHS) 78–1650

GIRLS 0–3 YEARS
WEIGHT PERCENTILE CHART

Reproduced with permission of the Pharmacia Growth Service

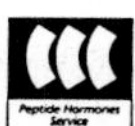

Weight should be taken in the nude, or as near thereto as possible. If a surgical gown or minimum underclothing (vest and pants) is worn, then its estimated weight (about 0.1 kg) must be subtracted before weight is recorded. Weights are conveniently recorded to the last completed 0.1 kg above the age of six months. The bladder should be empty.

DATE	AGE	LENGTH	WEIGHT	HEAD CIRCUM.

SIMPLIFIED CALCULATION OF BODY SURFACE AREA (BSA)

$$\text{BSA (m}^2\text{)} = \sqrt{\frac{\text{Ht (cm)} \times \text{Wt (kg)}}{3600}}$$

Ref: Mosteller R.D.
Simplified calculation of body surface area
N.Engl. J.Med. 1987; 317:1098.

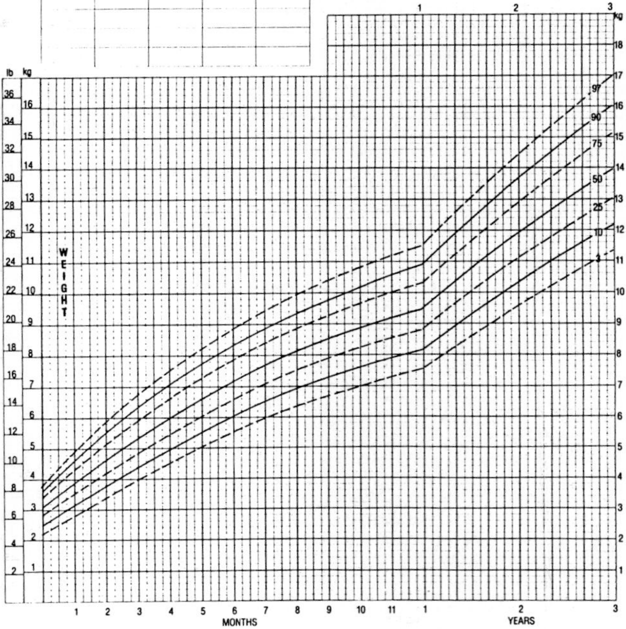

Data Source: Hamill P.V.V.: NCHS growth curves for children. DHEW publication (PHS) 78–1650

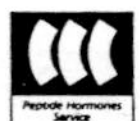

Reproduced with permission of the Pharmacia Growth Service

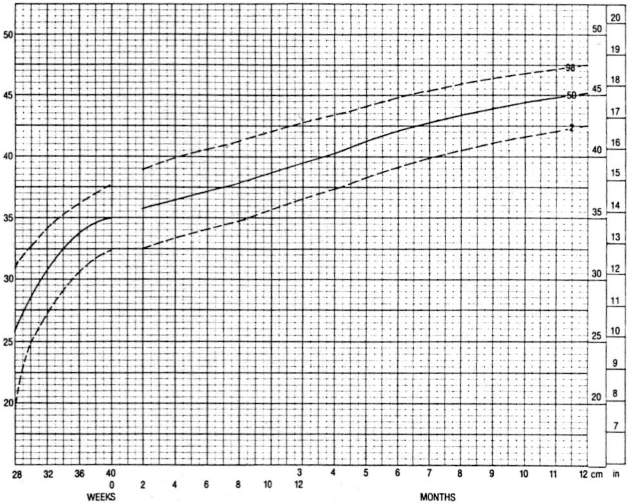

HEAD CIRCUMFERENCE
GIRLS
In utero 28–40 weeks, 0–12 months

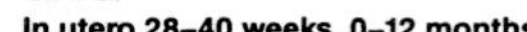

50 45 40 35 30 25 20

98 50 2

cm: 50 45 40 35 30 25 20
in: 20 19 18 17 16 15 14 13 12 11 10 9 8 7

28 32 36 40 WEEKS
0 2 4 6 8 10 12 (weeks)
3 4 5 6 7 8 9 10 11 12 MONTHS

1–3 years

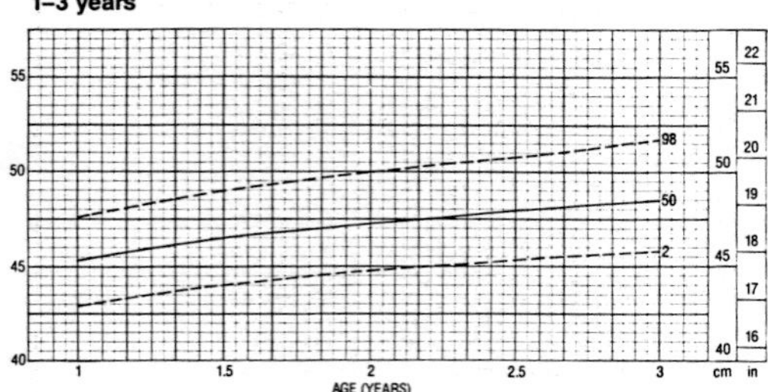

MEASURING TECHNIQUE HEAD CIRCUMFERENCE

The tape should be placed over the eyebrows, above the ears and over the most prominent part of the occiput taking a direct route. A paper tape is preferable to plastic which stretches unacceptably. Record to nearest 0.1 cm.

SOURCES

Head circumference 0–3 years from NSW Health Commission Publication (Jones DL and Hemphill W, 1974).

Head circumference 28–40 weeks gestation from Kitchen WH Aust. Paediatr. J. *(1983) 19:157–161).*

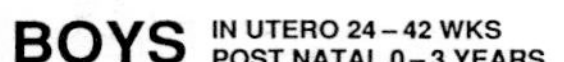

BOYS IN UTERO 24 – 42 WKS POST NATAL 0 – 3 YEARS

Reproduced with permission of the Pharmacia Growth Service

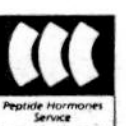

INTRAUTERINE GROWTH CURVES (COMPOSITE MALE/FEMALE)

Measuring techniques: (as for ages 0–36 months – see over page)

Additional Notes: Gestational ages are recorded in completed weeks from the first day of the mother's last menstrual period. Foetal growth is influenced by many factors including age, body weight, height, parity, ethnic origin of the mother and sex of the foetus. Corrections for some of these factors are found in the quoted reference.

Data Source: *W.H. Kitchen et al* ***Revised intrauterine growth curves for an Australian hospital population.*** **Aust. Paediatr. J.** *(1983) 19:157–161.*

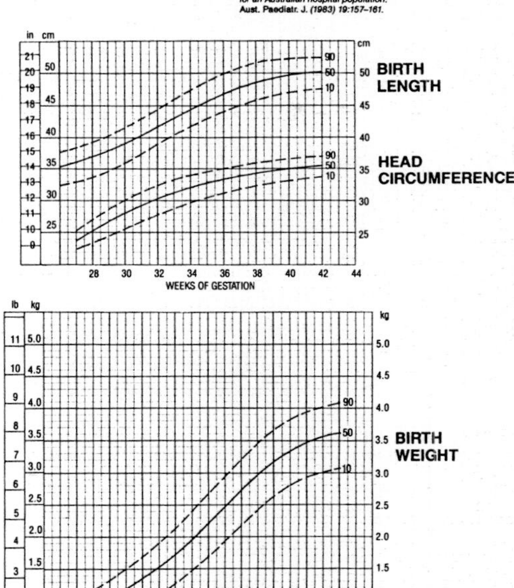

Designed by the Department of Endocrinology, The Adelaide Children's Hospital, 1989.

BOYS 0–3 YEARS
LENGTH PERCENTILE CHART

Reproduced with permission of the Pharmacia Growth Service

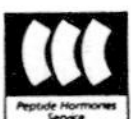

MOTHER'S HEIGHT________ FATHER'S HEIGHT________

Supine length (recommended up to the age of 3 so that there is overlap with standing height at 2 to 3) is taken on a flat surface, with the child lying on his back. One observer holds his head in contact with a board at the top of the table and another straightens the legs and turns the feet upward to be at right angles to the legs and brings a sliding board in contact with the child's heels.

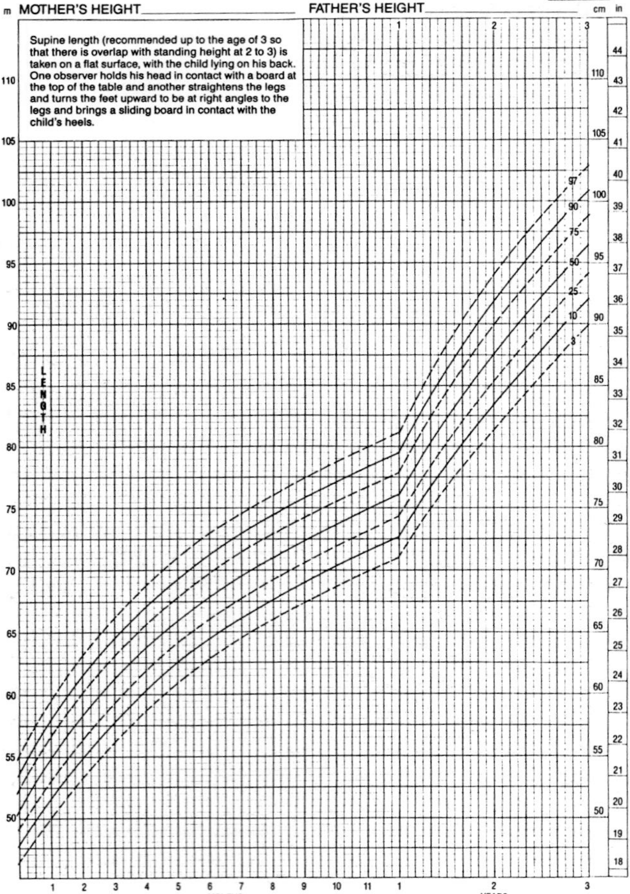

Data Source: Hamill P.V.V.: NCHS growth curves for children. DHEW publication (PHS) 78–1650

BOYS 0–3 YEARS
WEIGHT PERCENTILE CHART

Reproduced with permission of the Pharmacia Growth Service

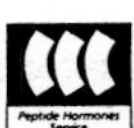

Weight should be taken in the nude, or as near thereto as possible. If a surgical gown or minimum underclothing (vest and pants) is worn, then its estimated weight (about 0.1 kg) must be subtracted before weight is recorded. Weights are conveniently recorded to the last completed 0.1 kg above the age of six months. The bladder should be empty.

DATE	AGE	LENGTH	WEIGHT	HEAD CIRCUM.

SIMPLIFIED CALCULATION OF BODY SURFACE AREA (BSA)

$$BSA\ (m^2) = \sqrt{\frac{Ht\ (cm) \times Wt\ (kg)}{3600}}$$

Ref: Mosteller R.D.
Simplified calculation of body surface area
N.Engl. J.Med. 1987; 317:1098.

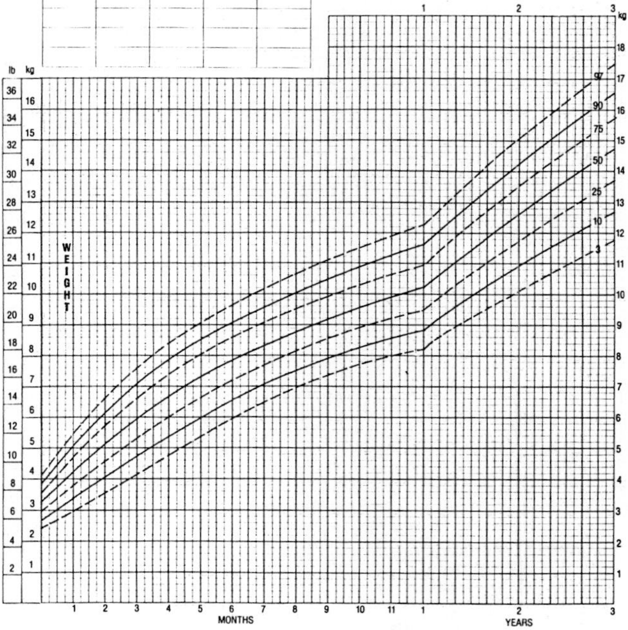

Data Source: Hamill P.V.V.: NCHS growth curves for children. DHEW publication (PHS) 78–1650

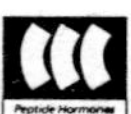

Reproduced with permission of the Pharmacia Growth Service

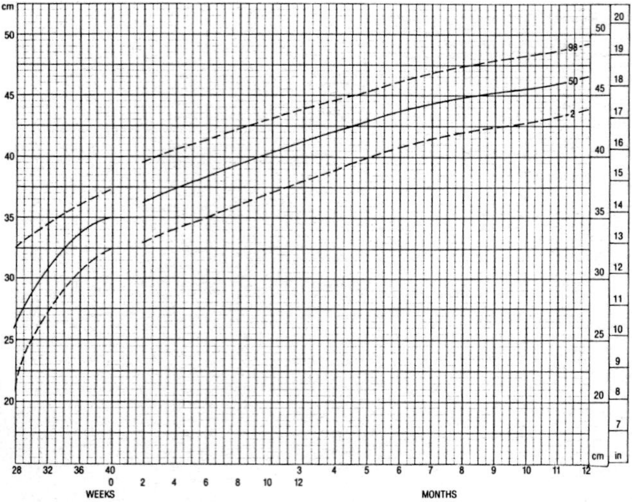

HEAD CIRCUMFERENCE
BOYS

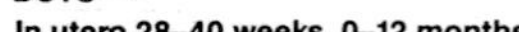

In utero 28–40 weeks, 0–12 months

cm 50 45 40 35 30 25 20

98 50 2

28 32 36 40 WEEKS

0 2 4 6 8 10 12 WEEKS

3 4 5 6 7 8 9 10 11 12 MONTHS

cm 50 45 40 35 30 25 20 cm

in 20 19 18 17 16 15 14 13 12 11 10 9 8 7 in

1–3 years

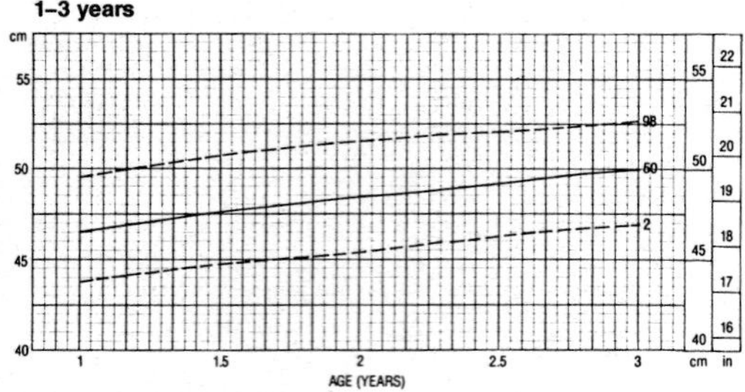

MEASURING TECHNIQUE HEAD CIRCUMFERENCE

The tape should be placed over the eyebrows, above the ears and over the most prominent part of the occiput taking a direct route. A paper tape is preferable to plastic which stretches unacceptably. Record to nearest 0.1 cm.

SOURCES

Head circumference 0–3 years from NSW Health Commission Publication (Jones DL and Hemphill W, 1974).

Head circumference 28–40 weeks gestation from Kitchen WH Aust. Paediatr. J. (1983) 19:157–161).

GIRLS: 2 TO 18 YEARS
HEIGHT PERCENTILE

Reproduced with permission of the Pharmacia Growth Service

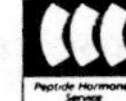

MOTHER'S HEIGHT________________ FATHER'S HEIGHT________________

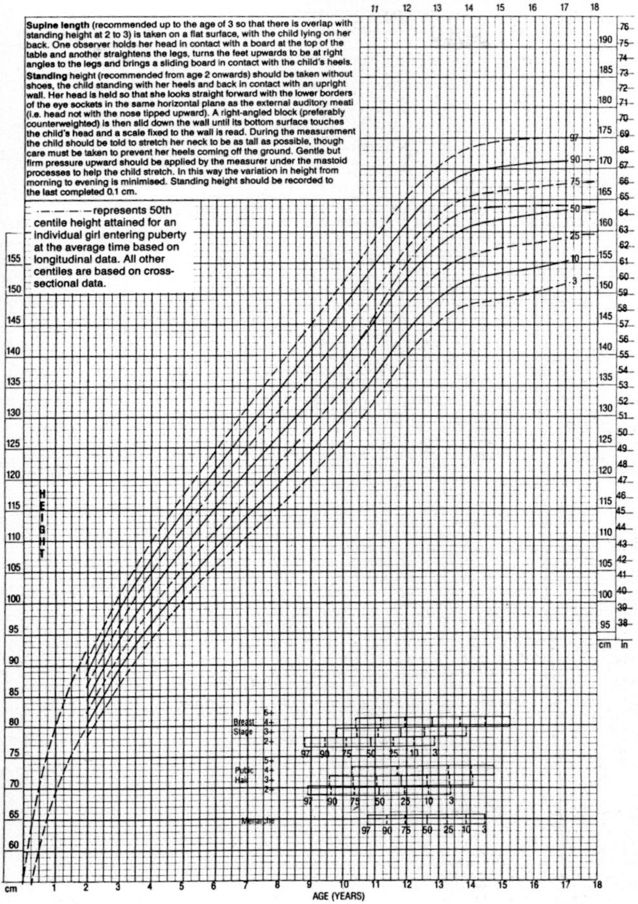

Supine length (recommended up to the age of 3 so that there is overlap with standing height at 2 to 3) is taken on a flat surface, with the child lying on her back. One observer holds her head in contact with a board at the top of the table and another straightens the legs, turns the feet upwards to be at right angles to the legs and brings a sliding board in contact with the child's heels. **Standing** height (recommended from age 2 onwards) should be taken without shoes, the child standing with her heels and back in contact with an upright wall. Her head is held so that she looks straight forward with the lower borders of the eye sockets in the same horizontal plane as the external auditory meati (i.e. head not with the nose tipped upward). A right-angled block (preferably counterweighted) is then slid down the wall until its bottom surface touches the child's head and a scale fixed to the wall is read. During the measurement the child should be told to stretch her neck to be as tall as possible, though care must be taken to prevent her heels coming off the ground. Gentle but firm pressure upward should be applied by the measurer under the mastoid processes to help the child stretch. In this way the variation in height from morning to evening is minimised. Standing height should be recorded to the last completed 0.1 cm.

—·—·— represents 50th centile height attained for an individual girl entering puberty at the average time based on longitudinal data. All other centiles are based on cross-sectional data.

HEIGHT

Breast Stage 2+ 3+ 4+ 5+ — 97 90 75 50 25 10 3

Pubic Hair 2+ 3+ 4+ 5+ — 97 90 75 50 25 10 3

Menarche — 97 90 75 50 25 10 3

Centiles: 97, 90, 75, 50, 25, 10, 3

cm: 60, 65, 70, 75, 80, 85, 90, 95, 100, 105, 110, 115, 120, 125, 130, 135, 140, 145, 150, 155, 160, 165, 170, 175, 180, 185, 190

in: 38–76

AGE (YEARS): 1–18

Source: Adapted from Hamill P.V.V.: NCHS growth curves for children. DHEW publication (PHS) 78–1650

GIRLS: 2 TO 18 YEARS WEIGHT PERCENTILE

Reproduced with permission of the Pharmacia Growth Service

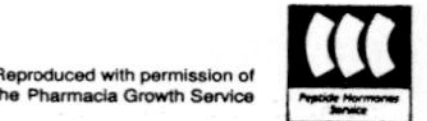

Weight should be taken in the nude, or as near thereto as possible. If a surgical gown or minimum underclothing (vest and pants) is worn, then its estimated weight (about 0.1 kg) must be subtracted before weight is recorded. Weights are conventionally recorded to the last completed 0.1 kg above the age of six months. The bladder should be empty.

DATE	AGE	HEIGHT	WEIGHT	HEAD CIRCUM.	PUBERTAL STAGES: BREAST	PUBERTAL STAGES: PUBIC HAIR	PUBERTAL STAGES: MEN-ARCHE

SIMPLIFIED CALCULATION OF BODY SURFACE AREA (BSA)

$$BSA\ (m^2) = \sqrt{\frac{Ht\ (cm) \times Wt\ (kg)}{3600}}$$

Ref: Mosteller R.D.
Simplified calculation of body surface area
N.Engl. J.Med. 1987; 317:1098.

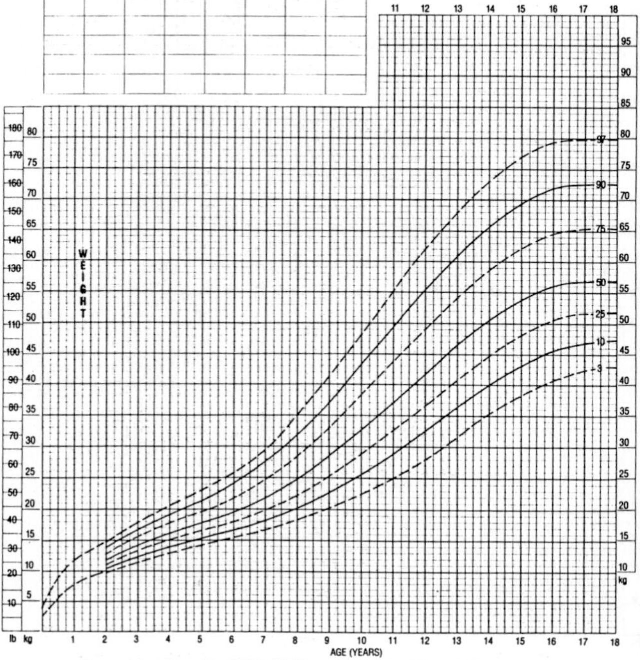

Source: Adapted from Hamill P.V.V.: NCHS growth curves for children. DHEW publication (PHS) 78–1650

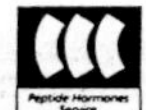

Reproduced with permission of the Pharmacia Growth Service

HEAD CIRCUMFERENCE, GIRLS

Head Circumference: The tape should be placed over the eyebrows, above the ears and over the most prominent part of the occiput taking a direct route. A paper tape is preferable to plastic, which stretches unacceptably under tension. The maximum measurement should be recorded to the nearest 0.1 cm.

Data Source: 2–5 yr. Jones DL (1973) NSW Health Comm. Publ. 5–18 yr Nellhaus G. Pediatrics (1968) 41:106–114

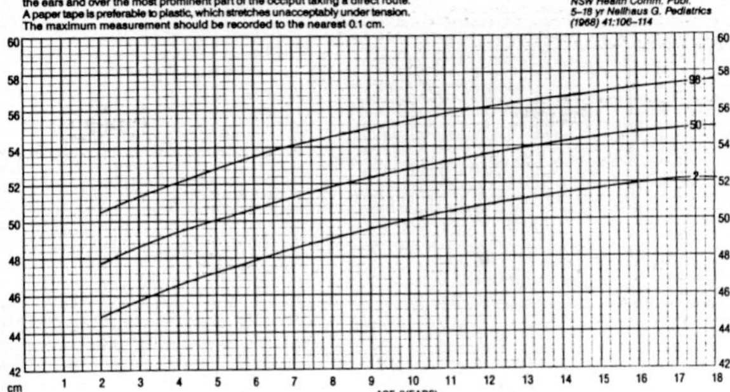

HEIGHT VELOCITY, GIRLS

The standards are appropriate for velocity calculated over a whole year period, not less, since a smaller period requires wider limits (the 3rd and 97th centiles for whole year being roughly appropriate for the 10th and 90th centiles over six months). The yearly velocity should be plotted at the mid-point of a year. The centiles given in black are appropriate to children of average maturational tempo, who have their peak velocity at the average age for this event. The red line is the 50th centile line for the child who is two years early in maturity and age at peak height velocity, and the blue line refers to a child who is 50th centile in velocity but two years late. The arrows mark the 3rd and 97th centiles at peak velocity for early and late maturers.

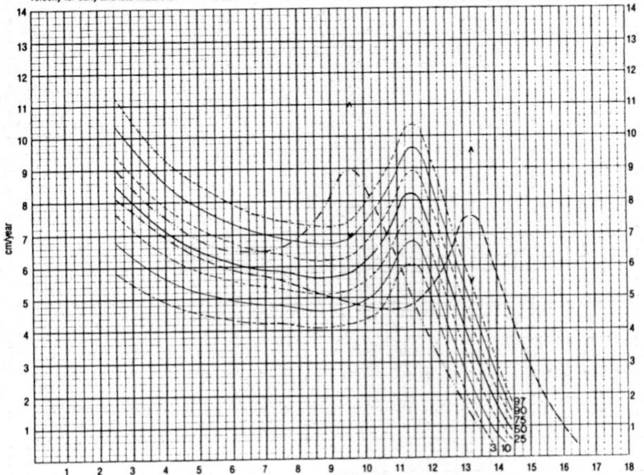

Reproduced by permission of
© Castlemead Publications

Data Source: Tanner J, Davis PSW, *Journal of Pediatrics* 1985:107

BOYS: 2 TO 18 YEARS
HEIGHT PERCENTILE

Reproduced with permission of the Pharmacia Growth Service

MOTHER'S HEIGHT__________________ FATHER'S HEIGHT__________________

Supine length (recommended up to the age of 3 so that there is overlap with standing height at 2 to 3) is taken on a flat surface, with the child lying on his back. One observer holds his head in contact with a board at the top of the table and another straightens the legs, turns the feet upwards to be at right angles to the legs and brings a sliding board in contact with the child's heels.
Standing height (recommended from age 2 onwards) should be taken without shoes, the child standing with his heels and back in contact with an upright wall. His head is held so that he looks straight forward with the lower borders of the eye sockets in the same horizontal plane as the external auditory meati (i.e. head not with the nose tipped upward). A right-angled block (preferably counterweighted) is then slid down the wall until its bottom surface touches the child's head and a scale fixed to the wall is read. During the measurement the child should be told to stretch his neck to be as tall as possible, though care must be taken to prevent his heels coming off the ground. Gentle but firm pressure upward should be applied by the measurer under the mastoid processes to help the child stretch. In this way the variation in height from morning to evening is minimised. Standing height should be recorded to the last completed 0.1 cm.

-·—·—·— represents 50th centile height attained for an individual boy entering puberty at the average time based on longitudinal data. All other centiles are based on cross-sectional data.

Source: Adapted from Hamill P.V.V.: NCHS growth curves for children. DHEW publication (PHS) 78–1650

BOYS: 2 TO 18 YEARS WEIGHT PERCENTILE

Reproduced with permission of the Pharmacia Growth Service

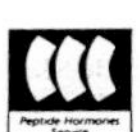

Weight should be taken in the nude, or as near thereto as possible. If a surgical gown or minimum underclothing (vest and pants) is worn, then its estimated weight (about 0.1 kg) must be subtracted before weight is recorded. Weights are conventionally recorded to the last completed 0.1 kg above the age of six months. The bladder should be empty.

DATE	AGE	HEIGHT	WEIGHT	HEAD CIRCUM.	PUBERTAL STAGES GENITAL	PUBIC HAIR	TESTES R	TESTES L

SIMPLIFIED CALCULATION OF BODY SURFACE AREA (BSA)

$$BSA\ (m^2) = \sqrt{\frac{Ht\ (cm) \times Wt\ (kg)}{3600}}$$

Ref: Mosteller R.D.
Simplified calculation of body surface area
N.Engl. J.Med. 1987; 317:1098.

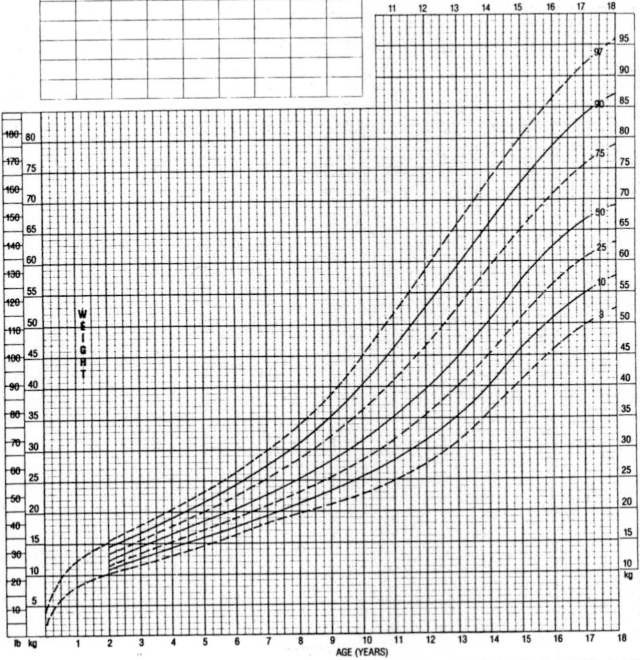

Source: Adapted from Hamill P.V.V.: NCHS growth curves for children. DHEW publication (PHS) 78–1650

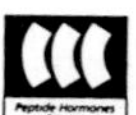

Reproduced with permission of
the Pharmacia Growth Service

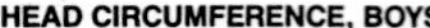

HEAD CIRCUMFERENCE, BOYS

Head Circumference: The tape should be placed over the eyebrows, above the ears and over the most prominent part of the occiput taking a direct route. A paper tape is preferable to plastic, which stretches unacceptably under tension. The maximum measurement should be recorded to the nearest 0.1 cm.

Data Source: 2–5 yr. Jones DL (1973) NSW Health Comm. Publ. 5–18 yr Nellhaus G. Pediatrics (1968) 41:106–114

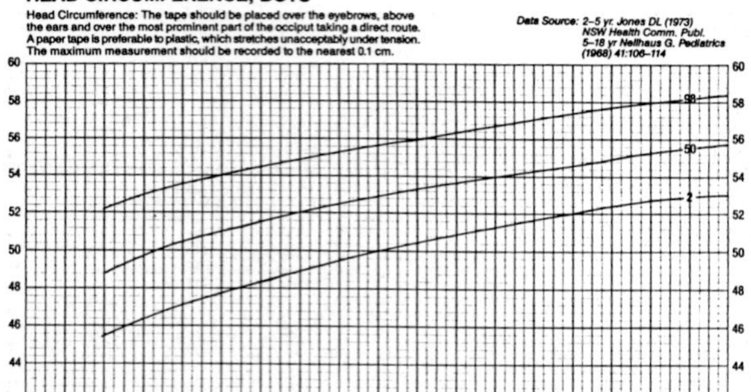

HEIGHT VELOCITY, BOYS

The standards are appropriate for velocity calculated over a whole year period, not less, since a small period requires wider limits (the 3rd and 97th centiles for whole year being roughly appropriate for the 10th and 90th centiles over six months). The yearly velocity should be plotted at the mid-point of a year. The centiles given in black are appropriate to children of average maturational tempo, who have their peak velocity at the average age for this event. The red line is the 50th centile line for the child who is two years early in maturity and age at peak height velocity, and the green line refers to a child who is 50th centile in velocity but two years late. The arrows mark the 3rd and 97th centiles at peak velocity for early and late maturers.

Centiles of whole-year velocity for maturers at average time — 97, 50, 3
97 and 3 centile at peak height velocity
Early (+2SD) maturers
Late (−2SD) maturers

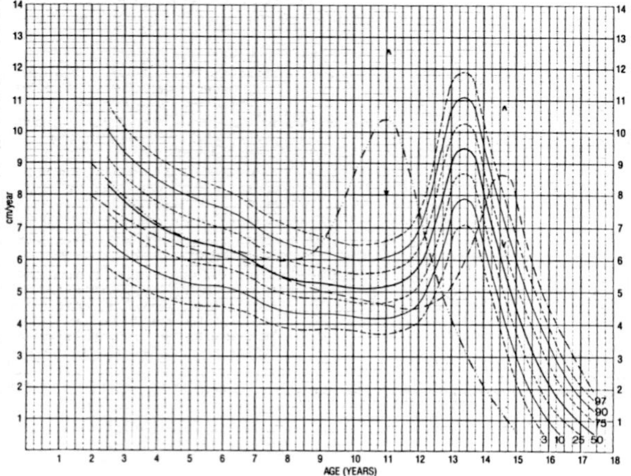

Reproduced by permission of
© Castlemead Publications

Data Source: Tanner J, Davis PSW, *Journal of Pediatrics* 1985:107

GIRLS 2–18

Reproduced with permission of
the Pharmacia Growth Service

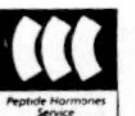

Breast Development

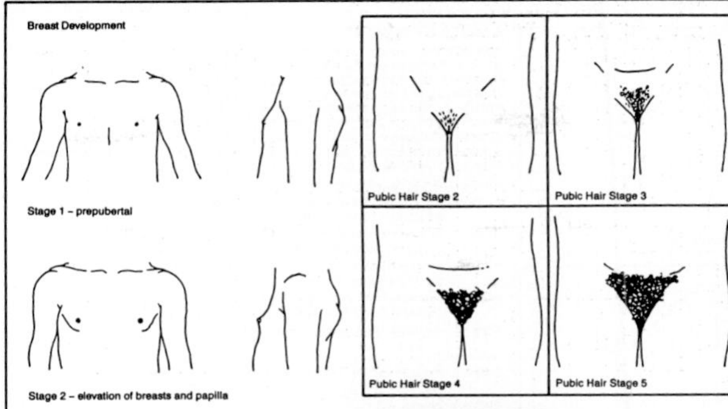

Stage 1 – prepubertal

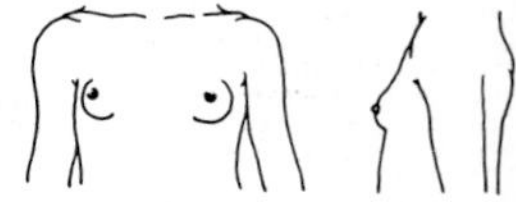

Stage 2 – elevation of breasts and papilla

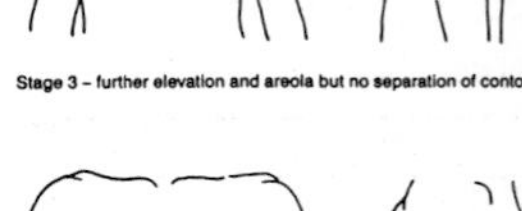

Stage 3 – further elevation and areola but no separation of contours

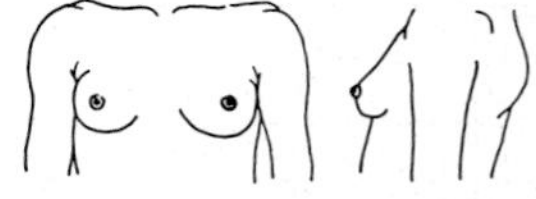

Stage 4 – areola and papilla form a secondary mound above level of the breast

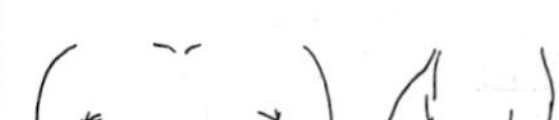

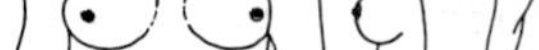

Stage 5 – areola recesses to the general contour of the breast

STAGES OF PUBERTY

Ages of attainment of successive stages of pubertal sexual development are given in the height centile chart overpage. The stage Pubic Hair 2+ represents the state of a child who shows the pubic hair appearance stage 2 but not stage 3 (see below). The centiles for age at which this state is normally seen are given, the 97th centile being considered as the early limit, the 3rd centile as the late limit. The child's puberty stages may be plotted at successive ages (Tanner, *Growth at Adolescence*, 2nd Ed., 1962).

Pubic hair:

Stage 1. Pre-adolescent. The vellus over the pubes is not further developed than that over the abdominal wall, i.e. no pubic hair.

Stage 2. Sparse growth of long, slightly pigmented downy hair, straight or slightly curled, chiefly along labia.

Stage 3. Considerably darker, coarser and more curled. The hair spreads sparsely over the junction of the pubes.

Stage 4. Hair now adult in type, but area covered is still considerably smaller than in the adult. No spread to the medial surface of thighs.

Stage 5. Adult in quantity and type with distribution of the horizontal (or classically 'feminine') pattern. Spread to medial surface of thighs but not up linea alba or elsewhere above the base of the inverse triangle (spread up linea alba occurs late and is rated stage 6).

Designed by the Department of Endocrinology, The Adelaide Children's Hospital, 1989.

BOYS 2–18

Reproduced with permission of the Pharmacia Growth Service

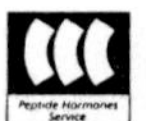

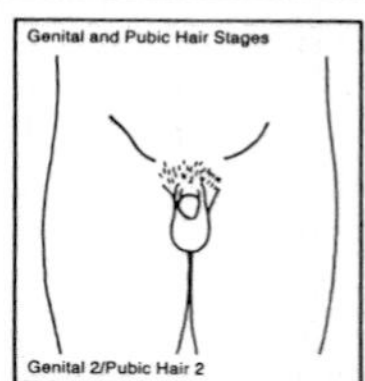

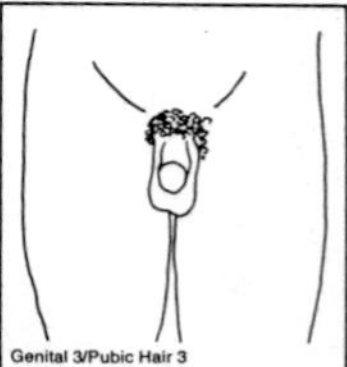

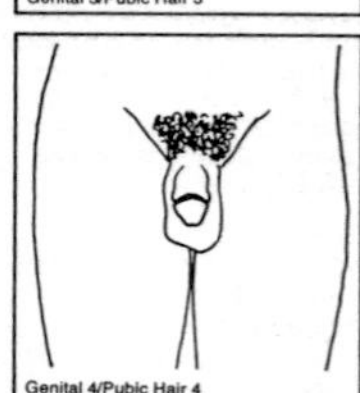

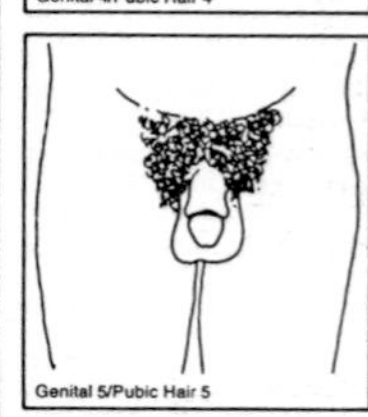

STAGES OF PUBERTY

Ages of attainment of successive stages of pubertal sexual development are given in the height centile chart overpage. The stage Pubic Hair 2+ represents the state of a child who shows the pubic hair appearance stage 2 but not stage 3 (see below). The centiles for age at which this state is normally seen are given, the 97th centile being considered as the early limit, the 3rd centile as the late limit. The child's puberty stages may be plotted at successive ages (Tanner, *Growth at Adolescence*, 2nd Ed., 1962). Testis sizes are judged by comparison with the Prader orchidometer (Zachmann, Prader, Kind, Haflinger and Budliger, *Helv. Paed. Acta.* 29, 61–72, 1974).

Genital (penis) development:

Stage 1. Pre-adolescent, testes, scrotum and penis are of about the same size and proportion as in early childhood.

Stage 2. Enlargement of scrotum and testes. Skin of scrotum reddens and changes in texture. Little or no enlargement of penis at this stage.

Stage 3. Enlargement of the penis which occurs at first mainly in length. Further growth of the testes and scrotum.

Stage 4. Increased size of penis with growth in breadth and development of glans. Testes and scrotum larger; scrotal skin darkened.

Stage 5. Genitalia adult in size and shape.

Pubic hair:

Stage 1. Pre-adolescent. The vellus over the pubes is not further developed than that over the abdominal wall, i.e. no pubic hair.

Stage 2. Sparse growth of long, slightly pigmented downy hair, straight or slightly curled at the base of the penis.

Stage 3. Considerably darker, coarser and more curled. The hair spreads sparsely over the junction of the pubes.

Stage 4. Hair now adult in type, but area covered is still considerably smaller than in the adult. No spread to the medial surface of thighs.

Stage 5. Adult in quantity and type with distribution of the horizontal (or classically 'feminine') pattern. Spread to medial surface of thighs but not up linea alba or elsewhere above the base of the inverse triangle (spread up linea alba occurs late and is rated stage 6).

Stretched Penile Length

Measured from the pubo-penile skin junction to the tip of the glans (Schonfeld and Beebe, *J. of Urology* 48, 759–777, 1942).

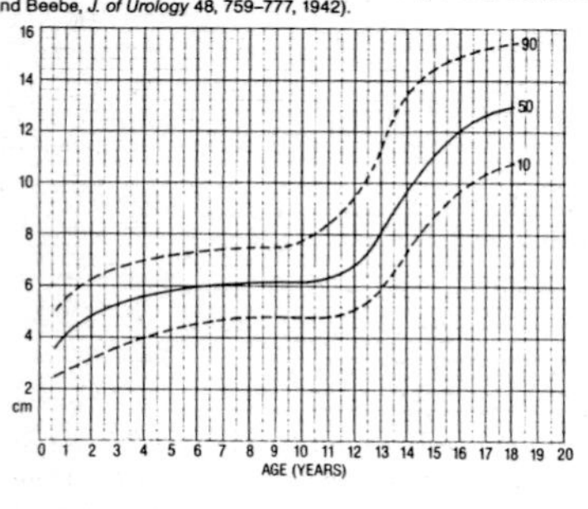

Designed by the Department of Endocrinology, The Adelaide Children's Hospital, 1989.

INDEX

B

D

E

F

G

J

K

L

M

N

T

U

V

W

Z